# UNDERSTANDING MENTAL DISORDERS

*Your Guide to DSM-5*®

# UNDERSTANDING MENTAL DISORDERS

*Your Guide
to DSM-5*®

## AMERICAN PSYCHIATRIC ASSOCIATION

With Foreword by Patrick J. Kennedy

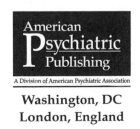

American **P**sychiatric Publishing

A Division of American Psychiatric Association

**Washington, DC
London, England**

Manufactured in the United States of America on acid-free paper

19  18  17  16  15          5  4  3  2

First Edition

Typeset in Adobe's Palatino LT Std and Helvetica Lt Std

American Psychiatric Publishing
A Division of American Psychiatric Association
1000 Wilson Boulevard
Arlington, VA 22209-3901
www.appi.org

**Library of Congress Cataloging-in-Publication Data**
Understanding mental disorders : your guide to DSM-5 / with foreword by Patrick J. Kennedy.—First edition.
    p. ; cm.
Includes index.
ISBN 978-1-58562-491-1 (alk. paper)
I. American Psychiatric Association, issuing body.
[DNLM: 1. Diagnostic and statistical manual of mental disorders. 5th ed.
2. Mental Disorders--Popular Works. WM 140]
RC467
616.89—dc23

2014047440

**British Library Cataloguing in Publication Data**
A CIP record is available from the British Library.

Text Design—Tammy J. Cordova
Writer—Glenda Fauntleroy

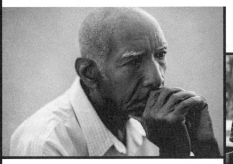

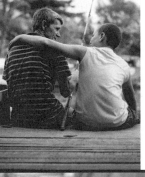

# Contents

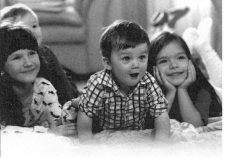

# Foreword

**M**ental illness touches everyone. Nearly half of all Americans have a risk of mental disorder in the course of their lifetimes. We all know someone—parent, partner, child, friend, coworker, neighbor—who has suffered or is suffering from a psychiatric condition. Mental illness costs our nation and our world trillions of dollars every year. Yet as devastating as the financial toll clearly is, the cost in lives lost or severely compromised by mental illness is incalculably greater.

Across the globe, depression robs more people of more years lost to disease than any other condition. Suicide is the third leading cause of death among young people ages 10–24 in the United States. Our veterans, who have given so much for their country, are among the most vulnerable: every day 22 American veterans take their own lives. Just as tragic are the stories of the many Americans living in pain who are never diagnosed or treated. Too frequently, our society's response to mental disorders is to assign blame, leaving millions of Americans marginalized, neglected, vilified, or incarcerated because of their illness.

But mental illnesses are not a question of character; they are illnesses that can be treated. And like most illnesses, mental illnesses respond best to treatments that are timely and effective. Yet often we ignore or dismiss these illnesses in their earliest, most treatable stages—and respond only when they have escalated to critical and potentially life-threatening conditions. Simply put, too few of us know the signs and symptoms of mental illnesses, and countless people suffer as a result.

This is why *Understanding Mental Disorders: Your Guide to DSM-5* makes such an important contribution. By translating the psychiatric profession's most recent *Diagnostic and Statistical Manual of Mental Disorders* (DSM) into clear, accessible language, it empowers family members and friends to help identify individuals who might be at risk or who are already suffering from a mental disorder and need treatment. This book gives those of us with these conditions the keys to better understand our own situations.

*Understanding Mental Disorders* also helps us address the great challenge of stigma. People with mental disorders often experience fear, shame, and a terrible sense of being alone because their condition is not discussed. This invaluable guide will equip patients and families with the tools they need to break through stigma, seek professional diagnosis and care, and stick with their treatment. Mental health is the right of every citizen, and this guide will help us better understand how to claim that right.

When I was in Congress, I worked for years with my father, Senator Edward M. Kennedy, and many others on both sides of the aisle to pass the Mental Health Parity and Addiction Equity Act because so many Americans were being denied access to the treatments that could help them lead happier, more productive lives. This parity law—the first ever to ensure equal care for people with mental illnesses and substance use disorders—requires insurance providers to cover mental health treatments the same way they cover treatments for all other medical illnesses. The mental health parity act is a tremendously important milestone, but its true value will only be realized if all of us are informed and know what services to seek and expect. Researchers must continue to search for new and effective treatments, and patients and payers must make sure doctors are held accountable for providing such treatments—and then make sure insurers pay for them. We must ensure compliance with the law and demand enforcement.

When we talk about "parity" for mental illnesses, we should think not only about insurance coverage but also about how our society approaches these common disorders. If it's unacceptable to withhold treatment until a cancer hits Stage IV or diabetes is claiming a patient's vision or limbs, surely it must be wrong to wait until a mental illness has become life threatening before making treatment available. Early intervention is as appropriate for mental illnesses as it is for all other conditions, and we should all expect our health care providers to monitor our mental health as carefully as they do our blood pressure or cholesterol levels.

Every routine physical exam should include a "check-up from the neck up." This guide gives us the language to use in sometimes critical discussions about mental health with all of the medical professionals we encounter.

Back in 1963, in the months before his assassination, my uncle, President John F. Kennedy, described the national lack of attention to mental health as a "situation that has been tolerated for too long" because too many Americans viewed mental illness "only as a problem, unpleasant to mention...and despairing of solution."

My belief is that Americans today are more ready than ever to step up and address mental health issues. As this guide shows, we have solutions to the problems caused by mental illness. Do we use these solutions effectively and get them to the people who need them most? Not yet, but this guide helps to point the way.

The struggle to change this perspective is gaining ground, but we need to accelerate the campaign to enhance mental health awareness. This guide is a valuable addition to a growing list of transformative approaches—recovery and wellness self-management strategies, family education, and mental health first-aid among them—that will empower us as individuals and, ultimately, change our society's understanding of mental illness. All of us can do our part. It is time to stop marginalizing people with mental disorders and to show greater compassion and love. You can't eradicate bigotry just by passing a law, but you can help create a new culture that embraces the need for treating those with mental illness in the same manner as those with physical illness. Remember: If you help just one person, you help the world.

*Understanding Mental Disorders* gives individuals with mental disorders and their loved ones something they have too long been denied: the power that comes from knowledge and understanding.

*Patrick J. Kennedy*
*Member, House of Representatives*
*Rhode Island, 1st District, 1995–2011*

# Preface

More than 450 million people worldwide, and over 61 million adults and over 7 million children in the United States, live with a mental disorder at some point in their lives. Although some people are at higher risk, anyone can develop a mental illness. Most everyone has had a friend, a coworker, or a loved one with a mental illness. It is for all of us that *Understanding Mental Disorders: Your Guide to DSM-5* has been written.

Key to overcoming a mental illness is to recognize its symptoms, to know when to seek help, and to get the right treatment. This may be hard for someone who is struggling with mental illness. *Understanding Mental Disorders* is designed to help these people, as well as their loved ones. It lets them know what to expect from the illness—and informs them about the major forms of treatment.

Good treatment is tailored by a health care provider for each person and his or her unique needs and symptoms. This book cannot replace such care and does not provide in-depth details on treatment of specific disorders. Rather, it gives an overview of the treatments for these conditions—both talking therapies and psychiatric medications.

*Understanding Mental Disorders* is based on the latest edition of the *Diagnostic and Statistical Manual of Mental Disorders,* known as DSM-5. The purpose of DSM-5 is to create a common language for health care providers who diagnose mental illnesses. First published in 1952, DSM has since become the primary tool used by mental health care providers and other health care providers to define and diagnose mental disorders.

*Understanding Mental Disorders* is a version of DSM-5 for the general public—although it is not meant for use in self-diagnosis. Rather, it describes most of the disorders contained in DSM-5. This book can be a helpful resource when talking with a health care provider before or after a diagnosis is received. The content of this book mirrors that of DSM-5—it describes symptoms, risk factors, and related disorders. It defines mental disorders based on their symptoms and explores special needs or concerns.

This book also includes ways to cope, personal vignettes, and additional resources—such as a glossary, table of medications, and list of organizations that can help. (The stories in the book are from real people whose names, ages, and other information have been changed to protect them so that others do not know who they are. If a real person matches any of these stories, it is by chance and is not the intent of the authors.)

As with any medical illness, early recognition and treatment improve the chances of a better outcome. *Understanding Mental Disorders* will help patients and caregivers to receive the care they need.

*Understanding Mental Disorders: Your Guide to DSM-5* was developed by a team of world-renowned psychiatrists and psychologists who were involved in writing DSM-5. To all of those involved in this book, as well as DSM-5, we extend our thanks for your commitment to improving the mental health of individuals around the world.

# Acknowledgments

This pioneering project would not have been possible without the valuable contributions of the Editorial Advisory Group, as well as the following colleagues: Glenda Fauntleroy, who wrote the crucial first draft; Darrel A. Regier, M.D., DSM-5 Task Force Vice-Chair, who reviewed all book chapters; Robert H. Chew, Pharm.D., for his creation of Appendix B: "Medications"; John M. Oldham, M.D., M.S., for his review of Chapter 18, "Personality Disorders"; Emily A. Kuhl, Ph.D., Senior Staff Writer in the Department of Research, American Psychiatric Association, for her review of chapters; and at American Psychiatric Publishing: Rebecca D. Rinehart, Publisher, for her pioneering vision for this book and selection of the editorial advisory group; Ann M. Eng, Senior Developmental Editor, for shepherding the process and helping to shape the book for our audience; Rick Prather, Production Manager, for designing the cover; and Tammy J. Cordova, Graphics Design Manager, for designing the book interior and special graphics.

# Photography Credits

*Table of Contents:* African American man, man and boy fishing, Copyright © Diego Cervo; happy children, Copyright © Olesia Bilkei; *chapter graphics:* notebook with pen, Copyright © Kae Deezign; *chapter images:* Chapter 1, "Disorders That Start in Childhood": Copyright © Diego Cervo; Chapter 2, "Schizophrenia and Other Psychotic Disorders": Copyright © bikeriderlondon; Chapter 3, "Bipolar Disorders": Copyright © ostill; Chapter 4, "Depressive Disorders": Copyright © Dereje; Chapter 5, "Anxiety Disorders": Copyright © Adam Gregor; Chapter 6, "Obsessive-Compulsive Disorders": Copyright © Marin Conic (under license from Dreamstime.com); Chapter 7, "Trauma and Stress Disorders": Copyright © Denizo71; Chapter 8, "Dissociative Disorders": Copyright © Yan-Lev; Chapter 9, "Somatic (Physical) Symptom Disorders": Copyright © Alice Day; Chapter 10, "Eating Disorders": Copyright © Diego Cervo; Chapter 11, "Elimination Disorders": Copyright © Federico Rostagno; Chapter 12, "Sleep-Wake Disorders": Copyright © Aseph; Chapter 13, "Sexual Dysfunctions": Copyright © wavebreakmedia; Chapter 14, "Gender Dysphoria": Copyright © Tveritinova Yulia; Chapter 15, "Disruptive and Conduct Disorders": Copyright © parinyabinsuk; Chapter 16, "Addictive Disorders": Copyright © Kamira; Chapter 17, "Dementia and Other Memory Problems": Copyright © Nadino; Chapter 18, "Personality Disorders": Copyright © Michal Kowalski; Chapter 19, "Paraphilic Disorders": Copyright © Oleg Golovnev; Chapter 20, "Treatment Essentials": Copyright © Africa Studio.

# Introduction

About 1 in 4 adults suffers from mental illness at some point in their lives, and nearly that many children are affected as well. It is a very common—and treatable—health problem that has a major impact on quality of life for both individuals and their families. In the past, the subject of mental illness was surrounded by mystery and fear. Today, there has been major progress in the understanding of and ability to treat mental illness. Unfortunately, the early signs of mental illness often go unnoticed and those who would most benefit from treatment do not receive it. They may be reluctant to admit to having a problem, or they may not be aware of the signs and symptoms that signal the presence of a mental illness. The difference between normal and abnormal—of mental health versus mental illness—is often not clear. For this reason, it is important to have a guide to knowing when to seek care early, when treatment is most effective.

The American Psychiatric Association (APA) developed *Understanding Mental Disorders: Your Guide to DSM-5* to help people whose lives have been touched by mental illness to better understand mental disorders and how to manage them. The APA is the official organization that represents approximately 35,000 psychiatrists and supports the delivery of high-quality mental health care. The APA also publishes the *Diagnostic and Statistical Manual of Mental Disorders.* DSM-5, as the fifth edition is known throughout the world, creates a common language for diagnosing mental disorders that is used by psychiatrists and other mental health care providers. *Understanding Mental Disorders* is a practical guide to the disorders described in DSM-5. It explains mental disorders, their diagnosis, and their treatment in basic terms for those seeking mental health care and for their loved ones.

DSM-5 specifies symptoms that must be present for a given diagnosis and organizes these diagnoses together into a classification system. The drive to organize such a system began during World War II, when it became clear that psychiatrists needed to communicate clearly with one another in describing mental disorders. First published in 1952, DSM has evolved to serve as the foundation for defining mental disorders in a variety of settings. The current edition reflects more than a decade of research and the expertise of hundreds of mental health care doctors and professionals who focus on the mental disorders that are their specialty. Psychiatrists, psychologists, other mental health care providers, other physicians, nurses, lawyers, and social workers use DSM-5 as a clinical guide and textbook. It is used in schools, hospitals, courtrooms, and the insurance industry to define what is a mental disorder.

A *mental disorder* is a major disturbance in an individual's thinking, feelings, or behavior that reflects a problem in mental function. Mental disorders cause distress or disability in social, work, or family activities. An expected response to a source of stress or loss, such as the death of a loved one, is not a mental disorder. Likewise, it is normal at times to have feelings of being down, anxious, fearful, or angry. Specific symptoms define mental disorders and help lead to a correct diagnosis. These symptoms, as well as other factors that could determine the diagnosis, are described in each chapter. They can be used to help explain thoughts and feelings to a mental health care provider. All the symptoms listed need not be present in order to diagnose a disorder. The degree of distress and effect on daily living also are important considerations.

In *Understanding Mental Disorders,* as in DSM-5, similar disorders are grouped on the basis of their symptoms and when they first appear in life. Thus, disorders that begin in childhood are found in the first chapter, while disorders that begin in adulthood appear later in the book. For ease of use, each chapter explains the major and most common DSM-5 disorders that occur within these groups. Disorder names are in *italics* to aid notice within chapters, and terms are defined within the text. A glossary of terms also is included near the end of the book, and a complete listing of all DSM-5 disorders is found in Appendix A.

Although self-diagnosis based on these symptoms is tempting, a mental health care provider is best equipped to provide an accurate diagnosis and treatment. Some of the same symptoms occur in many different disorders. For example, anxiety is a symptom that occurs in people with depression, schizophrenia, and posttraumatic stress disorder. Some mental disorders can be related to a medical problem, such as heart disease or diabetes. The mental health care provider will consider possible causes and then narrow it down to the most likely diagnosis. Communicating clearly about symptoms, including when they first arose and the problems they cause, will help in getting the most appropriate diagnosis and the very best care. Lab tests and other assessments are often used to help gather information about symptoms and progress. Some measures that assess symptoms can be found at www.psychiatry.org/practice/dsm/dsm5/online-assessment-measures.

Mental illness affects people of all ages. Children may be too young to clearly relay in words what is wrong. Likewise, an older person with dementia may be confused and not understand what is occurring. A mental health care provider can evaluate the many behaviors, symptoms, and in some cases biological causes to determine the correct diagnosis, and thus, best treatment.

Chapter 20, "Treatment Essentials," presents an overview of types of mental health treatments and how they work. It also reviews types of mental health care providers, what to expect from a first session, types of therapies and medications, and ways to support general mental health. Appendix B provides a list of medications often prescribed for mental disorders.

For most persons with mental illness, treatment is tailored to their symptoms and special needs. Some conditions increase the risk for other disorders (for instance, sometimes an anxiety disorder can develop into a depressive disorder). When one disorder improves, the relief in symptoms may help the treatment of the other illness. Often more than one type of treatment is used. Treatment options for specific disorders are discussed briefly in each chapter, along with information on what to expect—and when to look at other options.

Each person is unique; there is no single approach to diagnosing something as complex as a mental illness. People may express or describe mental disorders in different ways based on their culture or background. Each chapter includes personal stories that show how mental illness may have affected individuals, and their families and friends. (Names, ages, and other information have been changed to disguise each real-life person in these stories.)

This level of awareness is as important for caregivers as it is for a person with a mental disorder. In some cases, those caring for an individual with a mental illness—whether it is a spouse, sibling, or parent—can have more insight about the effects of the illness than the person with the disorder. Some mental illnesses can have an intense effect on the mind, clouding judgment and leading to harmful behaviors such as use of alcohol or other drugs. The person may be unable to think clearly enough to help himself or herself, and others must intervene.

Common warning signs of mental illness include a change in sleep (more or less than usually needed), changes in weight (gain or loss), changes in mood or attention, and feeling "not normal." Being alert to warning signs and knowing when to seek help and what to expect from treatment can be vital. The chapters in *Understanding Mental Disorders* highlight risk factors for certain disorders.

Living with a mental illness, whether it affects you or a loved one, can be very hard—but help is available. People can learn how to maintain a healthy mind and body, and to make positive changes that can improve quality of life and outlook. One way of dealing with mental illness is by seeking support from people who care. In addition to a helpful doctor or mental health care provider, support groups and other organizations can provide sound knowledge for coping with the disorder. Appendix C includes a listing of these additional resources.

A healthy lifestyle can promote optimal mental health. This involves getting sufficient exercise and adequate sleep, having a healthy diet, and learning to confide in friends and trusted family members. It also means learning how to better cope with life's stresses. Even small steps toward these goals help improve health and well-being. Tips for maintaining good mental health are found throughout *Understanding Mental Disorders*.

*Understanding Mental Disorders* is designed to help combat mental illness through education about the disorders and their symptoms, when to seek help, and what to expect from treatment. It can help caregivers serve as the "eyes and ears" of those who may not recognize symptoms in themselves. These disorders can be very painful, but as with any other health condition, most can be treated successfully. Treatment can relieve symptoms and reduce suffering. Overcoming mental illness will take some work and effort, but there is always hope—and help.

*The American Psychiatric Association (APA) is a national medical specialty society representing more than 35,000 physician members specializing in diagnosis, treatment, prevention, and research of mental illnesses, including substance use disorders. Visit the APA at www.psychiatry.org.*

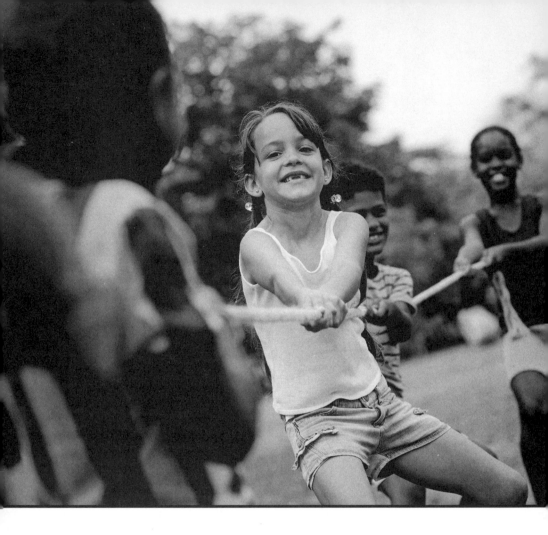

Autism Spectrum Disorder

Attention-Deficit/Hyperactivity Disorder (ADHD)

Intellectual Disability

Other Disorders That Start in Childhood

    Communication Disorders

    Specific Learning Disorder

    Motor Disorders

*For a complete list of DSM-5 disorders, see Appendix A.*

# CHAPTER 1

# Disorders That Start in Childhood

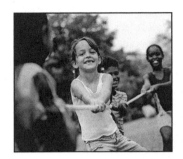

The disorders that begin during childhood featured in this chapter are also known as *neurodevelopmental disorders*. This means they affect the growth and development of the brain. They often begin before a child enters grade school and can impair personal, social, school, or work function. Some of these disorders may last only during childhood. They may get better on their own or with treatment. Others can last longer or may not be noticed or diagnosed until the teen or adult years. For all these disorders, symptoms begin at an early age, even if they are mild.

These disorders include *autism spectrum disorder, attention-deficit/hyperactivity disorder, intellectual disability, communication disorders* (such as problems with speech), *specific learning disorder* (such as reading, math, or writing problems), and *motor disorders* (such as tic disorders). A child may have more than one of these disorders—for instance, both autism spectrum disorder and intellectual disability.

These disorders can cause great distress and concern to parents and children, and the impact of the child's symptoms can affect the whole family. Seeking help from a doctor or mental health care provider will provide a diagnosis if there is indeed a disorder (versus just normal childhood struggles). Treatment can lead to learning new skills and ways to manage symptoms, resources for support and coping, and in some cases, medications to relieve symptoms. It also can offer hope. Many children with these disorders can go on to lead full and rewarding lives. Undiagnosed and untreated disorders increase the risk for more severe problems and hardships as the child grows.

In DSM-5, neurodevelopmental disorders have been regrouped and more clearly defined. *Autism spectrum disorder* is a new, single diagnosis that combines disorders that used to be separate conditions, such as autistic disorder (autism), Asperger's disorder, childhood disintegrative disorder, Rett's disorder, and pervasive developmental disorder not otherwise specified.

Another change was made to follow the wording used by the federal government and many special education and health care providers. *Mental retardation* is no longer used and has been replaced with *intellectual disability*. "Intellectual disability" is a better way to describe children who have problems in mental abilities at an early age. These abilities include reasoning, problem solving, and academic learning. These problems also may involve other types of thinking and behavior beyond just pencil-and-paper types of tests (sometimes called "formal intelligence testing" or IQ test scores).

# Autism Spectrum Disorder

*Autism spectrum disorder* is marked by two main symptoms: problems with the child's ability to relate to others, and having a fixed set of interests or repetitive behaviors. The disorder name reflects a range, or spectrum, of symptoms that vary greatly by age and person.

Many people with the disorder may not be able to handle changes in their daily routines. They may show a lack of eye contact, social response to others, and shared play. Signs of autism spectrum disorder begin during early childhood and often last through a person's lifetime. Some people with the disorder need a lot of help in their daily lives, and others need less. Symptoms can improve with treatment for children and adults with the disorder.

Autism spectrum disorder has been reported in about 1% of children and adults in the general public in the United States and non-U.S. countries. The rates may be rising, but it remains unclear whether this is due to increased awareness or different guidelines for the disorder across studies.

Symptoms are often seen in the first 2 years of life and can be seen before 12 months—or after 24 months if symptoms are milder. Babies who are less likely to smile and coo or babble back and forth with parents may be showing autism spectrum disorder symptoms. First symptoms also involve delayed speaking in toddlers and a low interest in social contact. Some children show a slow or sudden loss of speaking or social skills during the first 2 years of life. Such a loss of skills is rare for other disorders and may be a sign (or a "red flag") for autism spectrum disorder.

In other children with the disorder, symptoms may not appear until there is a change in their routine. This may include going to preschool or a new setting where they must try out new social skills. Sometimes children may learn ways to avoid social contacts that are a challenge for them, and their symptoms are not fully known. But over time, their symptoms are seen more clearly as social contact becomes a bigger part of daily life as they mature.

Symptoms of autism spectrum disorder can be more pronounced during childhood and early school years. Interest in social contact may increase in later childhood. Adults with the disorder may learn coping methods for their problems with social cues (such as when or how to join a conversation, or what not to say). This requires great effort on their part to think through how to engage with others. People with autism spectrum disorder may struggle to know how other people find such social contact to be natural or easy. The need to learn coping methods and build new skills to improve function can persist through life. People with autism spectrum disorder are able to keep learning over time and often have a sense of purpose about learning new social skills.

People with autism spectrum disorder may also have *intellectual disability, language disorder, attention-deficit/hyperactivity disorder, developmental coordination disorder, anxiety disorders,* and *depressive disorders.* Other medical conditions, such as epilepsy, sleep problems, and constipation, also may occur. *Avoidant/restrictive food intake disorder* is somewhat common, in which only a narrow range of foods is eaten.

---

 ## Autism Spectrum Disorder

There is a great range of abilities and traits in people with autism spectrum disorder, and no two people reflect the disorder in the same way.

The following symptoms must be present in the child's early developmental stage for a diagnosis of autism spectrum disorder:

- Frequent and sustained problems in social communication and interaction in many settings:
  - Limited back-and-forth exchange of sounds, expressions, or talking. For instance, there may be reduced sharing of feelings, thoughts, or interests; or failure to start or respond to social contact.

- Problems with nonverbal communication used in social contact, such as lack of eye contact, gestures like pointing or waving, or facial expressions like smiling or frowning. For instance, there may be a failure to look where someone is pointing.
- Problems with building, keeping, and understanding relationships. For instance, the child may have problems changing behavior to suit the setting, making friends, or sharing pretend play; or may have a lack of interest in peers.
- Fixed and repeating patterns of behaviors, interests, or tasks in at least two of the following:
  - Repeating body movements, use of objects, or speech. For instance, the child may often flap his or her hands, repeat sounds or phrases, spin coins, or line up toys again and again.
  - Insisting on the same routines and behaviors. For instance, there may be extreme distress with small changes, problems with shifting to another task, rigid routines in greeting, or a firm need to eat the same foods each day.
  - Having strongly fixed interests with extreme or intense focus beyond what is normal. For instance, the child may be attached to unusual objects (such as vacuum cleaners or fans).
  - Showing great response or no response to certain sights, sounds, smells, textures, and tastes. For instance, there may be no or dulled response to pain, heat, or cold; great dislike for certain sounds or textures; or high pleasure for lights or movement.

These symptoms can cause problems in social, school, and work function. They can range from mild to severe and can change over time or by setting (see Table 1).

Diagnosing and treating autism spectrum disorder early are important to reduce symptoms and improve the quality of life for children with the disorder and their families. Under federal law, any child suspected of having a developmental disorder can get a free evaluation. The Centers for Disease Control (CDC) recommends that all children be screened for autism spectrum disorder at well-child visits with their pediatrician at 18 and 24 months of age.

There is no medical test for autism spectrum disorder. Doctors often diagnose autism spectrum disorder by talking with the child, watching how the child talks and acts compared with others the same age, asking questions of parents and other caregivers, and using screening questionnaires or tools. They assess the type of behavior, how often it occurs, and how intense it is.

| Table 1. Levels of autism spectrum disorder | | |
|---|---|---|
| Severity level | Social communication | Restricted, repetitive behavior |
| **Level 3** "Requiring very substantial support" | Severe lack of verbal and nonverbal communication that causes severe problems in social interactions. Speaks few understandable words and rarely starts social contact. | Preoccupations, fixed rituals, and/or repetitive behaviors that disrupt all areas of function. Very distressed when rituals or routines are interrupted. |
| **Level 2** "Requiring substantial support" | Clear lack of verbal and nonverbal communication. Speaks in simple sentences and has very odd nonverbal communication. | Restricted and repetitive behaviors occur often enough to be noticed by the casual observer. Distress or frustration is clear when behaviors are changed or interrupted. |
| **Level 1** "Requiring support" | Without support in place, impaired social communication causes clear problems. Can speak in full sentences and engage in communication but fail in back-and-forth communication with others. | Repetitive behavior causes great interference with daily function. Trouble switching between tasks. Problems organizing and planning that hamper independence. |

In some cases, the primary care doctor may refer the child and family to a specialist to better assess any symptoms. These include developmental pediatricians (doctors who have special training in child development and children with special needs), child neurologists (doctors who work on the brain, spine, and nerves), and child psychologists or psychiatrists (doctors who know about the human mind).

## Risk Factors

There are no known causes of autism spectrum disorder. Risk factors include the following:

- **Environment.** Children born to older parents, born with low birth weight, or whose mothers used valproate, a medication used to treat seizures and *bipolar disorder*, during pregnancy are more likely to have autism spectrum disorder.

- **Genetics.** The risk of autism spectrum disorder is much greater if there is a family member with the disorder (about 1 in 5 later-born siblings will develop autism spectrum disorder, compared to nearly 1 in 100 young children in the general public). Genes play a major role in autism spectrum disorder, but they are not the only factors. About 15% of children with autism spectrum disorder have a genetic basis for the disorder.

Much debate has occurred over the belief that childhood vaccines cause autism spectrum disorder. This has focused mostly on vaccines that protect against measles-mumps-rubella (MMR) and that contain a preservative known as thimerosal. One reason people believe that autism spectrum disorder is linked to vaccines is that the signs of the disorder sometimes do not appear until around the same age the MMR vaccine is given. If a child is diagnosed shortly after getting the vaccine, this may seem like the vaccine caused the disorder.

Many studies have found no proof of a link between autism spectrum disorder and vaccines. In 2001, thimerosal was removed from or used in much smaller amounts in all vaccines except for one type of flu vaccine, according to the CDC. A flu vaccine without thimerosal also is available. Parents are strongly urged to have their child immunized to protect against serious childhood diseases.

## Adam's Story

Adam, a 12-year-old boy, was brought in by his mother for psychiatric evaluation. He had temper tantrums that were causing problems for him at school. She said that school had always been stressful for Adam and that it had become worse after he entered middle school.

Adam's sixth-grade teachers reported that he could do classroom work, but that he had a hard time making friends. He seemed to mistrust the motives of classmates who were sincere and nice to him. Instead, he believed others who laughed and faked interest in the toy cars and trucks that he brought to school. The teachers noted that he often cried and rarely spoke in class.

When interviewed one-on-one, Adam mumbled when asked questions about school, classmates, and his family. When asked if he liked toy cars, however, Adam lit up. He pulled out several cars, trucks, and airplanes from his backpack. He did not make good eye contact but talked at length about the vehicles, using their correct names, such as front-end loader, B-52, and Jaguar.

Adam spoke his first word at age 11 months and began to use short sentences by age 3. He had always been very focused on trucks, cars, and trains. His mother said that he had always been "very shy" and had never had a best friend. He struggled with childhood jokes and banter because "he takes things so literally." Adam's mother had always seen this behavior as "a little odd." She added that this behavior was like that of Adam's father, a successful lawyer, who had the same focus in his interests. Both of them were "sticklers for routine" who "lacked a sense of humor."

During the exam, Adam was shy and made below-average eye contact. The doctor diagnosed him with *autism spectrum disorder without intellectual impairment*. Adam has trouble interacting with classmates and holding a conversation—both symptoms of social communication problems. Adam also has fixed interests—he is interested in cars and trains and little else. Perhaps because his autism spectrum symptoms were like his father's behavior, his mother viewed Adam as "a little odd" but did not seek an evaluation and diagnosis.

## Treatment

In most cases, autism spectrum disorder is a lifelong disorder. Although there is no cure, children who are diagnosed and treated early can get better. There is no single treatment, but rather different approaches suited to each child to improve behavior and communication. These include intensive skill building and education sessions. They provide structure, direction, and organization for the child and family.

Methods of *applied behavior analysis* often are used. This technique involves types of rewards to support desired behavior and lessen those that can cause harm or block learning. These methods can improve skills such as listening, looking, reading, and relating with others. A child also may receive speech and language therapy, occupational therapy (to help with tasks of daily living), and social skills training. The child's family plays a key role in treatment.

There are no medications to treat the core symptoms (problems with social communication and repetitive behavior) of autism spectrum disorder. Some children and adults with autism spectrum disorder also have other disorders, such as an *anxiety* or *depressive disorder* or *attention-deficit/hyperactivity disorder* (ADHD). These disorders may improve with psychotherapy or medication. Improved or reduced symptoms of these disorders may help in the treatment of autism spectrum disorder.

Many types of special diets have been discussed and explored by those seeking to find better ways to help autism spectrum disorder. These diets often try to avoid foods or substances that might cause problems or allergies. These include excess sugar, gluten, casein, food additives (used to improve taste or flavor), and colorings. So far, it is not known whether any one ingredient can cause the disorder. An unproven treatment might help one child, but it may not help another. Nutrient supplements, such as antioxidants and flavonoids (luteolin), have become popular with many parents who believe that they help improve autism spectrum disorder symptoms. There is little scientific proof that these supplements work. Support groups for autism spectrum disorder caution against their use. Research has shown that the high amounts of flavonoid found in supplements can affect hormone levels and can be harmful to young children. Checking with a doctor before adding a supplement or changing the child's diet can benefit treatment and ensure the child receives the proper vitamins and nutrients for healthy growth.

## Ways to Cope

Having a child with autism spectrum disorder affects the whole family. It can be stressful and require much time to manage the disorder. Paying attention to the physical and emotional health of the entire family is important. The following steps can help:

- **Learn as much as possible.** Get trusted, reliable information about the diagnosis from organizations such as the Autism Society (www.autism-society) and Autism Speaks (www.autismspeaks.org).
- **Provide structure and routine.** Many who have autism spectrum disorder function better if the day is consistent and predictable. Stick to a schedule for daily activities, including mealtimes, schoolwork, and play.
- **Connect with other parents.** Talking to parents who share your experiences can help you cope with your child's challenges. The Autism Society and Autism Speaks offer online support groups for parents and families, as well as help finding resources around the country.
- **Know your child's rights.** A federal law known as the Individuals with Disabilities Education Act (IDEA) requires that special services be available for children with a disability. The services can include early treatment and support for birth through age 3, and "free and appropriate" special education funded by the government for ages 3 to 21. Read more about IDEA at http://idea.ed.gov.

## Attention-Deficit/Hyperactivity Disorder

*Attention-deficit/hyperactivity disorder* (ADHD) is one of the most common mental disorders in children. Although this disorder begins in childhood, it also can affect adults. Its main features include *inattention* (not being able to keep focus), *hyperactivity* (excess movement that is not fitting to the setting), and *impulsivity* (hasty acts that occur in the moment without thought). It can disrupt school, social, and work tasks or function and cause problems in development.

About 5% of children and 2.5% of adults have ADHD. It occurs twice as often in boys than in girls. Parents may notice symptoms in their toddlers, but most children cannot be diagnosed with ADHD until age 4. ADHD often is diagnosed during elementary school, when problems paying attention become clear. During the teen years, hyperactivity may be expressed as being fidgety, restless, or impatient. In adults, inattention, poor planning, restless feelings, and impulsivity may cause problems in all aspects of life.

People with ADHD also may have *oppositional defiant disorder* or *disruptive mood dysregulation disorder*. *Specific learning disorder* is also common.

---

 **ADHD**

Symptoms must be noticed before age 12 and last for at least 6 months. In children, at least six symptoms must be present. In older teens and adults (age 17 and older), at least five symptoms must be present. The symptoms are *not* due only to disobedience or rebellion, defiance, hostility, or failure to understand tasks or instructions. The symptoms clearly disrupt or reduce the quality of social, school, or work function.

ADHD occurs when there is a lasting and frequent pattern of inattention and/or hyperactivity or impulsivity that disrupts function or development, as shown in the following types of symptoms.

**Inattention:** Six (or five, for those 17 and older) of the following symptoms occur *often*:

- Doesn't pay close attention to details or makes careless mistakes in school or job tasks.
- Has problems staying focused in tasks or leisure, such as during lectures, conversations, or long reading.
- Does not seem to listen when spoken to (mind seems to be elsewhere).
- Does not follow through on instructions and doesn't finish schoolwork, chores, or job duties (may start tasks but quickly loses focus).
- Has problems bringing order to tasks and work (for instance, does not manage time well; has messy, disorganized work; misses deadlines).
- Avoids or dislikes tasks that require sustained mental effort, such as schoolwork or homework. Older teens and adults may avoid preparing reports and completing forms.
- Often loses things needed for tasks or daily life, such as school papers, books, keys, wallet, cell phone, and eyeglasses.

- Is easily distracted.
- Forgets daily tasks, such as doing chores and running errands. Older teens and adults may forget to return phone calls, pay bills, and keep appointments.

**Hyperactivity and impulsivity:** Six (or five, for those 17 and older) of the following symptoms occur *often*:

- Fidgets with or taps hands or feet or squirms in seat.
- Not able to stay seated (in the classroom, workplace).
- Runs about or climbs where it is inappropriate.
- Unable to play or do leisure activities quietly.
- Always "on the go," as if driven by a motor.
- Talks too much.
- Blurts out an answer before a question has been finished (for instance, may finish people's sentences, can't wait to speak in conversations).
- Has difficulty waiting his or her turn, such as while waiting in line.
- Interrupts or intrudes on others (for instance, cuts into conversations, games, or activities; or starts using other people's things without permission). Older teens and adults may take over what others are doing.

The symptoms must occur in two or more settings, such as school, home, or work, and with family and friends. They are not due to other disorders such as *schizophrenia, anxiety disorder,* or *substance intoxication.* The disorder can be mild, moderate, or severe based on the symptoms and how much there are problems in social, school, or work function.

ADHD is diagnosed based on the types of symptoms that occur over the past 6 months: *Combined type* is diagnosed when the required number of symptoms occurs for both inattention and hyperactivity or impulsivity. *Inattentive type* is diagnosed when the required number of inattentive symptoms is present, but not all required symptoms of hyperactivity or impulsivity occur. *Hyperactive/impulsive type* is diagnosed when the required number of hyperactivity or impulsivity symptoms is present, but not all required symptoms of inattention occur.

## Risk Factors

Some factors that may increase the risk of the disorder are as follows:

- **Environment.** Babies born weighing less than 3 pounds have a two- to three-fold increased risk of ADHD. A mother who drinks alcohol while pregnant may increase a child's risk. A history of infections and exposure to toxins, such as lead, also might play a role.
- **Genetics and physiology.** People with ADHD are much more likely to have a first-degree blood relative (parent or sibling) with ADHD.

# Josh's Story

Josh, a 19-year-old college student, came to a school clinic for help with academic problems. Since starting college 6 months earlier, he had done poorly on tests and could not manage his study schedule. His worries about flunking out of college were causing him poor sleep, poor focus, and lost hope. After a week of low grades, he returned home and told his family he should drop out of college. His mother brought him to the clinic where he and his older brother had been treated for ADHD when they were younger. She wondered if his ADHD might be causing his problems, or whether he had outgrown it.

Josh had been to the clinic when he was 9 years old and had been diagnosed with ADHD. Notes from that evaluation showed Josh had been in trouble at school for getting out of his seat, losing things, not following instructions, not completing homework, and not listening.

A psychologist also confirmed reading problems during the evaluation. Because Josh's problems did not meet the standards for a learning disability diagnosis, he could not receive special education services. Josh's primary care doctor had proposed medication, but his mother refused. Instead, she hired a tutor to help her son "with concentration and reading."

Since starting college, Josh said he often had trouble staying focused while reading and listening to lectures. Because of his stress at school, he had trouble falling asleep, had poor energy, and didn't "have fun" like his peers.

Josh's older brother had ADHD. His father, who died when Josh was 7, had dyslexia (a reading disorder). His father had dropped out of community college after one semester.

Josh was referred to a psychologist for more testing, and the doctor diagnosed him with *ADHD*. The report stated that Josh had certain problems with reading fluency and comprehension (reading quickly and knowing the correct meaning), as well as spelling and writing. When he was first assessed at age 9, the standards for ADHD required six of nine symptoms. He had been diagnosed with the *combined type* of ADHD, because the specialty clinic had found at least six symptoms in inattention and hyperactivity/impulsivity. With DSM-5, only five symptoms are needed for people age 17 and older. At age 19, Josh met the standards for ADHD and for a *specific learning disorder* (discussed later in this chapter). With the correct diagnosis, he was able to receive services for academic support for his college studies.

# Treatment

Behavior therapy and medication can improve the symptoms of ADHD. Both methods combined often work best.

- *Behavior therapy* focuses on managing the symptoms of ADHD and can help children learn how to control their behavior. It often consists of teaching parents and teachers how to give positive feedback for desired behaviors and negative results for undesirable ones.

- *Medication* helps children improve their attention span, perform tasks better, and control impulsive behavior. *Stimulants* increase the action of certain brain chemicals and have been safely used for decades when taken as the doctor prescribes. They include methylphenidate and amphetamines. *Nonstimulants* are prescribed as an alternative to stimulants and include atomoxetine and guanfacine. Between 70% and 80% of children with ADHD respond to medications. Others may have only some relief and may need changes in medications or doses.

It is key for children who have ADHD to receive a correct diagnosis and proper treatment for their symptoms. Children who are not treated are at greater risk for serious problems, such as school failure, behavior and discipline troubles, social problems, family problems, alcohol and drug use, depression, and later problems with work function. Adults with the disorder can benefit from psychotherapy, cognitive-behavior therapy, medication, and learning how to use tools such as electronic reminders.

## Ways to Cope

Being a parent of a child with ADHD can be a challenge. Along with regular treatment, these tips can help:

- **Keep routines.** Structure helps keep a child from becoming too disorganized and distracted. Set a consistent time for homework, meals, playtime, bedtime, and wake time.
- **Stay organized.** Put schoolbags, clothing, and toys in the same place every day so your child will be less likely to lose them.
- **Make sure instructions are understood.** Give brief, clear directions and set limits. Children who have ADHD need to know exactly what others expect from them.
- **Avoid distractions.** Turn off the TV, radio, and computer when your child is doing homework or needs to focus.
- **Limit choices.** Offer a choice between two things (this outfit, meal, toy, etc., or that one) so that your child isn't overwhelmed and overstimulated.
- **Have a plan for discipline.** Reward good behavior and respond to misbehavior with alternatives such as a time-out or loss of privileges.
- **Maintain communication with the child's teacher.** Being aware of how a child is doing each day with behavior and schoolwork is important to help track his or her progress.

- **Find support.** The group Children and Adults with Attention-Deficit/Hyperactivity Disorder (CHADD) provides online community discussions, resources, and a directory of local support groups in the United States (www.chadd.org).
- **Help your child find a talent.** All children need to have some success to feel good about themselves. Finding out what your child does well—and giving him or her support in these pursuits—can boost your child's social skills and self-esteem.
- **Know your child's rights.** The Individuals with Disabilities Education Act (IDEA) ensures children with ADHD receive care.

# Intellectual Disability

Children with *intellectual disability* (called "mental retardation" in the past) have problems both with their intellectual ability and with learning and doing the skills needed for day-to-day living. About 1% of the U.S. population has intellectual disability. By age 2, delayed motor skills (such as walking) and language (or speech) skills and social milestones may point to severe intellectual disability, which is found in about 6 of every 1,000 children. Mild intellectual disability may not be noticed until a child starts school and learning problems become clearer. See Table 2 for the levels of intellectual disability across types of function.

People with intellectual disability may struggle with communication and may not be able to express themselves clearly. Others may misunderstand what they mean, which can cause people with intellectual disability to lash out in an attempt to be understood. This may include yelling or trying too hard to communicate. They may become forceful toward others who don't know what they are trying to say. People with intellectual disability may also notice and feel awkward or ashamed that they are behind others their own age. As a result, they can act out, feel worried, or try to be alone and away from others. They may have symptoms of depression and problems with eating and sleeping because of the distress they feel. They may also be easily misled by others. This leaves them at risk for being victims of abuse and fraud, or being involved in crime without their knowledge or true consent.

After early childhood, the disorder tends to be lifelong, although how severe it is may change over time. Early and ongoing treatment and support may improve daily function through childhood and adult years. In some cases, these services result in major improvement of intellectual function, such that the diagnosis of intellectual disability no longer applies. For this reason, when doctors assess infants and young children, they often delay diagnosis of intellectual disability until proper support services are given for a certain amount of time. For older children and adults, support services may allow them to take full part in all daily living skills and greatly improve their function.

People with intellectual disability often have other mental, neurodevelopmental, and physical conditions. For instance, other disorders such as cerebral palsy and epilepsy may occur three to four times more often in people with intellectual disability than in the general public. The most common mental and neurodevelopmental disorders that occur with intellectual disability include *ADHD, depressive* and *bipolar disorder, anxiety disorders, autism spectrum disorder,* and *impulse-control disorders.*

---

 **Intellectual Disability**

Intellectual disability begins during child development and involves problems in thinking, social, and real-world functions. All of the following must occur for a diagnosis:

- Impaired *intellectual function* that may be seen in problems with reasoning, problem solving, planning, academic learning, and learning from experience (for instance, problems with memory, knowing word meanings, solving problems, math concepts).
- Impaired *adaptive function* that results in failure to meet standards for age in being independent and socially responsible (such as being able to master real-life tasks). Ongoing support is needed to function in at least one setting of school, work, home, or community.
- Both of the above types of problems begin in the *developmental period* (before age 18).

Intellectual disability is measured in part through a standardized intelligence test given by a psychologist. The average score on such tests, often termed an IQ, is 100. Scores between 65 and 75 (based on the test) fall in the range for intellectual disability. Test scores must be balanced with adaptive function. *Adaptive function* includes self-care and how the child handles common skills needed for life on his or her own as compared with other children of the same age. It includes three skill types: conceptual (academic learning), social, and practical (daily life skills). Problems in these areas must be present for a diagnosis. Intellectual disability occurs across a range of levels: mild, moderate, severe, and profound. Table 2 provides examples for each skill type across levels.

Children are diagnosed based on an exam by a doctor (such as a pediatrician or a child psychiatrist), a standardized intelligence test, and assessment of their behavior or adaptive function. Many health care providers may be involved in making a diagnosis. These include the fields of neurology (the brain and nervous system), special education, hearing, speech, and vision.

## Risk Factors

Anything that affects a baby's normal brain development before or after birth can cause or increase risk for intellectual disability:

- **Genetics.** Chromosomal (genetic) disorders, such as Down syndrome.
- **Environment.** A mother who has consumed or was exposed to alcohol, drugs, toxins, and certain infections or diseases.
- **Childbirth complications.** A baby deprived of oxygen or born before full term.
- **Illness or injury.** Brain injury, infections, seizure disorders, severe neglect or abuse, or exposure to toxins such as lead.

## Treatment

Treatment goals focus on helping the child stay in the family and take part in a fulfilling life. After intellectual disability has been diagnosed, parents work with a team of professionals to develop a plan for care. This includes certain services the child will need, such as speech therapy, occupational therapy, physical therapy, and family counseling. If the child's disability is mild, as in most cases, care is often given in the home by parents, along with outside support and special education. For children with more severe disabilities, health care providers may suggest a group home or specialized institution to provide more special care. Group homes and supported housing also may help adults with intellectual disabilities to reach their highest level of independence.

Children with intellectual disability qualify for special education services according to the Individuals with Disabilities Education Act (IDEA). The services can include early treatment and support for birth through age 3, and "free and appropriate" special education funded by the government for ages 3–21.

Parents of children with intellectual disability can benefit from learning as much as they can about the disorder and their child's rights under the law (such as IDEA). Talking with other parents who have children with intellectual disability can provide ideas and support, as well as help to maintain hope, build the child's skills at home, enjoy and learn from the child, and improve coping.

| Table 2. Levels of intellectual disability for each type of function (examples) | | |
|---|---|---|
| **Mild** | | |
| **Conceptual** | **Social** | **Practical** |
| For preschool children, there may be no clear problems.<br><br>For school-age children and adults, learning reading, writing, math, time, or money is hard. Help is needed in one or more of these areas to meet standards for their age.<br><br>In adults, planning, setting priorities, short-term memory, and use of academic skills in daily life (such as reading or dealing with money) are impaired. | Talking with others, knowing words, and picking up on social cues lag behind age standards.<br><br>There may be trouble keeping feelings and behavior under control in ways that match their peers. These problems are noticed by peers in social settings. | Full function in self-care and hygiene may be present.<br><br>In adults, help may be needed for grocery shopping, transportation, home and child care tasks, health care and legal choices, and banking and money management.<br><br>Adults may hold jobs and can learn skills for work. |
| **Moderate** | | |
| **Conceptual** | **Social** | **Practical** |
| For preschool children, delays in speech may occur.<br><br>For school-age children, progress in reading, writing, math, and understanding of time and money lags behind peers.<br><br>For adults, school skills (such as reading and math) remain at a grade school level. They need daily help for use of these skills in work and personal life. | They can form ties to family and friends, and they may have romantic bonds as adults. Caregivers must assist with life decisions. Help is needed to learn and apply social norms (such as manners and greetings). | By adult age, self-care and household tasks may be done with teaching and reminders.<br><br>Adults may hold jobs with ongoing help from others on the job, as well as from caregivers. Help is needed to manage job duties, schedules, transportation, health benefits, and money. |

## Table 2. Levels of intellectual disability for each type of function (examples) *(continued)*

### Severe

| Conceptual | Social | Practical |
|---|---|---|
| There is little understanding of written language or of concepts that involve numbers, amounts, time, or money. Caretakers provide much support for problem solving throughout life. | Speech may be single words or phrases. Simple speech and gestures are understood. Ties with family members and familiar others are a source of pleasure and help. | Help is required for all functions of daily living, such as meals, dressing, bathing, and using the bathroom. Care is needed at all times to ensure safety and well-being. In adult age, taking part in tasks at home, leisure, and work requires ongoing support and help. Learning skills involves long-term teaching and ongoing support. |

### Profound*

| Conceptual | Social | Practical |
|---|---|---|
| They may learn skills, such as matching and sorting based on size, shape, or color. | Simple instructions or gestures may be understood. They express desires and feelings mostly through nonverbal communication. They enjoy ties with well-known family members, caretakers, and familiar others, and start and respond to social contact through gestures and emotions. | Help from others is needed for all aspects of daily physical care, health, and safety, although they may take part in some of these activities as well. Those without severe physical impairments may assist with some daily work tasks at home, like carrying dishes to the table.<br><br>Leisure activities may involve listening to music, watching movies, going out for walks, or water activities, all with the support of others. |

*If present, motor and sensory (such as hearing or vision) problems may prevent taking part in activities in any area of function.

# Other Disorders That Start in Childhood

These disorders are diagnosed when they cause distress, prevent progress, or create other problems with the child's self-care, home, social, or school tasks. They include *communication disorders, specific learning disorder,* and *motor disorders*. These disorders are not due to the effects of a drug or medication, brain condition, or any other mental disorder, although other conditions or mental disorders may also occur with these disorders. Without treatment or care, these disorders can cause greater problems for the child. Treatment for some disorders can allow complete recovery. Treatment also can relieve symptoms and lead to better coping to aid the child's present and future.

## Communication Disorders

*Communication disorders* are problems in language, speech, or communication (any verbal or nonverbal behavior) that begin early in a child's development. They include *language disorder, speech sound disorder, stuttering,* and *social (pragmatic) communication disorder.*

### Language Disorder

Children with *language disorder* have chronic problems with learning and using language. They have trouble knowing what others' words mean (*receptive language*) and using words or gestures to express themselves (*expressive language*). Their language skills are well below what is normal for their age. Their first words and phrases are often delayed. Problems following instructions may result from struggles to recall new words and phrases. A family history of language disorders is often present. The disorder is lifelong, but speech therapy can improve skills. Psychotherapy can help relieve any problems with emotions or behavior that might result from the disorder. Key symptoms are as follows:

- Reduced vocabulary (for instance, trouble learning new words or often using the same words and phrases).
- Limited sentence structure (uses words and word endings incorrectly when forming sentences).
- Problems using vocabulary to have a conversation with someone or to explain a topic.

### Speech Sound Disorder

With *speech sound disorder,* the child has not learned enough about sounds or is unable to make correct speech sounds with the jaw, tongue, or lips. These problems result in speech that cannot be understood well by others or problems in verbal communication of messages. The disorder is diagnosed when the child's speech is at lower than normal standards for his or her age. For instance, by age 4, most children's speech can be understood—and by age 7 or 8, most children speak clearly. The sounds *l, r, s, z, th,* and *ch* are often the latest for children to learn. A family history of speech or language disorders is often present. Most children with the disorder respond well to treatment with speech therapy, and problems with speech can improve over time. These are the key symptoms:

- Frequent problems with making speech sounds that cause speech to be unclear or that prevent verbal communication.
- The problem limits how well the person can express himself or herself and hinders social, school, or work function.

## Stuttering

People with *stuttering* have frequent problems with the flow and timing of speech. The problem does not go away quickly, but it may end on its own in children. Stuttering that starts in childhood often occurs by age 6. The problem can start slowly or have a sudden onset. Once the problem starts, it becomes more frequent. Stress and anxiety can worsen the symptoms (such as for a school report or job interview). The risk of stuttering among first-degree blood relatives (parents, siblings) is three times higher than in the general public. Treatment includes speech therapy or cognitive-behavior therapy to address thoughts about speaking. The patience and support of parents to remind the child to take more time to speak greatly helps. The disorder is diagnosed when at least one of the following occurs:

- Repeated sounds and syllables ("W-W-W-Where did you go?").
- Lengthened consonant and vowel sounds ("SSSave me a seat").
- Broken words (pauses within a word).
- Pauses in speech that may be silent or filled with sound.
- Replaced words to avoid those that cause problems ("um um").
- Great physical tension with produced words.
- Repeated single-syllable whole words ("I-I-I-I see him").

## Social (Pragmatic) Communication Disorder

A new diagnosis in DSM-5, *social (pragmatic) communication disorder* involves problems in the social use of verbal and nonverbal communication. Problems can be seen by age 4 or 5 years. Milder forms of the disorder may not be known until the early teens, when social communication becomes more complex. Some children greatly improve with speech, language, and behavior therapies that involve the family, special education teachers, and mental health care providers. Other children may still have some struggles in social relationships that persist into adult years.

Because of the problems in social communication, this disorder might look like *autism spectrum disorder*, but those with this disorder do not have fixed interests or repeating behaviors. Those who had a prior diagnosis of *Asperger's disorder* or *pervasive developmental disorder not otherwise specified* (PDD-NOS) based on their problems in social communication might better fit this new diagnosis of social communication disorder. A family history of *autism spectrum disorder*, other *communication disorders*, or *specific learning disorder* increases risk for the disorder. All of the following must be shown for a diagnosis:

- Problems communicating for social reasons, such as greeting or chatting with someone just met.
- Problems changing communication to match the setting (such as a playground or classroom) or the needs of the listener (such as a child or adult).
- Problems with keeping the rules of conversation and storytelling, such as taking turns to speak or listen, and knowing how to use verbal and nonverbal signals to guide contact.
- Trouble understanding humor, figures of speech, what is not stated, and words that might have different meanings in other settings.

## Specific Learning Disorder

Children with a *specific learning disorder* have frequent problems learning one or more key academic skills despite receiving extra help to master them. The diagnosis includes problems with reading, writing, or math that are well below grade level. These problems can impair school or job function and success. If the disorder remains undiagnosed and untreated, a child may begin to dislike or feel upset by schoolwork, which can lead to low self-esteem, depression, and other problems. The learning problems are not due to *intellectual disability*, sight or hearing problems, low income, adverse home life, chronic absence from school, lack of education, brain or mental disorders, or lack of knowledge of the English language.

The diagnosis is made through standardized tests and an evaluation by a team that may include a psychologist, special education expert, and reading and speech-language specialists. Risk factors for a learning disorder include premature birth, low birth weight, and being exposed to nicotine (such as cigarette smoke) while in the womb. Having a first-degree blood relative (parent or sibling) with a learning disorder increases risk four to eight times. The disorder occurs more often in boys, whose risk is at least two times higher than in girls. The disorder can be mild, moderate, or severe based on how hard it is for the child to learn the needed skills. Treatment includes learning new strategies and tools to grasp concepts and build on the child's strengths.

Specific learning disorder is diagnosed when one or more of the following symptoms has lasted for at least 6 months:

- Incorrect or slow reading that requires great effort (for instance, reads words aloud incorrectly, often guesses at words, has problems sounding out words).
- Problems understanding the meaning of what is read.
- Problems with spelling (such as adding letters or leaving them out).
- Problems with writing (for instance, problems putting ideas in order, many grammar and punctuation mistakes).
- Poor understanding of numbers (counts on fingers, gets confused with math problems).
- Problems with mathematical reasoning (applying math facts or concepts).

# Motor Disorders

*Motor disorders* begin early in the developmental years and involve problems with movement. They include *developmental coordination disorder, stereotypic movement disorder,* and *tic disorders.*

## Developmental Coordination Disorder

Children with *developmental coordination disorder* sit, crawl, walk, climb stairs, button shirts, use zippers, or ride a bike later than others their age. Even when the skill is achieved, the movements may appear awkward, slow, or less precise than those of peers. Older children and adults may display slow speed or mistakes with tasks such as self-care skills or playing ball games, writing, typing, and driving.

The disorder is often not diagnosed until after age 5. Boys are twice as likely to have the disorder as girls. In children ages 5–11 years, 5%–6% may have the disorder. Low birth weight, premature birth, or mothers who drink alcohol while pregnant can also increase the risk. In 50%–70% of children affected, problems persist into the teenage years. There may be poor self-esteem, poor physical fitness, reduced physical activity, and behavior problems along with the disorder. Although the disorder is lifelong, treatment can include physical education (exercise), perceptual motor training (helps train the brain and body to improve coordination), and occupational therapy (helps adapt skills for daily life and self-care). Key symptoms for the disorder include the following:

- Learning and doing motor skills lags greatly behind that of peers and standards for age. The person may appear clumsy, drop or bump into things, and seem slow or make mistakes using scissors or writing.
- Symptoms often prevent or greatly delay doing normal daily tasks at home and school, lessen the amount of work that can be done, and hinder leisure and play tasks. For instance, there are challenges in getting dressed, eating meals, and using scissors, pencils, or rulers during class.
- Symptoms are not due to *intellectual disability*, vision problems, or brain disorders that affect movement (such as cerebral palsy).

## Stereotypic Movement Disorder

*Stereotypic movement disorder* begins in the first 3 years of life. The child repeats movements such as hand shaking or waving. Some types of movement may cause self-injury, such as self-biting or head banging. Symptoms before age 3 may be a sign of another neurodevelopmental problem. In children with normal development (that is, meeting age standards for growth and skills), the movements resolve over time or can be stopped when the child is given attention, is asked to stop, or changes focus to another task. Being left alone for a long time or other stress in the child's home may increase risk for the behavior. In children with *intellectual disability*, 4%–16% may have symptoms. In these children, the behavior can last for years.

Treatment should focus on the cause, symptoms, and child's age. Settings around the child can be made safer to prevent harm. Behavior therapy and psychotherapy often help. Some medications, such as antidepressants or naltrexone, may help reduce symptoms.

The disorder may be mild, moderate, or severe. When mild, the child can stop the behavior. When moderate, measures are needed to protect the child and change the behavior. When severe, constant watching and safety measures are needed to prevent great harm. Key symptoms include the following:

- Frequent movements that repeat over and over, such as hand shaking or waving, body rocking, head banging, self-biting, eye poking, face slapping, or hitting one's own body.
- Movement that disrupts social, school, or other tasks and may result in self-harm (such as bruises, cuts, loss of fingers).

## Tic Disorders

*Tics* are quick, sudden movements or vocal outbursts that the child may repeat over and over. They are not done on purpose. Often the person cannot control them but may be able to stop them for a certain amount of time before they occur. Tics get worse with worry, excitement, and fatigue. They may stop or lessen during times of calm or relaxing, or doing school or work tasks.

*Tic disorders* occur two to four times as much in boys as in girls. They often begin between ages 4–6 years and reach their peak at ages 10–12. Symptoms lessen during the teen years, and a small number of people may have tics worsen or last into adult years. Treatment includes behavior therapy, parent training, and if needed, medications.

Although few or many tics may occur, tic disorders are diagnosed when the tic has been present for at least 1 year. The different types of tic disorders all begin before age 18. (If Tourette's disorder is present, none of the other tic disorders can be diagnosed.)

- *Tourette's disorder*—a person has both multiple motor tics (such as blinking eyes, turning head, shrugging shoulders) and at least one vocal tic (such as grunting, clearing throat, repeating words, or unintentionally blurting out offensive words).
- *Persistent (chronic) motor or vocal tic disorder*—a person has one or more motor tics or one or more vocal tics, but not both.
- *Provisional tic disorder*—Motor and/or vocal tics have been present for less than 1 year.

# Key Points

- *Neurodevelopmental disorders* affect the growth and development of the brain and begin during childhood. Once these disorders are diagnosed, they can be treated. A range of support services may be available. With treatment and support, many children with these disorders can go on to lead full and rewarding lives. Untreated disorders increase the risk for more severe problems and hardships as the child grows.

- Many of these disorders (such as *autism spectrum disorder, attention-deficit/hyperactivity disorder, intellectual disability,* and *specific learning disorder*) will qualify a child for special services. A federal law known as the Individuals with Disabilities Education Act (IDEA) requires that special services be available for children with a disability. The services can include early treatment and support for birth through age 3, and "free and appropriate" special education funded by the government for ages 3–21. Read more about IDEA at http://idea.ed.gov.

- Treatment goals should focus on helping the child take part in life as fully as possible. Treatments should help find and build the child's strengths, as well as improve skills that lag behind those of peers or age standards. In most cases, the child will be able to reach these goals while staying with his or her family.

- If treated, some of these disorders may last only during childhood. Others may be lifelong. The need to learn coping methods and build new skills can last through life—and lead to lasting gains.

- The treatment plan for the child's disorder should also include helping parents and families to learn new skills to adapt to the child's disorder. The physical and emotional health of the entire family are important. Learn as much as possible about the disorder and connect with other parents whose children also have these disorders. See Appendix C, "Helpful Resources," for support groups and organizations.

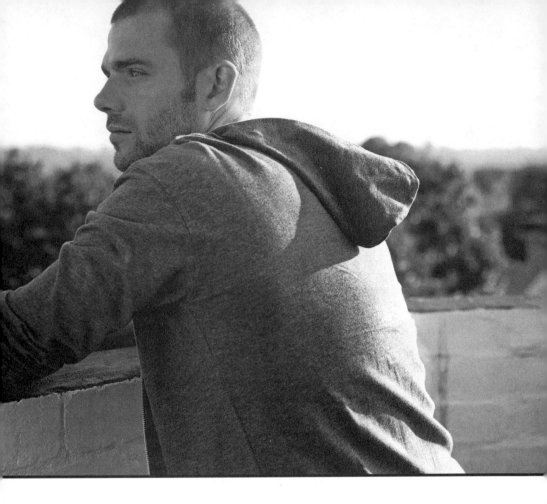

Schizophrenia

Schizoaffective Disorder

Delusional Disorder

Other Psychotic Disorders

    Brief Psychotic Disorder

    Schizophreniform Disorder

    Catatonia

*For a complete list of DSM-5 disorders, see Appendix A.*

CHAPTER 2

# Schizophrenia and Other Psychotic Disorders

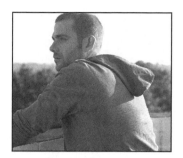

**S**chizophrenia and other psychotic disorders are illnesses that disrupt how someone thinks and understands what he or she sees or hears. These disorders involve a *psychosis:* symptoms that make it very hard or impossible for a person to know what is real, to think clearly, to communicate and relate with others, and to feel normal emotions. When these symptoms occur, it can be hard to get through to the person or to understand what he or she is trying to say. With treatment, many people with these disorders do get better and can work and live on their own.

*Schizophrenia* is the most common of the psychotic disorders. Less common disorders discussed in this chapter are *schizoaffective disorder, delusional disorder, brief psychotic disorder, schizophreniform disorder,* and *catatonia.*

The symptoms of these disorders differ from person to person, yet one or more of these five key features must be present:

- *Delusions* are false beliefs that do not change even with proof that the beliefs are not true, no matter what others may say. Delusions are

**29**

called *bizarre* if they are clearly far-fetched, cannot occur in real life, or are not based on beliefs of the person's culture. There are several types of delusions:

- *Persecutory delusions* are the most common. With these, the person believes that he or she is being harmed or harassed by another person or group (such as the government). People with these delusions may believe that others are stealing from them or mocking them in some way. When people have persecutory delusions, they may be described by friends and family as "paranoid" (that is, suspicious of others).
- *Referential delusions* are also common. People with these false beliefs think that certain gestures and words from others are directed at them. Believing that people on television are sending special messages to them is a common referential delusion.
- *Grandiose delusions* involve the belief that one has exceptional abilities, wealth, or fame.
- *Erotomanic delusions* center on the false belief that another person is in love with him or her.
- *Nihilistic delusions* lead a person to believe that a major crisis will happen or that he or she is doomed, dying, or already dead.
- *Somatic delusions* involve having false ideas about one's health or bodily functions, such as a belief that one's organs are rotting away.

- *Hallucinations* refer to seeing, smelling, feeling, or hearing things that are not there. They appear real to the person having them. The more common type of hallucination is hearing voices. There may be one or more voices speaking to the person or speaking about the person. When people have these *auditory hallucinations*, they may appear to be talking to themselves when they are actually responding to what they are hearing. These voices may say bad things, such as "kill yourself," or they may give constant comments on what the person is doing, such as "John is brushing his teeth....John is going out to the street now."
- *Disorganized thinking and speech* describes scattered or jumbled thoughts and speech. The person is not thinking clearly and does not sound logical when he or she talks (is not "making sense"). People with disorganized speech may appear alert and engaged in a conversation, but their words and sentences may not connect in a way that a listener can follow.
- *Disorganized or abnormal motor behavior* describes movements that seem nervous, restless, or frantic, or that repeat without a clear purpose. Or

the person may be *catatonic* (in a daze, not moving or speaking for hours, even when asked questions). For persons with schizophrenia, the term *grossly disorganized* conveys severe problems in being able to complete routine daily tasks or behave in a normal way, beyond disorganized (scattered, inefficient, extra) movement.

- *Negative symptoms* refer to what is absent in a person with schizophrenia as opposed to what is present, such as delusions and hallucinations. A person with negative symptoms has little energy, may not speak as much as usual, has little interest in past pursuits that were once enjoyed, and has no desire to meet daily goals, have social contact, or express feelings. The person may seem as if he or she has no interest in the outside world and is not bothered at all by this lack of interest. These negative symptoms are unlike depression symptoms because those with psychotic disorders are not bothered or distressed by not meeting (or not having) daily goals.

Schizophrenia and other psychotic disorders almost always begin during the late teen years or early 20s. These disorders also may first occur at around age 40 or much later in life, even in elderly persons, although this is rare. They also can occur rarely in children. When the main symptoms of the disorders appear, getting help quickly is key.

When diagnosing schizophrenia and other psychotic disorders, mental health care providers look at factors such as culture, religion, ethnic background, and socioeconomic status. These factors can play a big role in what a person may consider a delusion or hallucination. For example, a belief in witchcraft might appear to be a delusion, but some cultures believe in witchcraft, and this belief would not be a sign of a psychotic disorder in someone who belongs to that culture. "Hearing God's voice" is also a normal part of some religions, and this is not considered a psychotic symptom in those who belong to these groups.

Although there is no complete cure for these disorders, treatment can improve symptoms. Many go on to live full and meaningful lives.

# Schizophrenia

*Schizophrenia* is a brain disorder that can disturb normal thoughts, speech, and behavior. It tends to remain for life once it begins and to cause problems with day-to-day living. Schizophrenia occurs in about 0.3%–0.7% of people during their life, and rates differ across countries. It affects men and women equally.

Schizophrenia can have a sudden or slow start. For most people with the disorder, it begins slowly over time. A person might have a normal childhood and function very well until symptoms start in the late teens or early adult years. Men tend to have symptoms a little earlier than women. Most men have their first psychotic episode (that is, delusions or hallucinations) in their early to mid-20s. For most women, the first episode is in their late 20s.

It is rare for symptoms to start before the teen years. Children may have daydreams or fantasies that are not delusions or hallucinations. Symptoms of schizophrenia in children (such as disorganized speech or behavior) are the same as some symptoms of other disorders that start in childhood (see Chapter 1, "Disorders That Start in Childhood"). These childhood disorders should be ruled out with care before schizophrenia is diagnosed in childhood.

People with schizophrenia are at high risk to abuse alcohol or other drugs. Over half of people with schizophrenia are regular cigarette smokers. A person with schizophrenia may use alcohol, marijuana, or other drugs to help cope with some of the symptoms of schizophrenia. These can make the illness worse and treatment more difficult. The rates of *obsessive-compulsive disorder* and *panic disorder* are high in people with schizophrenia as well.

Suicide is another major risk for those with schizophrenia. There may be voices telling the person to take his or her own life, and drug use and symptoms of depression also can increase risk. About 5%–6% of people with the disorder take their own lives, and about 20% have attempted suicide at least once. Suicide risk is reduced with treatment, close support, and supervision. For this reason, finding a caring and skilled mental health care provider for treatment as soon as possible is vital.

Schizophrenia often requires treatment with medications throughout life, and most people find relief from their symptoms with treatment. Psychotic symptoms tend to lessen with age. About 20% of people with schizophrenia have a good outcome, where their symptoms become less severe over time, and a small number of people recover completely. Most people with the disorder will need lifelong support and some level of assistance with daily needs.

---

 **Schizophrenia**

Schizophrenia occurs when a person has at least two of the following symptoms for 1 month:

- Delusions
- Hallucinations
- Disorganized speech

- Grossly disorganized or catatonic behavior
- Negative symptoms

A person must have at least one of the first three symptoms. For most of the time since the symptoms began, the person's day-to-day function has worsened in one or more major areas, such as work, relationships, or personal hygiene. The signs of his or her troubled behavior also have lasted for at least 6 months; they have not been temporary. A mental health care provider should rule out other disorders, such as *schizoaffective, depressive,* and *bipolar disorders.* If the symptoms are caused by a drug, medication, or other medical condition, schizophrenia cannot be diagnosed. If there is a history of *autism spectrum disorder* or a *communication disorder* that began in childhood, schizophrenia is only diagnosed if a person has had delusions or hallucinations and the other symptoms of the disorder for at least 1 month.

## Risk Factors

These factors seem to play a role in the start of schizophrenia:

- **Genetics.** Genes play a strong role in risk for schizophrenia. However, many with the disorder do not have a family history of the disease.
- **Pregnancy and childbirth complications.** Problems during childbirth may increase risk. Health problems for a mother during pregnancy, such as stress, infection, malnutrition (poor diet), diabetes, and other medical conditions, also have been linked with the disorder. At the same time, most women who have these conditions do not have children who go on to have schizophrenia.

### Myles' Story

Myles was a 20-year-old man who was brought to the emergency room by the campus police of the college from which he had been suspended several months ago. A professor had called and reported that Myles had walked into his classroom, accused him of taking his tuition money, and refused to leave.

Although Myles had much academic success as a teenager, his behavior had become increasingly odd during the past year. He quit seeing his friends and no longer seemed to care about his appearance or social pursuits. He began wearing the same clothes each day and seldom bathed. He lived with several family members but rarely spoke to any of them. When he did talk to them, he said he had found clues that his college was just a front for an organized crime operation. He had been suspended from college because of missing many classes. His sister said that she had often seen him mumbling quietly to himself and at times he seemed to be talking to people who were not there. He would emerge from his room and ask his family to be quiet even when they were not making any noise.

Myles began talking about organized crime so often that his father and sister brought him to the emergency room. On exam there, Myles was found to be a poorly groomed young man who seemed inattentive and preoccupied. His family said that they had never known him to use drugs or alcohol, and his drug screening results were negative. He did not want to eat the meal offered by the hospital staff and voiced concern that they might be trying to hide drugs in his food.

His father and sister told the staff that Myles' great-grandmother had had a serious illness and had lived for 30 years in a state hospital, which they believed was a mental hospital. Myles' mother left the family when Myles was very young. She has been out of touch with them, and they thought she might have been treated for mental health problems.

Myles agreed to sign himself into the psychiatric unit for treatment. His story reflects a common case, in which a high-functioning young adult goes through a major decline in day-to-day skills. Although family and friends may feel this is a loss of the person they knew, the illness can be treated and a good outcome is possible. In the case of Myles, he was having persecutory delusions, auditory hallucinations, and negative symptoms that had lasted for at least 1 year. All of these symptoms fit with a diagnosis of *schizophrenia*. It is key for the treating doctor to quickly rule out other causes of the problem, such as substance use, a head injury, or a medical illness. Treatment for these conditions differ from that for schizophrenia and may be lifesaving.

## Treatment

There is no cure for schizophrenia, but treatments can relieve its symptoms. Medication and psychotherapy can help people with schizophrenia lead productive and rewarding lives. Some people with the illness may have more lasting problems in daily living despite treatment and family support. For most people with schizophrenia, recovery includes managing the illness with medication. Recovery may mean that although some symptoms are still present, there is no major disability.

Treatment often begins with medications to get delusions and hallucinations reduced or stopped. When these are under control, other types of therapy and services can help those with schizophrenia (see "Key Support Options" later in this section). Taking care of general health and wellness (such as eating a healthy diet, quitting smoking, and getting exercise) is a key part of caring for the illness.

Family members and loved ones can play a key role in helping someone with schizophrenia get and stay better. Along with the person who has schizophrenia, they should learn as much as possible about the disorder. With the help of a mental health care provider, family members can learn coping strategies and problem-solving skills. When needed, family members can help make sure their loved one sticks with treatment and stays on his or her medication.

A mental health care provider can help family members to know about warning signs after treatment has started (for instance, if the person stops taking medication, seems to stop eating or sleeping, or otherwise doesn't seem to get better) and how best to understand and interact with their family member with schizophrenia.

## Before Treatment Begins

Before treatment can begin, a doctor must conduct a thorough medical exam to rule out substance use or other medical illnesses whose symptoms are similar to schizophrenia. Many persons with schizophrenia may also have problems with drug use, so it may take a while for the diagnosis to be fully clear. For a person to have schizophrenia, the symptoms must still be clearly present even when the person is not under the influence of a substance and has not used the substance for a long time, such as a month or more. Also, symptoms that first appear to be due to schizophrenia may later turn out to be those of a manic episode (a time of extreme energy, risky behavior, or little sleep) or depression (feeling hopeless or sad, or having little energy). The source of the problem may be *bipolar disorder* or *major depressive disorder* (see full discussions in Chapter 3, "Bipolar Disorders" and Chapter 4, "Depressive Disorders").

The mental health care provider should ask about alcohol or drug use. If a person shows signs of addiction, treatment for substance abuse should be pursued along with other treatment for schizophrenia. An alcohol or drug problem can make schizophrenia symptoms worse and cause problems with medications prescribed to treat schizophrenia. Treatment for an alcohol or drug problem is helpful and can occur along with treatment for schizophrenia.

Sometimes it can be hard to figure out how much of the problem is due to substance use and how much is due to schizophrenia. In general, substance use causes symptoms like hallucinations or delusions for only a brief time. If all alcohol or drug use is fully stopped for several weeks or a month, then any symptoms that occur after that would be from schizophrenia.

## Medications

*Antipsychotic medications* are used to treat schizophrenia. These medications are most often taken every day on a regular basis to keep symptoms under control—in the same way that many people need to take medicines every day to keep their blood pressure or cholesterol under control. Taking the medicine every day helps reduce delusions and hallucinations and prevents them from coming back. If the medication is stopped, the problem is likely to return or become worse.

Two types of antipsychotic medications can help with schizophrenia symptoms. One type is called a *first-generation* or *typical antipsychotic* (some of these have been available since the mid-1950s). Some of the more common typical antipsychotics include haloperidol, fluphenazine, and perphenazine. The other type is called a *second-generation* or *atypical antipsychotic* (these became available in the 1990s). Common atypical antipsychotics prescribed include risperidone, olanzapine, and quetiapine.

Sometimes, people with symptoms of schizophrenia may not be able to understand that they have an illness. They perceive their beliefs and their hallucinations as real, and so they don't understand the need for medication. This can be hard for loved ones and care providers who want to be sure that needed medication is taken. In some cases, it is useful for a family member to remind the person about the need for medicines and to make sure the medicines are taken. In other cases, antipsychotic medicines that can be given in a shot (injection) form once or twice a month might ease treatment for the person. Learning about the different types of medications and their effects is also helpful (see box).

## Key Support Options

After the symptoms of schizophrenia are under control, support services can help people improve skills that may have declined during the illness or were never attained. Services can provide training to help in coping with day-to-day stresses, building social skills, learning early warning signs of relapse, and learning how to manage symptoms before they worsen.

Because schizophrenia often strikes in early adult years, those with the disorder may need support and guidance to help build life skills, complete school or training, and hold a job. For instance, supported-employment programs help people with schizophrenia prepare for, find, and keep jobs in real-world settings.

Rehabilitation and community support programs can include counseling, job counseling and training, teaching skills to manage money, help in using public transport, and chances to practice communication skills. Rehabilitation programs work well when they include both job training and therapy designed to improve thinking skills. Programs like this help people with schizophrenia hold jobs, remember important details, and improve their function.

Many people living with schizophrenia receive emotional and material support from their family. Therefore, families must receive educa-

## Medication Tips

The medications used for schizophrenia are each very different in their side effects. If problems arise with one of the medicines, ask the doctor about other choices. Here are some more tips:

- Take the medication as the doctor directs.
- Know what to expect with side effects (weight gain or fatigue may be common side effects with some medications). Ask about how best to cope with side effects.
- Set a helpful routine to make sure the medications are taken every day.
- Do not stop a medication right away or decrease the dose without checking with a doctor first. If some medications are stopped right away or the dose is reduced, they may cause unhealthy and unpleasant symptoms—or can make symptoms worse.
- Pay close attention to how the medicines are working or not working, even as time passes. After a while, the body can adjust to medications, symptoms can improve or worsen, and the doctor may need to adjust the dose or switch medications.
- Even when symptoms improve—or side effects are unpleasant—know that medications help symptoms improve.
- Be sure to keep in touch with your doctor. Medicines can cause health changes over time (for instance, in cholesterol, blood pressure, and blood sugar). Any of these problems can be handled safely as long as you see the doctor regularly.

tion and assistance on how best to manage their loved one's illness. This type of help has been shown to help prevent relapses and improve the overall mental health of the family, as well as the person with the illness.

Cognitive-behavior therapy (CBT) is a type of psychotherapy that focuses on thinking and behavior. CBT helps people with schizophrenia to test the reality of their thoughts and perceptions, how to "not listen" to their voices, and how to manage their symptoms overall. Along with medication, CBT can help reduce the severity of symptoms and reduce the risk of relapse.

People with schizophrenia often can receive care for their illness in the community where they live. If symptoms become severe, hospital care may be needed. When living alone or with family is not an option for someone with schizophrenia, supportive housing (such as halfway houses, group homes, and monitored cooperative apartments) is often available.

It is important that caregivers for a person with schizophrenia get support for themselves and understand how best to help their friend or family member. Talking with a mental health care provider can benefit and comfort those caring for their loved one. Appendix C, "Helpful Resources," contains a list of support groups that may also help.

*Schizophrenia and Other Psychotic Disorders*     **37**

# Schizoaffective Disorder

People with *schizoaffective disorder* suffer from a mix of symptoms of *schizophrenia* and a mood disorder, such as a *depressive* or *bipolar disorder*. Schizoaffective disorder is less common than schizophrenia. About 0.3% of people will have the disorder in their lifetime, and it appears more often in women than men. Most often, people with this disorder have symptoms that are like schizophrenia. They often have a decline in day-to-day living skills and achieve less than they could without the disorder. This means they may have a life course similar to Myles, above, in that they may not finish college as expected or reach a high level of success in their work. Schizoaffective disorder may begin with symptoms of delusions and hallucinations much like schizophrenia. In people with schizoaffective disorder, there are also times of having problems with a low mood (as in depression) or an extreme high or euphoric mood (as in a manic episode).

People with schizoaffective disorder have a 5% risk for suicide. The risk is higher for people who have depressive symptoms. This risk can be managed by getting care for the illness and appropriate treatment.

Many with the disorder are also diagnosed with other mental disorders, especially a *substance use disorder* or an *anxiety disorder.*

---

 **Schizoaffective Disorder**

Schizoaffective disorder is diagnosed when someone has:

- A major depressive mood or manic mood while also having periods of time with at least one of the following symptoms of *schizophrenia:* delusions, hallucinations, disorganized speech, grossly disorganized or catatonic behavior, or negative symptoms.
- Delusions or hallucinations for at least 2 weeks without a major depressive or manic mood.

Mood symptoms must exist for most of the total length of the illness (more than half the time). The symptoms of schizoaffective disorder cannot be related to a drug, medication, or any other medical condition.

---

## Risk Factors

The causes of schizoaffective disorder are unknown, but genes likely play a role. People with a first-degree blood relative (parent or sibling) with *schizophrenia, bipolar disorder,* or *schizoaffective disorder* may be at higher risk for schizoaffective disorder.

## Treatment

Treating schizoaffective disorder is much like treating schizophrenia. Treatment may include antipsychotic medication, as well as antidepressant medication to improve depressive moods that may occur with the disorder. Often people with schizoaffective disorder also have problems with manic symptoms, so medications that stabilize mood and prevent extreme "highs" are needed. These medications may include lithium carbonate or valproate. In addition to medication, the same types of therapy and rehabilitation support used to help those with schizophrenia also enable those with schizoaffective disorder and their families to better manage the condition.

# Delusional Disorder

*Delusional disorder* involves a false belief (delusion) in something that is not true, just as someone with schizophrenia may have. The disorder differs from schizophrenia because it does not include the other schizophrenia symptoms of hallucinations; disorganized thought, speech, or movement; or negative symptoms. Like people with schizophrenia, people with delusional disorder may have nonbizarre or bizarre delusions. *Nonbizarre delusions* are false beliefs about events that could occur in real life but are unlikely. These include beliefs about being followed, poisoned, deceived, or conspired against, or that a stranger or famous person is in love with them. *Bizarre delusions* are false beliefs that are not possible to occur (for instance, a stranger has removed their organs and replaced them with someone else's without leaving any wounds or scars).

People with a delusional disorder may seem to function close to normal in the world. They may not appear to others to be ill or abnormal in any way, unless they begin to talk about or act on their delusions.

Delusional disorder is less common than the other psychotic disorders—about 0.2% of adults will have it in their lifetime. Because people with the disorder often do not have other severe schizophrenia symptoms aside from their false beliefs, they are more likely to hold a job and may not seek care for their problem. Delusional disorder can occur in young people but tends to strike in middle to late adult life. It affects men and women equally. The mental health care provider should ask about faith and culture to assess whether the belief is a part of these systems or a delusion.

**Delusional Disorder**

Delusional disorder is diagnosed when someone:

- Has one or more delusions that have lasted at least 1 month.
- Does not have hallucinations, disorganized speech, disorganized behavior, or negative symptoms.

Although the person has delusions and may have problems relating with others due to the false beliefs, in general the person can do fine in day-to-day life and does not show bizarre or odd behavior. Other symptoms such as depression or manic symptoms tend not to occur along with delusional disorder. If they do occur, these symptoms would be only a brief part of the illness, because the delusions are the main problem. The disorder also cannot be caused by a drug, medication, another medical condition, or another mental disorder, such as *obsessive-compulsive disorder.*

## Risk Factors

The cause of delusional disorder is unknown, although risk increases with older age. The disorder may be affected by changes in the brain that occur with aging.

## Treatment

Getting someone with delusional disorder to accept treatment can be very hard. Those with the disorder often deny they have a problem and can mistrust other people and their motives. If they agree to treatment, one-on-one psychotherapy may help them notice and change their false beliefs and manage stressful feelings. In general, people with delusional disorder can manage their daily lives fairly well because they do not have other schizophrenia symptoms, such as negative symptoms. Medications often do not have a useful effect on their beliefs, which often remain strong and never fully go away.

# Other Psychotic Disorders

This brief review of other psychotic disorders that can occur (but are less common than schizophrenia) includes *brief psychotic disorder, schizophreniform disorder,* and *catatonia.* These disorders differ in their symptom profiles. Catatonia is a medical emergency and can occur with other medical and mental disorders.

# Brief Psychotic Disorder

People with *brief psychotic disorder* have sudden, short periods of psychotic behavior that last at least 1 day but less than 1 month. They often recover quickly afterward, and the symptoms fully go away. Symptoms may appear to be like *schizophrenia*. People with brief psychotic disorder may be greatly confused and upset, and have extreme moods that change quickly. They have severe problems with self-care and with home, school, work, and life function. Because of delusions or hallucinations, they may be at risk for suicide and have poor judgment.

This is not a common disorder, although it occurs twice as often in women as in men. Antipsychotic medications may be used, but only for a short time until the episode is over. The disorder may occur during pregnancy or 4 weeks after giving birth. It may be a response to a major stressful life event, but sometimes there is no clear reason for the disorder. There are often no warning signs that suggest schizophrenia, such as negative symptoms, or any decline from daily living skills before the brief episode occurs. Once the brief episode is over, often within a few days, the person returns to his or her daily life, and there is no longer any sign of a problem. At least one of the first three symptoms below must be present for at least 1 day but less than 1 month:

- Delusions
- Hallucinations
- Disorganized speech
- Grossly disorganized behavior or catatonic behavior

The disorder is not due to any drug or medication, another medical condition, or *major depressive, bipolar,* or other *psychotic disorders.*

# Schizophreniform Disorder

*Schizophreniform disorder* has the same key symptoms as *schizophrenia,* but the symptoms last for a shorter time—at least 1 month, but less than 6 months. Once the symptoms last at least 6 months, the diagnosis is changed from schizophreniform disorder to schizophrenia. With schizophreniform disorder, the person loses daily living skills and often begins having frequent problems with school or work. People with schizophreniform disorder also can have negative symptoms. They may stop joining in usual activities and may stop caring for themselves, and yet may interact with others in a normal way. Most often, schizophreniform disorder is diagnosed when someone may have schizophrenia, but 6 months have not yet passed to meet the schizophrenia diagnosis. Key symptoms are at least two of the items below. At least one of the symptoms must be delusions, hallucinations, or disorganized speech:

- Delusions
- Hallucinations
- Disorganized speech
- Grossly disorganized behavior or catatonic behavior
- Negative symptoms

The disorder is not due to any drug or medication, another medical condition, or *major depressive, bipolar,* or other *psychotic disorders.*

## Catatonia

*Catatonia* can occur as a symptom of other medical conditions (such as head trauma and brain diseases) and several mental disorders, such as *neurodevelopmental, psychotic, bipolar,* and *depressive disorders*. It can occur at any age. Most of the time, it happens fairly quickly, over a few days or weeks. The problem is often very serious and urgent. It requires a doctor's care, most often with a stay in the hospital. The main features include decreased response to others and decreased, extreme, or strange movement. Symptoms may switch between decreased and extreme movement. In severe stages, safety measures and watching are needed to prevent harm to self or others. A person with catatonia has at least three of the following symptoms:

- Stupor (that is, unable to move, not responding to the settings around him or her)
- Rigid muscles or fixed posture
- Waxy flexibility (a person's limbs stay in any position they are put in by another person)
- No or little verbal response to others
- Extreme resistance (not responding to instructions)
- Sudden holding of a position for a long time against gravity
- Strange movements or mannerisms
- Frequent, repeating movements that do not have a purpose
- Agitation (restless movement, moving in an excited manner)
- Grimacing (face shows pain, disgust, or displeasure)
- Repeating someone else's words
- Copying someone else's movements

People with catatonia cannot respond to their surroundings and may stop eating and drinking. Treatment for catatonia varies based on other illnesses that may be present. Sometimes getting fluids and nutrition in the hospital is needed to maintain health until the best treatment is decided. Treatments such as electroconvulsive therapy (ECT) can sometimes improve symptoms quickly. The person begins to "wake up," respond to others, and be aware of what is going on around him or her after just a short time of treatment. (See Chapter 20, "Treatment Essentials," for more about ECT.)

## Key Points

- People with a *psychotic disorder* lose touch with reality, and they have problems knowing what is real and thinking clearly. With treatment, they do get better and many can work and live on their own. Recovery may mean that although they still have some symptoms, they are not impaired or disabled in a major way.
- Many times, people with symptoms of *schizophrenia and other psychotic disorders* may not be able to understand that they have an illness. They perceive their beliefs and their hallucinations as real, and so they do not see a need for treatment.
- Family members and loved ones play a key role in helping someone with schizophrenia or another psychotic disorder get and stay better. Along with the person who has the disorder, they should learn as much as possible about the disease. With the help of a mental health care provider, family members and loved ones can learn coping strategies and problem-solving skills. When needed, they can help make sure needed treatment is received.
- A doctor should be contacted at any time with concerns or questions about medications or side effects. If some medications are stopped right away or the dose is reduced, they may cause unhealthy and unpleasant symptoms—or can make symptoms worse. Alcohol or drug use also makes symptoms worse and can disrupt the way medications work.
- Mental health care providers can help people with these disorders better handle their feelings. They can teach how to test the reality of thoughts and perceptions, how to "not listen" to voices, and how to manage their symptoms in all parts of life. Psychotherapy can help reduce the risk of relapse.

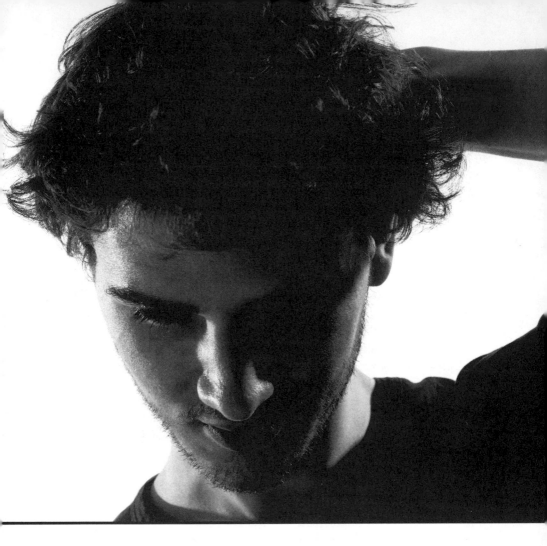

Bipolar I Disorder
Bipolar II Disorder
Cyclothymic Disorder

*For a complete list of DSM-5 disorders, see Appendix A.*

# CHAPTER 3

# Bipolar
# Disorders

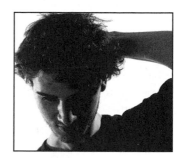

**B**ipolar disorders are brain disorders that cause marked shifts in a person's mood, energy, and ability to function. People with these disorders have extreme and intense emotional states that occur in distinct periods called *mood episodes*. These differ from the normal ups and downs in mood that occur in daily life.

The symptoms of bipolar disorder can damage relationships, cause problems with work or school, and even lead to suicide. People with the disorder may feel out of control or ruled by their extreme moods and behaviors. Although there may be periods of normal mood as well, people with a bipolar disorder will often continue to have these mood episodes if the condition is left untreated.

More than 10 million Americans suffer from a bipolar disorder. The bipolar disorder class includes three different conditions: *bipolar I, bipolar II,* and *cyclothymic disorder.* They share many of the same symptoms, but differ in severity and intensity, and thus need somewhat different treatments.

Although these disorders are lifelong once they begin, treatment can relieve symptoms and bring hope. People with these disorders benefit most from a combination of medications, psychotherapy ("talk therapy"), and healthy lifestyle habits. With the right treatment, people with bipolar disorders can lead full and productive lives.

# Bipolar I Disorder

*Bipolar I disorder* can cause dramatic and wild mood swings—from high spirits that lead the person to feel on top of the world, to being quickly annoyed or angry, to feeling sad and hopeless, often with periods of normal moods in between. The high spells are called episodes of *mania*, and the low spells are episodes of *depression. Hypomanic* episodes can also occur. These are like manic episodes but only last a few days and are not as intense as a manic episode.

An older name for bipolar disorder is "manic-depressive disorder." It is normal for most people to have a very good mood some of the time and a lower mood at other times. For those with bipolar disorder, severe mood swings create great problems in day-to-day life and being able to go to work or school.

More than 90% of people who have one manic episode will have more episodes. Sometimes manic episodes happen right after a major depressive episode, but the reverse can also be true. Four or more major depressive, manic, or hypomanic episodes in the same year are a form of bipolar I disorder known as *rapid cycling*.

Bipolar I disorder affects about 0.6% of the U.S. population each year. The average age for a person to have a first manic or depressive episode is 18 years, although the illness can start in early childhood or older adulthood, such as in the 60s and 70s. Men and women are just as likely to have bipolar I disorder. Women are more likely than men to have rapid cycling and depressive symptoms.

It is common to have other mental disorders along with bipolar I disorder, such as an anxiety disorder (*panic disorder, social anxiety disorder*), *attention-deficit/hyperactivity disorder* (ADHD), or a *substance use disorder*. In fact, more than half of the people with a bipolar I disorder also have an alcohol or drug use disorder.

The risk of suicide is estimated to be about 15 times higher in people with bipolar I disorder than in the general population. People with the illness may make up as much as 25% of all suicide deaths. Getting proper treatment for bipolar disorder can help the person feel more in control of emotions and his or her life.

---

 **Bipolar I Disorder**

Bipolar I disorder is diagnosed when a person has had a manic episode. The manic episode can come before or after a hypomanic episode or a major depressive episode. The symptoms are not due to psychotic disorders such as *schizoaffective disorder, schizophrenia, schizophreniform disorder,* or *delusional disorder.*

## Manic Episode

A distinct period lasting at least 1 week (or less if the person receives hospital care for the symptoms) in which a person is very happy, in high spirits, or irritable in an extreme way nearly every day for most of the day; is much more active or has more energy than usual; and has at least three of the following symptoms that reflect a clear change in behavior:

- Inflated self-esteem or grandiosity (such as believing he or she is better than others and deserves special treatment, believing he or she has a special talent that does not exist).
- Less need for sleep (for instance, feels rested or full of energy after only 3 hours of sleep).
- Talking more than usual (for instance, talking loudly and quickly, without stopping or concern for others' wishes).
- Racing thoughts or quickly changing ideas or topics that don't have any link to each other.
- Being easily distracted (for instance, not able to block out minor details such as someone's clothes or background noise, so that he or she cannot talk with others or follow instructions).
- Doing many activities at once (for instance, planning more events in the day than can be done or taking on new projects that overlap each other, often with little knowledge of the topic and at strange hours of the day).
- Increased risky behavior (reckless driving, spending sprees, out-of-character or careless sex).

Symptoms are severe enough to cause problems with social or work function. Someone with these symptoms may require hospital care to prevent harm to self or others. The changes are obvious to friends and family members. (For instance, have people told the person that he or she is not acting normal?) They are not due to the effects of a drug of abuse, a medication, or another medical condition.

## Hypomanic Episode

These episodes are similar to manic episodes, but the symptoms need only last 4 days in a row (rather than the 1 week with mania). The key difference between mania and hypomania is that while the mood changes are noticed by others, the hypomanic symptoms are not severe enough to cause such problems as getting arrested for speeding, getting into fights, or losing a valued relationship because of something reckless said or done—and are not severe enough to require hospital care. Symptoms are not due to the effects of a drug of abuse or a medication.

## Major Depressive Episode

A person with a major depressive episode has at least five of the following symptoms for 2 weeks, has a decline from his or her normal social or work function, and must have one of the first two symptoms on the list:

- Depressed mood or sadness lasting most of the day, nearly every day (feels sad, empty, or hopeless).
- Great loss of interest or pleasure in all or almost all activities that were once enjoyed.
- Sudden change in appetite, with weight gain or loss.
- Insomnia or hypersomnia (sleeping too little or too much).
- Feeling restless or agitated (as seen in pacing or hand-wringing) or having slowed speech and movements (behavior must be noticed by others).
- Fatigue or loss of energy.
- Feeling worthless or guilty.
- Trouble keeping focused or making decisions.
- Frequent thoughts of death or suicide, a suicide plan, or suicide attempt.

These depressive symptoms cause extreme distress or impair social or work function. They are not due to the effects of a drug of abuse, a medication, or another medical condition.

# Risk Factors

A family history of bipolar I disorder is a strong risk factor. The risk is 10 times higher than in the general population in adults who have first-degree blood relatives (parents, siblings) with bipolar I or bipolar II disorders.

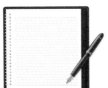

## Anthony's Story

Anthony, a man in his 30s, was brought to a city emergency room (ER) by the police. He spoke rapidly and referred to himself as the "New Jesus." He declined to offer another name.

He refused to remain in his exam room and kept walking into the special desk area for nurses and doctors. He became upset when he was led back to his exam room, raised his voice, and kept talking rapidly to the ER staff.

When asked when he last slept, he said he no longer needed sleep, saying that he had been "touched by heaven." The doctors took blood samples and gave him a drug test. They also noticed blisters on his feet. A review of his electronic medical record showed he had behaved this way 2 years earlier. At that time, a drug test was negative.

Anthony's sister soon arrived and said he had seemed strange a week ago. He had argued all night about religion with relatives at a holiday party, which he had never done before. She knew their father had bipolar disorder, but she had not seen their father since she was a child. She said that Anthony did not use drugs. She told the ER team that Anthony was a middle school math teacher who had just finished a semester of teaching.

Over the next 24 hours, Anthony became calmer, but he still spoke rapidly and loudly. His thoughts jumped from idea to idea. When the blood and drug tests came back, they showed that he had not been using drugs or alcohol.

Anthony was diagnosed with *bipolar I disorder* and with having a *current, severe manic episode*. He arrived at the ER with classic symptoms of mania: irritable mood, grandiosity, less need for sleep, racing thoughts, and restless movement. The blisters on his feet showed that he had likely been walking nonstop when he was brought to the ER. He fully met DSM-5 criteria for a manic episode.

# Treatment

Bipolar I disorder is very treatable. In almost all cases, treatment must be maintained throughout life to avoid relapse. Symptoms improve and can change over time, so keeping in touch with a mental health care provider will ensure the treatment that best suits the person and his or her life and needs.

## Medications

Medications called *mood stabilizers* are often prescribed to help control bipolar disorder. Lithium, the oldest and best-known mood stabilizer, is still widely used. *Anticonvulsant medications* (often prescribed for epilepsy seizures) are also used as mood stabilizers and include valproate, lamotrigine, and carbamazepine. For most people with bipolar disorder, treatment with medication is a daily need in the same way that people take medicine every day to lower high blood pressure.

If people with bipolar disorder stop taking their prescribed medications, the risk for another episode of mania or depression is high. Medications can work so well that some people with bipolar disorder feel no more symptoms, think they are cured, and believe medication is no longer needed. They stop taking the medication even when they know they had severe episodes in the past. They may do well for a time at work or school, but at some point they are likely to have another disabling episode.

Checking with the doctor or mental health care provider before changing or stopping medication is needed for good treatment. Share any thoughts or concerns about medications with him or her as a way to learn more about the disorder, one's own symptoms, and the medications. For information about medication and treatment, see Chapter 20, "Treatment Essentials."

## Psychotherapy

Like all major illnesses, bipolar disorder can disrupt life and relationships with others, especially with spouses and family members. People receiving medication for bipolar disorder often benefit from psychotherapy. They can learn more about the illness, work on the problems the illness has created, and renew close bonds damaged by the illness.

Several forms of psychotherapy focus on those with bipolar disorder. These include family-focused therapy, interpersonal and social rhythm therapy, the life goals program, and cognitive-behavior therapy that has been adapted to the needs of those with bipolar disorder. These forms of therapy share a number of common elements. They involve education about the illness, setting sleep and other daily routines, and a focus on the present and future. These therapies have been shown to help bipolar depression and prevent the return of symptoms.

## Electroconvulsive Therapy

In severe cases of bipolar I disorder, when medication and psychotherapy have not helped, a treatment known as *electroconvulsive therapy* (ECT) can be used. (It is also used to treat severe *major depression* and some cases of *schizophrenia* and *schizoaffective disorder*.)

With modern techniques, ECT is safely and widely used to help relieve severe episodes of illness. ECT may be chosen when medicines have failed to work or in times of very urgent need (such as constant thoughts of suicide or failure to eat and drink during a severe depressive episode). With ECT, a brief electrical current is applied to the scalp while the patient is under anesthesia. There is no pain, and muscles do not jerk or shake. The procedure takes about 10 to 15 minutes. A patient often receives ECT two or three times a week for a total of 6 to 12 treatments. How often ECT is used depends on how severe the symptoms are and how quickly symptoms improve.

ECT will help resolve an episode of illness, but daily medication is needed afterward. Without medication, a person with bipolar disorder will likely have another episode. Bipolar I disorder is much better controlled if treatment persists after a normal mood is restored. Even with no breaks in treatment, mood changes can still occur, but they are much less likely to happen with medication. Working closely with the doctor and talking openly about symptoms and concerns can help make treatment work best.

### Family Therapy and Support Groups

Bipolar disorder can create a stressful home life and cause serious trouble not just for people with the illness, but for those they love. The whole family may benefit from mental health care services, either through formal family therapy, or through a mental health advocacy or support group. Families can learn how best to cope with the illness and its impact. They can become an active part in their loved one's treatment. For people with bipolar I disorder who are married, marriage counseling can help repair the damage caused by the illness.

---

## A Healthy Mind and Body

Along with treatment, a healthy lifestyle can also help ease some of the symptoms of bipolar I disorder:

- **Keep a regular routine.** Getting out of bed, eating meals, and going to sleep at just about the same time every day, 7 days a week, have been shown to help maintain wellness in those with bipolar disorder.
- **Make healthy choices.** Eating well-balanced meals, exercising, and getting plenty of sleep can improve mood.
- **Connect with peers.** Getting support from people who are coping with similar challenges is a key part of feeling better. A treatment center or mental health care provider can provide a referral to a local group, or one can be found online at the Depression and Bipolar Support Alliance Web site (www.dbsalliance.org).
- **Learn personal warning signs.** Figure out what symptoms signal the start of a manic or depressive episode and notify your mental health care provider when they appear.

---

# Bipolar II Disorder

People with *bipolar II disorder* have had at least one major depressive episode and at least one hypomanic episode (see definitions in "Bipolar I Disorder"). The main difference between bipolar I and bipolar II disorder is that there is no period of mania in bipolar II disorder.

Hypomanic episodes do not cause as many problems as manic episodes. For instance, they do not require hospital care (if so, the diagnosis changes from a hypomanic episode to a manic episode). Many people with bipolar II disorder return to full function between episodes. Hypomanic symptoms can cause random mood changes, disrupt social or work function, or change the person's normal behavior in ways that others notice. But they do not greatly impair the person, as can occur with mania. Close friends or family can provide useful information to help the mental health care provider conclude whether a hypomanic episode is present or has occurred.

Although bipolar II disorder often begins in the late teens or the early 20s, it can start later in life. This onset is a bit later than bipolar I disorder.

Bipolar II disorder affects 0.8% of people in the United States each year. The disorder tends to begin with a major depressive episode. It is not clear until later that the person has bipolar II disorder—when the hypomanic symptoms first appear. In 12% of people with *major depressive disorder,* hypomanic symptoms appear later, and the diagnosis becomes bipolar II disorder.

People with bipolar II disorder often first seek treatment from a mental health care provider because of depressive symptoms (feeling low, worthless, or guilty), which can be quite severe. The depressive symptoms tend to cause more problems than symptoms of hypomania, which may not bother them. People with bipolar II disorder tend to have longer episodes of depression than those with bipolar I disorder.

Other disorders often occur with bipolar II disorder. About 75% of people with bipolar II disorder have an *anxiety disorder*, and about 37% have a *substance use disorder*. Eating disorders such as *binge-eating disorder* are also very common. About 60% of people with bipolar II disorder have three or more other mental disorders.

Another concern for those with bipolar II disorder is the risk of suicide. They may be more prone to acting on impulse, which can increase risk. About one-third of people with the illness will attempt suicide at least once. Getting help for any symptom of bipolar II disorder is vital to reduce life problems and the risk of suicide.

---

 **Bipolar II Disorder**

In bipolar II disorder, at least one hypomanic and one depressive episode have occurred (as described for *bipolar I disorder*). Hypomanic symptoms do not lead to the major problems (such as arrests, broken relationships, lost jobs) that mania often causes. A manic episode has never occurred for this diagnosis. Someone with bipolar II disorder has had:

- A hypomanic episode (see above) lasting at least 4 days in a row.
- An episode of major depression (see above) lasting at least 2 weeks.

The symptoms are not due to the effects of a drug of abuse, a medication, another medical condition, or other psychotic disorders such as *schizoaffective disorder, schizophrenia, schizophreniform disorder*, or *delusional disorder*.

## Risk Factors

People with blood relatives who have bipolar II disorder are at highest risk of also developing the condition. In 10%–20% of women, childbirth may be a trigger for a hypomanic episode. It may occur early in the postpartum period (shortly after giving birth) and may precede a depressive episode. Being alert to this risk and getting treatment for depression can relieve symptoms.

### Chelsea's Story

Chelsea was a 43-year-old married librarian who came to an outpatient mental health clinic with a long history of depression. She described being depressed for a month since she began a new job. She had concerns that her new boss and colleagues thought her work was poor and slow and that she was not friendly. She had no energy or enthusiasm at home. Instead of playing with her children or talking to her husband, she watched TV for hours, overate, and slept long hours. She gained 6 pounds in just 3 weeks, which made her feel even worse about herself. She cried many times through the week, which she reported as a sign that "the depression was back." She also thought often of death but had never attempted suicide.

Chelsea said her memory about her history of depression was a little fuzzy, so she brought in her husband, who had known her since college. They agreed that she had first become depressed in her teens and that she had had at least five different periods of depression as an adult. These episodes involved depressed mood, lack of energy, deep feelings of guilt, loss of interest in sex, and some thoughts that life wasn't worth living. Chelsea also sometimes had periods of "too much" energy, irritability, and racing thoughts. These episodes of excess energy could last hours, days, or a couple of weeks.

Chelsea's husband also described times when Chelsea seemed excited, happy, and self-confident—"like a different person." She would talk fast, seem full of energy and good cheer, do all the daily chores, and start (and often finish) new projects. She would need little sleep and still be up the next day.

Because of her periods of low mood and thoughts of death, she had seen mental health care providers since her mid-teen years. Psychotherapy had given some help. Chelsea said that it "worked okay"—until she had another depressive episode. She could then not attend sessions and would just quit. She had tried three antidepressants. Each gave short-term relief from the depression, followed by a relapse. An aunt and grandfather had been in the hospital for mania, although Chelsea was quick to point out that she was "not at all like them."

Chelsea was diagnosed with *bipolar II disorder* and as having a *current depressive episode*. Her husband's information about her moments of hypomania helped in making the diagnosis.

## Treatment

Bipolar II disorder often responds to many of the same treatments as *bipolar I disorder* (see the "Treatment" section for that disorder). The medications for bipolar I disorder are often used to steady moods, and these medications can help prevent episodes of hypomania. These include either mood stabilizers or antidepressant medications. The symptoms that are the most serious in the current hypomanic or depressive episode will affect which medication is chosen.

Checking with the doctor about how long to keep taking the medication is important. It may be safest to take the medications daily for a long time to prevent more episodes. Each person is unique, and the doctor and patient should talk about symptoms and needs to find the best course. Stopping or changing the dose of medication without checking with a doctor first can cause problems and make symptoms worse.

People with bipolar II disorder can have severe depressive episodes. Treatment for these severe depressions can require care in a hospital. If medications cannot relieve depression, then ECT may be chosen as needed.

Some of the same types of psychotherapy and the healthy lifestyle tips that ease bipolar I disorder symptoms can help those with bipolar II disorder. The goal is to live a full and meaningful life, prevent relapse, and improve coping when symptoms are present.

# Cyclothymic Disorder

*Cyclothymic disorder* is a milder form of bipolar illness in which many mood swings with hypomania and depressive symptoms occur often and on a fairly constant basis. There are not enough symptoms to be full hypomanic and major depressive episodes (as defined in "Bipolar I Disorder"). People with this disorder may appear to others as moody. Even though the symptoms are not severe enough to require care in a hospital, the disorder can cause great distress and impair social, work, and other key aspects of function. Those with the disorder may seek treatment to help reduce their constant mood swings.

Cyclothymic disorder affects about 0.4%–1% of people in the United States. It often begins in the teen or early adult years. Children diagnosed with the disorder are often as young as 6 or 7 years old when they have their first symptoms. The disorder tends to begin without prior signs or symptoms of a problem.

Men and women share a similar risk for the disorder. Between 15% and 50% of people diagnosed with cyclothymic disorder may later progress to *bipolar I* or *bipolar II disorder. Substance use disorder* and *sleep disorders* can also be common in people with cyclothymic disorder. Children with the disorder may also have *attention-deficit/hyperactivity disorder* (ADHD).

---

 **Cyclothymic Disorder**

Cyclothymic disorder occurs when:

- For at least 2 years (or 1 year in children and teens), many periods of hypomanic symptoms and depressive symptoms have occurred. These have never reached the guidelines that define hypomanic and major depressive episodes (as described in *bipolar I disorder*).
- During the same 2 years (or 1 year in children and teens), the hypomanic and depressive mood swings have lasted for at least half the time (1 year for adults, 6 months for children and teens). Symptoms have never stopped for more than 2 months.
- Manic episodes have never occurred (as defined in *bipolar I disorder*).

The symptoms cause great distress and problems with social, work, and other key aspects of function. They are not due to the effects of a drug of abuse, a medication, another medical condition (such as thyroid problems), or other psychotic disorders such as *schizoaffective disorder, schizophrenia, schizophreniform disorder,* or *delusional disorder.*

---

## Risk Factors

People with first-degree blood relatives (parents or siblings) who have *bipolar I disorder* are at higher risk for cyclothymic disorder than those in the general population. *Major depressive disorder* and *bipolar II disorder* are also common in first-degree blood relatives of those with cyclothymic disorder.

# Treatment

Treatment for cyclothymic disorder that includes psychotherapy, medicine, and lifestyle change seems to help achieve the best quality of life. People with the disorder and their mental health care providers should work together to find the best mix of treatments over a lifetime of the disorder. For cyclothymic disorder, it is best to think about what symptoms cause the most trouble—whether it is the hypomanic or the low mood symptoms—and choose the treatment from there.

People with cyclothymic disorder may stop and start treatment throughout their lives. They may not be troubled enough by their symptoms to seek care. They may still function, although not as well, when symptoms are active. When having hypomanic symptoms, some people may feel they can get more done and be happy with the results. They need to be careful not to overdo their activity in a way that causes problems with their work or relationships. During their low or depressive moods, some people can withstand their symptoms, and they may prefer not to take medications. Psychotherapy may be a helpful option for them.

People with the disorder may benefit from the same types of one-on-one psychotherapy used for those with *bipolar I disorder* (as described in that "Treatment" section). Couples and family therapy, such as family-focused therapy, may be helpful for problems that result from the ups and downs of the disorder. Very often, the best treatment plan includes psychotherapy to help with daily stresses linked with the high and low moods.

The same medicines for bipolar I disorder are often helpful for cyclothymic disorder. Among these, lithium is one of the main medications that help. It may take 3–4 months to have a good effect for cyclothymic disorder, and as long as a year may be needed for the best results. The other medicines for mood swings—valproate, carbamazepine, and lamotrigine—may also be used. After a couple of years of medications, some people may try stopping them under the care and advice of a doctor. They and their doctor should then watch to see if they can do well in daily life without the medication.

The same healthy lifestyle tips that are useful in bipolar I disorder are also likely to help improve symptoms of cyclothymic disorder. These lifestyle habits include keeping regular daily routines; getting regular sleep, daily exercise, and careful sunlight exposure; having a healthy diet; and avoiding use of drugs and alcohol.

# Key Points

- People with *bipolar disorders* have extreme and intense moods (for instance, switching between being very happy and active—or feeling very low and out of energy). These are unlike the normal ups and downs in mood that occur in daily life.
- People with these disorders may feel out of control or ruled by their extreme moods and behaviors. The disorder can damage relationships, cause problems with work or school, and even lead to suicide.
- The bipolar disorder class includes three different conditions: *bipolar I, bipolar II,* and *cyclothymic disorder.* They share many of the same symptoms, but differ in severity and intensity, and thus need somewhat different treatment.
- Although these disorders are lifelong once they begin, they are very treatable. People with these disorders benefit most from a combination of medications, psychotherapy ("talk therapy"), and healthy lifestyle habits. With the right treatment, people with bipolar disorders can lead full and productive lives.
- Symptoms improve and can change over time, so keeping in touch with a mental health care provider will ensure that treatment best suits the person and his or her life and needs.

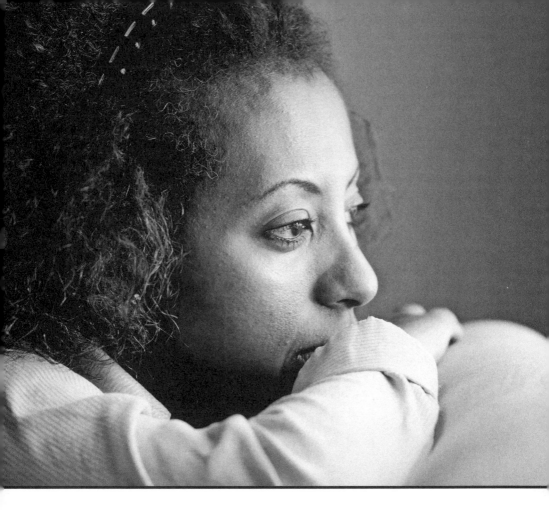

Major Depressive Disorder

Persistent Depressive Disorder

Premenstrual Dysphoric Disorder

Disruptive Mood Dysregulation Disorder

*For a complete list of DSM-5 disorders, see Appendix A.*

# CHAPTER 4

# Depressive Disorders

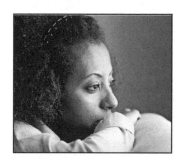

In everyday life, the word "depression" or "depressed" is often used to express when someone is unhappy or sad for a moment. For example, people might say "I'm depressed" when they feel let down that their sports team lost a game. In contrast, real depression is a major medical problem that can have a deep and profound impact on a person's safety and well-being. *Depressive disorders* share the common feature of causing a person to feel sad, empty, or irritable (easily annoyed or in a bad mood). Someone with depression may have trouble sleeping, thinking, or doing once-normal daily functions. The disorders in this group differ in how long symptoms last, when they arise, and their causes.

Depressive disorders include *major depressive disorder, persistent depressive disorder, premenstrual dysphoric disorder,* and *disruptive mood dysregulation disorder.* Depressive disorders can sometimes be caused by certain medications, alcohol and other drugs, and some medical conditions, such as thyroid disease.

Depression is not the same as normal sadness and grief. The death of a loved one, the loss of a job, or the ending of a relationship may be painful to endure, but they do not trigger major depression in most people. Depression can cause someone to feel hopeless, worthless, or guilty for weeks, months, and even years. The good news is that depression is often relieved with treatment. About 80%–90% of those with depression gain some relief from symptoms with treatment. Treatment can include medication, psychotherapy ("talk therapy"), or both. For many people, both treatments combined have shown to work better than either one alone. Some people may need to try several different medications before finding what works best for them.

# Major Depressive Disorder

*Major depressive disorder* is a serious illness that causes a person to feel deeply sad (or wholly absent of feeling) most of the day, nearly every day, for at least 2 weeks. This disorder is different from "the blues," which last for just a few days. Many people feel blue from time to time. People with major depressive disorder often lose interest in what they once enjoyed. They may have changes in sleep, find it hard to think or focus, and feel worthless. People with a major depressive disorder may describe it as "feeling down in the dumps." For those with major depression, this feeling remains over time, and they are not able to simply shake it off.

About 7% of people in the United States have a major depressive disorder in any given year. Young adults ages 18–29 are three times more likely to have the disorder than people over age 60.

More women than men have major depressive disorder. Starting in the early teen years, the chance that women will have the disorder is 1.5–3 times higher than for men, but the symptoms and how they are treated are the same for both men and women.

Anyone having symptoms of a major depressive disorder should get help. The mental pain and loss of hope that occur with it may lead to thoughts of suicide or even attempts. Feelings of being nervous or panic may also occur. Older persons are more prone to feeling anxious or worried. They may be more aware of physical symptoms when they have a major depressive disorder.

Major depressive disorder sometimes occurs along with other disorders. These include *substance use disorders* (sometimes called "addictions"), *panic disorder, obsessive-compulsive disorder, anorexia nervosa,* and *bulimia nervosa.*

---

 **Major Depressive Disorder**

Major depressive disorder occurs when a person has five or more of the symptoms below almost every day for at least 2 weeks:

- Depressed mood or sadness.
- Loss of interest or pleasure in activities that were once enjoyed.

- Sudden or recent weight gain, weight loss, or change in appetite.
- Insomnia (trouble sleeping) or hypersomnia (sleeping too much).
- Feeling restless or stirred up (such as pacing or hand wringing), or having slowed speech and movements.
- Fatigue or loss of energy.
- Feeling worthless or guilty.
- Trouble staying focused or making decisions.
- Regular thoughts of death or suicide, planned suicide, or attempted suicide.

One of the first two symptoms above must be present, and the changes in behavior cause great distress or impair social, work, or other key aspects of function. Children and teens may be irritable instead of sad. The symptoms cannot be caused by a drug, medication, *psychotic disorder,* or any other medical condition. A manic or hypomanic episode (see Chapter 3, "Bipolar Disorders," for more detail) has never occurred. The disorder may be mild, moderate, or severe, based on the number of symptoms and level of impaired function. Although a major loss may cause feelings like those of depression, normal grieving differs from depression (see box).

## Risk Factors

Although major depressive disorder can affect anyone, several factors can play a role:

- **Temperament.** People with low self-esteem, who have problems coping with stress, or who have a downbeat attitude may be at more risk for the disorder.
- **Environment.** A stressful childhood or life events such as violence, neglect, abuse, or low income can lead to major depressive disorder.
- **Genetics.** A person with a close blood relative with major depressive disorder (such as a parent, sibling, or child) has a two to four times higher risk of also having the disorder.
- **Biochemistry.** Although much is not known about how chemicals in the brain cause depression, it's believed that two chemicals, serotonin and norepinephrine, might play a role.

A major depressive episode may also occur when a person has a *bipolar disorder.* With a bipolar disorder, *manic episodes* also are present. Symptoms of a manic episode include extremes in feeling happy, irritable, or active; the person may need less sleep to do more tasks, or talk more or faster than is normal for him or her (see Chapter 3 for more detail).

Grieving the death of a loved one can cause feelings of emptiness and loss that often come in waves and become less frequent as weeks and months pass. These waves of feelings, sometimes called "pangs of grief," are focused on the lost loved one. Often, there are also moments of good thoughts and happy memories.

In contrast, someone with a *major depressive disorder* has feelings of sadness and despair that last longer and few, if any, pleasant or enjoyable thoughts. Grief usually does not cause the sense of low self-worth or guilt that often occurs with major depressive disorder. If these feelings are present with grief, they may focus on how one might have failed the deceased, such as not visiting often enough or not telling the deceased how much he or she was loved. In this case, the guilty feelings are about certain actions not taken, not a total sense of low self-worth as occurs in depression. Frequent thoughts of one's own death and wishing to die because of feeling worthless or hopeless do not often happen during grief as they do with major depressive disorder. When a grieving person has had at least four or five symptoms of major depression (as opposed to symptoms of grief) for at least 2 weeks, the person should think about seeing a doctor.

## Trish's Story

Trish was a 51-year-old woman who was brought to the emergency room by her husband. She said, "I feel like killing myself." She had lost her interest in life about 4 months before. During that time, she reported depression every day for most of the day. Symptoms had been getting worse for months. She had lost 14 pounds without dieting because she did not feel like eating. She had trouble falling asleep almost every night and woke at 3:00 A.M. several mornings a week (she normally woke at 6:30 A.M.). She had low energy, trouble staying focused, and less ability to do her office job at a dog food–processing plant. She was convinced that she had made a mistake that would lead to the deaths of thousands of dogs. She expected that she would soon be arrested and would rather kill herself than go to prison.

Trish showed all nine symptoms of major depression for at least 2 weeks: depressed mood, loss of interest or pleasure, weight loss, insomnia, restlessness, loss of energy, extreme guilt, trouble staying focused, and thoughts of suicide. Her doctor diagnosed her with *major depressive disorder.*

## Treatment

Major depressive disorder is among the most treatable of mental disorders. Most people respond well to treatment and almost all gain some relief from their symptoms.

Trish's condition is a severe case of major depressive disorder because she had the false belief (a delusion) that she caused the deaths of thousands of dogs. This type of depressive disorder with delusions or thoughts of suicide requires urgent care. The person may need a hospital stay for his or her own safety, as well as for treatment.

Before a doctor suggests a certain treatment, he or she will fully assess the problem and the symptoms the person is having. This includes asking questions about the problem and symptoms. A physical exam or discussion with the person's primary care doctor may also occur. Psychotherapy and medication are useful in treating moderate and severe major depressive disorder. Mild major depressive disorder often can be treated with psychotherapy alone. See Chapter 20, "Treatment Essentials," to learn more about the types of treatments discussed below.

Psychotherapy, or "talk therapy," may be one-on-one with the mental health care provider or may include others. Certain types of psychotherapy have been shown useful in the treatment of major depressive disorder and include the following:

- *Interpersonal psychotherapy* aims to enhance relationships and interpersonal skills.
- *Supportive psychotherapy* aims to maintain or restore the highest level of function possible with problem solving, advice, and other methods.
- *Cognitive-behavior therapy* finds and changes patterns in unhelpful thinking and behavior.
- *Family or couples therapy* may help address issues that can arise within families or couples.
- *Group therapy* involves people who have similar illnesses.

Medications also help reduce the symptoms of major depressive disorder. Antidepressants may be used to adjust the chemicals in the brain believed to be "out of balance" from the depression. The types of antidepressants most often used are as follows:

- Selective serotonin reuptake inhibitors (SSRIs)
- Serotonin-norepinephrine reuptake inhibitors (SNRIs)
- Dopamine-norepinephrine reuptake inhibitors
- Tricyclics
- Monoamine oxidase inhibitors (MAOIs)

These antidepressants work in slightly different ways. When choosing one that will likely work best, the doctor will look at factors such as a person's symptoms, other health issues, special concerns (such as weight gain), side effects, and cost.

Antidepressants can cause some side effects, such as nausea, weight gain, tiredness, and loss of sexual desire. The doctor can change the dose or type of medication if these side effects become a problem. With some antidepressants, the amount of medicine must be slowly reduced because sudden stopping can cause depression to worsen. Side effects may go away or lessen as the body adjusts to the medication. The doctor may prescribe a few different medications before finding one that works best, and can advise on the benefits and risks.

Most people start feeling better 2–4 weeks after starting treatment. Full benefits may not be felt for 2–3 months, or even longer in older adults. If there is little or no progress after several weeks, the doctor will change the dose of the medication or will add or replace it with another antidepressant. It is important to keep taking the medication as prescribed and allow it time to work, even after symptoms start to improve, to prevent depression from returning. Doctors usually recommend that patients keep taking the medication for 6 months or more once symptoms have improved.

Having one bout of depression greatly increases the risk of having another one, but treatment can reduce this risk. Psychotherapy may lessen the chance of depression coming back or being as intense if it recurs. For those who have had at least two episodes of depression, taking the medication after the second episode lowers the risk that depression will return. After two or three episodes of major depression, long-term maintenance treatment may be suggested.

Unlike the first stage of treatment, which aims to help the person get well, the goal of *maintenance treatment* is to keep the person well. This can be done using medication, psychotherapy, or both. With any of these approaches, during maintenance treatment, the person sees his or her mental health care provider less often, while the person and his or her family members and friends remain alert for signs of possible relapse between visits.

---

## A Healthy Mind and Body

The support of family and friends can help someone to prevent or overcome depression. They can encourage a depressed loved one to stay with treatment and practice the coping techniques and problem-solving skills he or she is learning through therapy. A healthy lifestyle also can help ease some of the suffering from major depressive disorder:

- **Exercise.** Although it can be very hard for people with major depression to feel motivated to exercise, regular exercise can help in coping with depression. Most types of exercise, such as walking, jogging, dancing, and yoga, improve the body's ability to fight pain and can reduce stress, boost self-esteem, and improve sleep in people of all ages.
- **Eat healthy.** Eating well-balanced meals is key to staying healthy during treatment. Meals with vegetables, fruits, and low-fat protein supply good nutrition and can help offset some of the side effects of treatment. Drinking alcohol can worsen depression. While alcohol can initially take the edge off the anxiety that often goes along with depression, it later makes the anxiety worse. It also disrupts the deep middle-of-the-night sleep needed to relieve depression.
- **Join a support group.** Being with others dealing with depression can go a long way in reducing the feeling of being "all alone." Support group members can encourage each other, get advice on how to cope, and share similar experiences. A treatment center or doctor can provide a referral to a local group, or one can be found online at the Depression and Bipolar Support Alliance's Web site (www.dbsalliance.org).
- **Be social.** Although being alone may feel more comfortable, isolation and loneliness make depression even worse. Close ties with family and friends can provide comfort, and being involved in social activities offers a way to have some pleasure or fun.
- **Get virtual help.** Attending face-to-face support group meetings is not for everyone. Some organizations offer support for patients and family members who prefer to meet with others in online forums. The National Alliance on Mental Illness (www.nami.org) and the Depression and Bipolar Support Alliance offer virtual community groups and classes that teach coping skills for depression.

# Persistent Depressive Disorder

*Persistent depressive disorder,* once called "dysthymic disorder," refers to a chronic or long-lasting type of depression in which a person's moods are often low for a long time. Symptoms last for least 2 years—and can last much longer. Persistent depressive disorder can begin early in childhood or in the teen or early adult years. If these symptoms become a part of a person's day-to-day life, he or she may not tell loved ones or mental health care providers about the feelings, assuming that's just how life is.

In any given year, about 1.5% of adults in the United States have persistent depressive disorder. People whose symptoms appear before age 21 are at higher risk for also having a *personality disorder* or *substance use disorder*. These disorders can be treated along with depression.

**Persistent Depressive Disorder**

Persistent depressive disorder occurs when symptoms for *major depressive disorder* are often present for 2 years. The disorder also is likely when a person:

- Has a depressed mood on most days for at least 2 years.
- While depressed, has two or more of the symptoms below:
  - Poor eating habits: eating too much or too little.
  - Trouble sleeping or sleeping too much.
  - Low energy.
  - Low self-esteem.
  - Difficulty staying focused or making decisions.
  - Feeling hopeless.
- Has symptoms without any relief for more than 2 months at a time.

The symptoms cause great distress or impair social, work, or other key aspects of function. Children and teens may be irritable instead of depressed, and their symptoms last for at least 1 year. The symptoms are not caused by a drug, medication, *psychotic disorder,* or any other medical condition. A manic or hypomanic episode or *cyclothymic disorder* (see Chapter 3, "Bipolar Disorders," for more detail) has never occurred. The disorder may be mild, moderate, or severe, based on the number of symptoms and level of impaired function.

## Risk Factors

Factors that play a role in persistent depressive disorder are:

- **Temperament.** People who have a downbeat attitude and problems with social or work life (such as no or few friends, not able to work or keep a job, trouble getting along with others) have a higher risk for long-term depression.
- **Environment.** Stressful childhood events, such as losing or being separated from a parent.
- **Genetics.** A person with a close blood relative with *major depressive disorder* (such as a parent, sibling, or child) is more likely to have the disorder.

## Heather's Story

Heather, 35, was referred to psychiatric treatment by her employer after she became tearful while being mildly criticized during an otherwise positive annual performance review. She told the psychiatrist that she had been "feeling low for years." Hearing what she felt were negative comments about her work had been "just too much." Heather left graduate school before getting her doctoral degree in chemistry and began work as a laboratory technician. She felt frustrated with her job, which she saw as a "dead end," yet feared that she lacked the talent to find more satisfying work. As a result, she struggled with guilty feelings that she "hadn't done much" with her life. Heather at times had trouble falling asleep. Although her romantic relationships tended to "not last long," she felt that her sex drive was normal. She noted that her symptoms would increase and decrease, but they had been unchanged over the past 3 years. Growing up, Heather had a close relationship with her father and became depressed for the first time in high school when he was often in the hospital for leukemia treatment. At that time, she was treated with psychotherapy and responded well.

Heather was diagnosed with *persistent depressive disorder.* Her symptoms had lasted for more than 2 years and were harming both her social and work life. After several months of treatment, she revealed that she had been sexually abused by a family friend during her childhood. It also emerged that she had few women friends and a pattern of unhealthy and often abusive relationships with men.

## Treatment

As with *major depressive disorder,* the two main treatments for persistent depressive disorder are medications and psychotherapy.

Most people start feeling better 2–4 weeks after starting medication. Full effects of the medication, however, may not be felt for 2–3 months, or longer in older adults. If there is little or no progress after several weeks, the doctor will change the dose of the medication or will add or replace it with another antidepressant. The person should keep taking the medication even when symptoms start to improve.

Psychotherapy can also be a key tool in getting better. A form of psychotherapy called *cognitive behavioral analysis system of psychotherapy* (CBASP) has been shown to be of great help to those with persistent depressive disorder. CBASP combines methods of cognitive, behavior, and interpersonal forms of psychotherapy. Other kinds of psychotherapy may also be useful (see Chapter 20, "Treatment Essentials").

The nature of persistent depressive disorder is that it can last for years. While many people fully recover, others may still have some symptoms—even during treatment. The best way to cope with the disorder is to stay with the treatment plan developed by the mental health care provider. Meanwhile, people who have persistent depressive disorder can practice some of the same lifestyle tips that help improve mental and physical health in those who have major depression.

# Premenstrual Dysphoric Disorder

*Premenstrual dysphoric disorder* (PMDD) is now recognized as a disorder after more than 20 years of scientific research. A woman with PMDD has severe symptoms of depression, irritability, and tension 1 week before menstruation (bleeding) begins. These symptoms lessen a few days after menstruation begins, and they end 1 week after menstruation stops. The main symptoms include problems with mood, anxiety, and sleep. Women with the disorder can also have physical symptoms, such as breast tenderness or bloating.

PMDD can arise at any point during a woman's menstruating years. Between 1.3% and 1.8% of women have the disorder, and some say their symptoms get worse as they near menopause. Symptoms stop once a woman's menstrual cycles end at menopause.

Some women may have PMS, or "premenstrual syndrome." This condition describes a range of broad emotional and physical symptoms that occur before menstruation, but these symptoms are not severe enough to disrupt daily life. In contrast, a diagnosis of PMDD requires that a number of certain symptoms be severe enough to lead to problems with relationships and work, school, or social function.

---

 **Premenstrual Dysphoric Disorder**

Women with PMDD have five of the symptoms below (at least one of the first four must be present):

- Sudden mood swings.
- Irritability, anger, or increased conflict with others.
- Depressed mood or feelings of hopelessness.
- Anxiety or tension.
- Decreased interest in usual activities.
- Difficulty staying focused in attention or thinking.
- Fatigue.
- Change in appetite, or food cravings.
- Trouble sleeping or sleeping more than usual.
- Feeling overwhelmed or out of control.
- Physical symptoms, such as breast tenderness, joint or muscle pain, weight gain, and bloating.

The diagnosis requires that symptoms have occurred for most menstrual cycles in the preceding year. Symptoms occur during the week before the start of menstruation (the day bleeding begins) and start to get better a few days after menstruation begins. They should go away the week after menstruation stops. The symptoms must cause great distress or disrupt work, school, usual activities, or relationships, and must not be due to the worsening of another disorder, such as *major depressive disorder*. The diagnosis can be confirmed by daily self-ratings of symptoms noted for at least two menstrual cycles, such as depressed mood, anxiety or tension, feeling moody or irritable, lack of energy, and sleep changes.

## Risk Factors

The risk of PMDD is increased by:

- **Environment.** Stress, history of trauma, seasonal changes, and cultural beliefs about distinct roles for women.
- **Genetics.** Between 30% and 80% of those with premenstrual symptoms have a close relative who has also had them.

## Treatment

Antidepressants may be used to relieve the mood symptoms. In many cases, women find relief from psychotherapy to learn how to best cope with the stress and anxiety caused by the disorder. Oral contraceptives and other hormone treatments may be helpful for some women. Most women with PMDD will find their symptoms go away or decrease with treatment.

## A Healthy Mind and Body

During treatment, changes in lifestyle may help relieve symptoms:

- **Eat healthy.** Making diet changes to reduce the intake of caffeine, salt, and sugar may help relieve symptoms.
- **Try over-the-counter relief.** Pain relievers such as aspirin and ibuprofen may help ease breast tenderness, backache, and cramping. Diuretics, or water pills, can help with bloating.
- **Exercise.** Although it's unclear whether exercise can relieve more severe symptoms of PMDD (and it may be hard to exercise when symptoms are at their worst), regular aerobic exercise—such as walking or bicycling—can help ease fatigue, boost moods, and improve sleep.

- **Keep a diary.** Writing down the type of symptoms, how severe they are, and how long they last can help the health care provider diagnose the disorder and choose the best treatment.

# Disruptive Mood Dysregulation Disorder

*Disruptive mood dysregulation disorder* is diagnosed in children who are severely irritable or angry and have frequent temper outbursts. This condition was added to DSM-5 because many children had these severe symptoms. They did not fit the pattern for any other disorder, which led to treatment that was not suited for children.

Children with disruptive mood dysregulation disorder have temper outbursts that are unique and differ from a normal temper tantrum. These outbursts are of greater force and length than the type of situation that triggers them. With disruptive mood dysregulation disorder, these outbursts happen as often as three times a week for over a year. People who are in close contact with the child witness the behavior. When not having an outburst, children with the disorder are still irritable or angry nearly every day.

Symptoms of the disorder must start before the child reaches age 10. It is only diagnosed for the first time in children who are at least 6 years old but not yet age 18. It is estimated that 2%–5% of children and teens suffer from disruptive mood dysregulation disorder. It is more common in males and school-age children than in females and adolescents.

---

 **Disruptive Mood Dysregulation Disorder**

Disruptive mood dysregulation disorder is diagnosed when a child has the symptoms below for at least 12 months:

- Severe and frequent temper outbursts, such as verbal rages and physical aggression toward people or property.
- Outbursts that are inappropriate for the child's developmental stage.
- Outbursts that occur about three times or more each week.
- Irritable or angry mood almost every day.
- Temper outbursts and angry mood occur in two different settings, such as at home, at school, and with friends.

During the year of temper outbursts and angry mood, the child must not have gone 3 or more months in a row without these symptoms. The symptoms are not due to a drug, medication, or other medical condition. Parents should be aware that some of the symptoms of disruptive mood dysregulation disorder may look like those of other disorders, such as *depression, bipolar disorder,* and *oppositional defiant disorder.* Some children with disruptive mood dysregulation disorder also have a second disorder, such as problems with attention or anxiety.

## Treatment

If a child is having symptoms of disruptive mood dysregulation disorder, parents should seek help for the child from a mental health care provider as soon as possible. Getting a diagnosis and starting treatment are key to the child's future normal development. A positive family relationship also helps support treatment.

Disruptive mood dysregulation disorder can be treated with success. The type of treatment will depend on the specific needs of the child and his or her family. Psychotherapy for the child alone as well as with the family is the first step. Medication can sometimes help to address certain symptoms, although the advice on the use of some medications for children may differ based on the care provider. The support of parents and other family members is key to the relief of symptoms and learning how to cope with behavior problems.

## Ways to Cope

Having a child with disruptive mood dysregulation disorder can be challenging. The best way to help the child cope with the condition is to follow the treatment plan set by the mental health care provider. It can also help to:

- **Learn as much as possible.** Ask the provider for any extra information that may be available about the condition. Do not delay asking questions if you have concerns about the risks and benefits of specific treatment options before deciding which is best.
- **Talk to other parents.** Joining a support group with other parents can help you feel less alone. Sharing experiences and getting advice from each other can go a long way in easing the stress and frustration in your home. If a support group is not offered in your area, try finding a virtual group that connects online. The National Alliance on Mental Illness (www.nami.org) offers support for parents and family members of children with mental illness.

# Key Points

- Depression is more than "the blues" that all people feel from time to time. Depression can cause someone to feel hopeless, worthless, or guilty for weeks, months, and even years. It is a major medical problem—but it is also among the most treatable of mental disorders.
- Finding help quickly can prevent the disorder from getting worse or lasting longer. Treatments often found to be helpful include psychotherapy ("talk therapy"), medications, or both.
- Common symptoms of *depressive disorders* include loss of pleasure in what the person once enjoyed, sleep problems (too much or too little), eating too much or too little, low energy or feeling tired, problems staying focused, and often feeling worthless, sad, or guilty.
- Someone with depression may not seem sad or hopeless. Children, teens, or older adults may seem worried, angry, or irritated much of the time.
- Being social, building close bonds with friends and family, eating healthy foods, and getting exercise can all help improve depression. Although it can be very hard for someone with a depressive disorder to engage in these healthy lifestyle habits, even small steps can benefit health. Drinking alcohol can worsen depression.

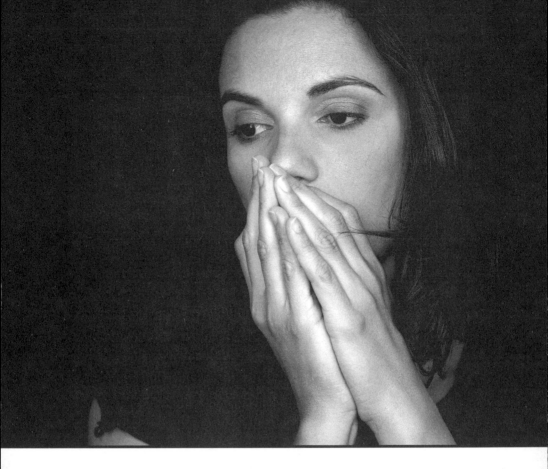

Panic Disorder

Agoraphobia

Generalized Anxiety Disorder

Specific Phobia

Social Anxiety Disorder

Separation Anxiety Disorder

*For a complete list of DSM-5 disorders, see Appendix A.*

# CHAPTER 5

# Anxiety Disorders

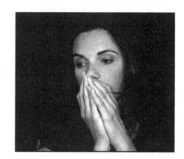

**E**veryone has worried during brief times of stress—or can be nervous at first when going to a party or facing new problems. Children may have normal fears when they are away from parents that often subside after a short time. *Anxiety disorders* differ from these normal feelings of at times being worried, ill at ease, or afraid. People with these disorders have extreme fear or worry that impairs their life function and goes beyond what is normal for their age or the setting.

The most common anxiety disorders are discussed in this chapter: *panic disorder, agoraphobia, generalized anxiety disorder, specific phobia, social anxiety disorder,* and *separation anxiety disorder.* The anxiety disorders differ from one another in the types of objects or settings that cause intense fear or anxiety. Unlike brief times of stress and worry, symptoms for anxiety disorders often last for 6 months or more. People may limit their job choices, prospects for promotion, daily routines, social life, and where they live because of their fears.

All anxiety disorders share symptoms of extreme fear and anxiety. The symptoms may be felt strongly even if the real threat or danger is not as grave as the person expects. At times, there may be no true danger at all. States of fear and anxiety overlap, but they also differ:

- *Fear* is felt when there is danger. Fear is often linked with physical symptoms that involve the *fight-or-flight response.* This response occurs with a real or perceived threat to life or safety. It causes a faster heartbeat, faster breathing, and sweating.

- These physical fear symptoms also occur in *panic attacks*. Panic attacks are a sudden surge of intense fear that can occur with anxiety and other mental disorders. Panic attacks may occur with thoughts of sudden danger and feeling an urgent need to escape.
- *Anxiety* is felt when someone expects future danger. These symptoms differ from fear because they often include muscle tension, a feeling of dread, or a sense of getting ready for future danger. Sometimes people with anxiety will tend to avoid settings that trigger or worsen their symptoms, such as being in public places alone.

A few major changes were made in the chapter on anxiety disorders in DSM-5. For one, *separation anxiety disorder* has been moved here from its prior place in the chapter on disorders that begin in childhood. While symptoms of separation anxiety disorder often begin before age 12, adults also can have the disorder even when they did not have it as children. Another change among the anxiety-related disorders in DSM-5 was moving *obsessive-compulsive disorder* and *posttraumatic stress disorder* into their own chapters, as in this book. Anxiety is a key symptom in these disorders, but they have distinct features that divide them from anxiety disorders. These include obsessions (repetitive and upsetting thoughts or worries), compulsions (repetitive actions to manage the obsession, such as hand washing), or having lived through a traumatic or stressful event.

# Treatment

Most anxiety disorders respond well to treatment. Often treatment for anxiety disorders involves a mix of psychotherapy ("talk therapy") and medications. Treatment can provide great relief from symptoms and teach healthy coping skills, but it may not always provide a complete cure. People with anxiety disorders also benefit from healthy lifestyle habits. See the section "A Healthy Mind and Body" on the next page for tips.

## Cognitive-Behavior Therapy

This form of psychotherapy (also called CBT) involves helping to change unhealthy thinking and behavior patterns. The mental health care provider may work with the person to develop a plan of action to help reduce fears and improve habits of thinking. CBT may include relaxation methods, breathing exercises, and ways to distract or refocus worries and fears. Many anxiety symptoms can improve greatly with CBT. People may learn how to stop avoiding feared situations by going into settings that frighten them, under the guidance of the mental health care provider. When a person has a certain fear, such as seeing spiders or being in high places (described later in this chapter in "Specific Phobia"), CBT may include techniques to practice being near the feared object. This method can help someone manage a fear response when there is no urgent danger.

## Medications

Treatment with medication often requires several weeks or more before people begin to get relief from their symptoms. The doctor needs to follow the person's progress with care and adjust the medication as needed.

Medicines that treat depression also can help anxiety disorders. These medications are *antidepressants*. The term "antidepressant" is somewhat misleading, in that these medications could easily be called anti-anxiety medications. Several different types of antidepressants can be prescribed. These include selective serotonin reuptake inhibitors (SSRIs), such as fluoxetine and paroxetine, and serotonin-norepinephrine reuptake inhibitors (SNRIs), such as venlafaxine.

Other types of medications may be used for anxiety symptoms because they have a stronger "calming" effect that can reduce the symptoms of fear, panic, anxiety, tension, and stress. These are *benzodiazepines* and include alprazolam, diazepam, and lorazepam. These medications may be called different names, such as *sedatives* or *tranquilizers*. Because these can become habit forming, the doctor may prescribe them for short-term use.

## A Healthy Mind and Body

Making these healthy lifestyle choices can help ease some of the suffering caused by anxiety disorders:

- **Learn basic relaxation techniques.** Relaxation may help in the treatment of phobias and panic disorder. Several types of techniques help people cope with stress, such as meditation, visualization, and massage. These techniques may be included in a CBT program.
- **Exercise.** Regular aerobic exercise (walking, biking, dancing) is one of the best ways to reduce symptoms of anxiety and stress. People who are physically active have lower rates of anxiety and depression than people who are less active. Yoga is a popular mind-body exercise that can also help with relaxation and stress management.
- **Avoid caffeine.** The caffeine found in coffee, tea, cola drinks, and even some over-the-counter cold medications can make anxiety symptoms worse.
- **Join a support group.** Being with others who have anxiety disorders can be very helpful. Support group members can encourage each other, get advice on how to cope, and share similar experiences.

# Panic Disorder

The core symptoms of *panic disorder* are panic attacks that recur without warning. *Panic attacks* are sudden spells of intense fear and discomfort that can include chest pains and shortness of breath. They can occur whether someone is calm or anxious, and may at first seem like a heart attack. When the first panic attack strikes, it causes great alarm and often a rushed visit to the emergency room (ER). At the hospital, tests show normal results. Panic attacks sometimes wake someone from sleep. They often peak within a few minutes of their onset.

People often first seek care for panic attacks for the physical symptoms, which mimic those that can threaten life, such as a heart attack. When the panic attacks recur, they cause many types of distress. This includes social concerns from being embarrassed by the symptoms, concerns about mental function (feeling like one is "going crazy"), concerns about being able to function at work, and changing routines to avoid being in public if an attack should occur.

How often panic attacks recur can vary. They can occur once per week for months at a time, or happen every day for a few weeks and then months may pass without any attacks.

Panic disorder affects about 6 million American adults and is twice as common in women as in men. Panic attacks often begin in the late teen or early adult years. They are rare before age 14 and after age 64. Although panic attacks are the main symptom for the disorder, not everyone who has a panic attack will go on to have panic disorder. Many people have just one attack and never have another.

People with panic disorder are more likely to have other mental disorders, such as other *anxiety disorders, major depressive disorder,* and *bipolar disorder*.

---

 **Panic Disorder**

The disorder is diagnosed when the following occur:

- More than one panic attack that recurs without warning. A panic attack is a sudden surge of intense fear or discomfort. During an attack, at least four of the following symptoms occur:
  - Pounding heart
  - Sweating
  - Trembling or shaking
  - Shortness of breath

- Feelings of choking
- Chest pain
- Nausea or abdominal pain
- Dizziness or feeling light-headed
- Chills or hot flashes
- Numbness
- Feeling unreal or disconnected
- Fear of losing control or "going crazy"
- Fear of dying

- After a sudden panic attack, a person has at least 1 month of one or both of the following:
  - Constant worry about having another attack and what will happen when it does (such as concern about losing control, "going crazy").
  - A major change in normal behavior in an effort to avoid having another attack (such as no longer exercising or going to unknown places).

The panic attacks are not due to another medical condition; the use of a drug, alcohol, or medication; or another mental disorder, such as *obsessive-compulsive disorder, posttraumatic stress disorder,* and other *anxiety disorders*.

---

## Risk Factors

The causes of panic disorder are unknown. The following factors may increase risk:

- **Temperament.** People who often worry, have downbeat thinking styles, or believe that anxiety symptoms are harmful have a greater risk of panic attacks.
- **Environment.** Childhood physical and sexual abuse are common in those with panic disorder. Smoking increases the risk for panic attacks and panic disorder. Stressful life events linked to physical health and well-being (such as the illness or death of a loved one) may also increase risk for a panic attack.
- **Genetics.** There is an increased risk for those whose first-degree blood relatives (parents, siblings) have *anxiety, depressive,* or *bipolar disorders*.

### Laura's Story

Laura was a 23-year-old single woman who was referred for psychiatric evaluation by her cardiologist. In the past 2 months, she went to the ER four times with complaints of heart pounding, shortness of breath, sweating, and the fear that she was about to die. Each of these events had a sudden start. The symptoms peaked within minutes, leaving Laura scared, exhausted, and convinced she had just had a heart attack. In the ER, all the exams and lab results came back as normal.

Laura said she had had five of these attacks in the last 3 months, while at work, at home, and driving a car. During the attacks, she was certain that her health was in danger because she could feel the symptoms of a heart attack. When the symptoms ended and she saw the normal test results, she knew that she was not in danger and felt embarrassed that she had hurried to the ER. Because the attacks were so scary, she became afraid of having other attacks, which led her to take many days off work and to avoid exercise, driving, and drinking coffee. When she had a panic attack while asleep in the middle of the night, she agreed to see a psychiatrist.

Laura said she had no history of psychiatric disorders except for a history of anxiety during childhood that had been diagnosed as a "school phobia."

Her mother had been in the hospital with *major depression* when Laura was a child. She has taken medications for many years and sees a mental health care provider on a regular basis. Laura denied that she was depressed but worried about how these attacks might affect her career and job function.

Laura was diagnosed with *panic disorder.* She has panic attacks, and she has 5 out of 13 panic symptoms: pounding heart, sweating, trembling, chest pain, and a fear of dying. The diagnosis of panic disorder also requires that the panic attacks affect the person between episodes. Not only does Laura have frequent worries about another panic attack, she avoids settings and tasks that might trigger another one. She also has a childhood history of anxiety and "school phobia." Her mother's long-term depression also would have had an effect on Laura.

# Agoraphobia

People with *agoraphobia* have intense fear or anxiety about real or expected problems that might occur in a wide range of places outside their homes. This includes places where they fear escape may be hard, they may not receive help, or they may have embarrassing health or panic symptoms (see "Panic Disorder" for symptoms). They begin to avoid settings that trigger their fear, such as public transportation, open spaces (such as parking lots or bridges), or crowds. They often change their daily lives to avoid being in these settings.

Without treatment, people who have agoraphobia can have symptoms so severe that they may refuse to leave their home. They then depend on others for basic tasks, such as grocery shopping. They often can venture into the feared setting with a trusted friend or a mental health care provider.

If they have another medical condition, such as inflammatory bowel disease or Parkinson's disease, the fear or avoidance is very extreme. In the case of bowel diseases, they may avoid leaving their homes due to an extreme fear that they may be unable to reach a restroom when needed and may lose control of their bowels in public. If they have Parkinson's disease, they may fear being away from medication in the event of a "freezing" episode from the disease. Or they may fear being unable to move quickly enough to depart a bus or train at the right exit.

Every year about 1.7% of teens and adults in the United States are diagnosed with agoraphobia. Women are twice as likely to have the disorder than men. Most cases of agoraphobia start before age 35, with the highest risk for first symptoms in the late teen and early adult years. Agoraphobia rarely starts in childhood.

Most people with agoraphobia also have other mental disorders, such as other *anxiety disorders, depressive disorders, posttraumatic stress disorder,* and *alcohol use disorder.*

---

 **Agoraphobia**

The disorder is diagnosed when the following symptoms occur:

- Intense fear or anxiety about at least two of the following:
  - Using public transportation (cars, trains, ships, planes)
  - Being in open spaces (parking lots, bridges)
  - Being in enclosed spaces (shops, theaters)
  - Standing in line or being in a crowd
  - Being outside of the home alone
- The person fears or avoids these settings because of concern that escape might be hard or help not ready in the event of embarrassing health (vomiting, losing bladder control) or panic (sweating, shaking) symptoms.
- The settings require the presence of a trusted companion or are endured with intense fear or anxiety.
- The fear or anxiety exceeds the true risk of danger in the setting.

The fear, anxiety, or avoidance must persist, often for at least 6 months, before a diagnosis is made. The fear, anxiety, or avoidance cause major distress and impair social, work, or other key aspects of function. If a medical condition is present, the fear, anxiety, or avoidance clearly exceed the normal range of concerns. The symptoms cannot result from another mental disorder, such as other *anxiety* or *obsessive-compulsive disorders.*

---

## Risk Factors

The following factors may increase risk of agoraphobia:

- **Temperament.** People who often withdraw from or avoid unknown settings, who worry often, have downbeat thinking styles, or perceive harm in anxiety symptoms may have an increased risk for the disorder.
- **Environment.** Childhood adverse events (such as death of a parent), other adverse life events (such as being attacked or mugged), or a childhood home life with little warmth and high levels of parental control may increase risk.
- **Genetics.** Agoraphobia has a strong genetic link; 61% of people with agoraphobia also have parents with the disorder.

# Generalized Anxiety Disorder

People with *generalized anxiety disorder* have severe anxiety or worry about a number of topics, events, or tasks. These frequent and intense worries exceed the real impact of the expected events. The constant worries disrupt daily function, making it hard to focus on tasks. People with the disorder feel unable to control these worries. The worries shift from one concern to another and include worries about their job, family, health, and money matters. The disorder often occurs with trouble sleeping, muscle aches and tension, and headaches.

About 0.9% of adolescents and 2.9% of adults (6.8 million people) in the United States have symptoms of generalized anxiety disorder each year. Women are twice as likely as men to be affected. The disorder often is diagnosed in those around age 30. It occurs rarely before the teenage years. When it does, the worries tend to focus on doing well in schoolwork and sports.

The symptoms of generalized anxiety disorder can begin slowly. Symptoms can come and go throughout life. The key symptoms of feeling worried differ in how they are expressed across cultures. For instance, some people may express more symptoms linked to worried thoughts and fears. Others may express more physical symptoms linked to lack of sleep or muscle tension when the disorder is first diagnosed. People with generalized anxiety disorder are more likely to have another *anxiety disorder* or *major depressive disorder*. The disorder also may overlap with physical symptoms that are common in middle age and older adults, such as poor sleep.

**Generalized Anxiety Disorder**

The disorder is diagnosed when the following symptoms occur:

- Severe anxiety or worry about a number of topics, events, or tasks (such as health, family, and work) that occurs most days for at least 6 months.
- The person finds it hard to control the worry.
- The anxiety or worry occurs with at least three of the following symptoms for most days in the past 6 months (only one symptom is needed for children):
  - Restlessness
  - Fatigue
  - Trouble keeping thoughts focused
  - Irritability
  - Muscle tension
  - Sleep problems

The anxiety, worry, or physical symptoms cause major distress or impair social, work, or other key aspects of function. The symptoms are not due to another medical condition; the use of a drug, alcohol, or medication; or another mental disorder, such as other *anxiety disorders, obsessive-compulsive disorders, posttraumatic stress disorder, anorexia nervosa,* or *delusional disorder*.

## Risk Factors

The exact cause of generalized anxiety disorder is unknown, but a few factors may play a role:

- **Temperament.** People who often withdraw from or avoid unknown settings and have downbeat thinking styles are at higher risk.
- **Environment.** Adverse childhood events and overprotective parenting may have occurred in those with generalized anxiety disorder.
- **Genetics.** People with a first-degree blood relative (parents, siblings) with *anxiety* or *depressive disorders* have an increased risk for generalized anxiety disorder.

# Specific Phobia

People with a *specific phobia* have an extreme fear of a certain object, place, or setting that is often not as harmful as they perceive. They may know their fear exceeds any real danger, but they have trouble calming it.

Specific phobias can focus on a fear of animals, insects, heights, thunder, needles (or getting a shot), flying, and elevators. While many people may feel uneasy during an airplane takeoff, people with a specific phobia may refuse to travel by plane. The intense fear causes people with the disorder to change their lives and daily routines to avoid the fear of being in the setting or near the object. For instance, someone with a phobia for flying may decline job offers if the work requires air travel. Others may move away or commute longer routes to avoid the feared object.

While specific phobias can occur after a traumatic event (such as nearly choking or drowning), many people with the disorder cannot recall why the phobias started. For most, specific phobias began in childhood before age 10. Fleeting fears are common in children as a part of normal growth, but the extreme fears in a phobia are long-lasting.

About 7%–9% of adults in the United States have a specific phobia. Women are two times more likely than men to be affected. Specific phobias also occur in 3%–5% of older adults in the United States. In this group, phobias are more likely to center on medical concerns, such as breathing problems and choking, and be linked to medical illness. These extreme fears combined with medical illness can greatly reduce quality of life. About 75% of people with a specific phobia have more than one feared object or setting (such as fear of thunderstorms and fear of flying).

Suicide is a major concern for people with specific phobia, as they are 60% more likely to attempt suicide than people without the disorder. Those with the disorder are also more likely to have other disorders, such as *depressive disorders* and other *anxiety disorders*. These other disorders may explain the high rate of suicide attempts in those with specific phobias. These facts are good reasons to seek mental health care.

---

 **Specific Phobia**

The disorder is diagnosed when the following symptoms occur:

- Extreme fear or anxiety about a certain object (such as needles, animals) or setting (such as flying, heights). Children may cry, have tantrums, freeze, or cling to an adult.
- Instant fear or anxiety almost always occurs with the feared object or setting.
- The feared object or setting is strongly avoided, or endured with intense fear or anxiety.
- The fear or anxiety exceeds the true risk of danger.

The fear, anxiety, or avoidance must persist, often for at least 6 months, before a diagnosis is made. The symptoms of fear, anxiety, or avoidance cause major distress and impair school, work, or other key aspects of function. The symptoms are not due to another mental disorder, such as *agoraphobia,* or *separation anxiety, social anxiety, obsessive-compulsive,* or *posttraumatic stress disorder.*

## Risk Factors

The causes of specific phobia are unknown. The following factors may increase risk for the disorder:

- **Temperament.** People who often withdraw from or avoid unknown settings, who worry often, or have downbeat thinking styles are more likely to have specific phobias.
- **Environment.** Being raised by overprotective parents, losing a parent to death or separation, or physical or sexual abuse can increase risk for the disorder. Traumatic events that involve the feared object or setting may also lead to a specific phobia.
- **Genetics.** People with a first-degree blood relative (parent or sibling) with a specific phobia are more likely to have that same phobia.

# Social Anxiety Disorder

People with *social anxiety disorder*—also called *social phobia*—have an intense fear of social settings in which others may watch, study, or judge them. This can involve public speaking, meeting new people, eating with others, or using public restrooms. They fear they may offend others, be embarrassed, or be looked down upon. They have an intense concern that others will reject them or not like them. These fears include thinking that others will find them to be nervous, weak, crazy, stupid, boring, or dirty. The degree of fear exceeds the real risk or result of any such negative judgments.

Because of these intense fears, people with the disorder often avoid social settings where they fear such judgments. This behavior can limit the fullness of their life because of fewer choices in activities they will do (such as not going to parties or other social events) and a reduced range of friendships. They may avoid jobs that require meeting people or giving talks—or endure these tasks with great dread and anxiety. They may have few friendships and romantic relationships.

About 15 million American adults (about 7% of adults) have social anxiety disorder. The average age for the first symptom to appear is age 13, and 75% of people have their first symptoms between ages 8–15.

Social anxiety disorder often occurs in people who are shy or have endured a stressful or embarrassing event, such as being bullied or vomiting during a public speech. The disorder also can occur more slowly, with symptoms building over time. In adults, it occurs more rarely. It is linked to major role changes, such as a higher-level job or marrying someone from a higher social class. Those with the disorder are more likely to also have other *anxiety disorders* and *substance use disorder*. (For instance, drinking before a party to calm nerves may increase to drinking in excess to dampen frequent social fears.) With social anxiety disorder, being often alone and without support can lead to *major depressive disorder.*

---

 **Social Anxiety Disorder**

The disorder is diagnosed when the following occur:

- Extreme fear or anxiety about one or more social settings in which others may watch, study, or judge the person. This may include talking with others, meeting new people, eating with others, or giving a speech. Children will show symptoms with their peers and not just with adults. They may cry, have tantrums, freeze, or cling to an adult.
- The person fears acting in a way that will lead to being ashamed or rejected by others, or will show anxiety symptoms (such as sweating or shaking).
- The social settings almost always cause fear or anxiety.
- The social settings are avoided or endured with intense fear or anxiety.
- The fear or anxiety exceeds the real threat posed by the social setting.

The fear, anxiety, or avoidance must persist, often for at least 6 months, before a diagnosis is made. The symptoms of fear, anxiety, or avoidance cause major distress and impair social, work, or other key aspects of function. The symptoms are not due to another medical condition; the use of a drug, alcohol, or medication; or another mental disorder, such as *panic disorder, body dysmorphic disorder,* or *autism spectrum disorder*.

---

## Risk Factors

The following factors may increase risk for social anxiety disorder:

- **Temperament.** People who often withdraw from or avoid unknown settings are at higher risk.
- **Environment.** Childhood abuse, neglect, or other adverse life events.

- **Genetics.** People with a first-degree blood relative (parent, sibling) with a social anxiety disorder are two to six times more likely to also have the disorder.

# Separation Anxiety Disorder

*Separation anxiety* is the feeling of discomfort a child has when separated—or when he or she expects separation—from a loved one, such as a parent or other caregiver. This anxiety is a normal part of growth in very young children who are ages 10–15 months. When the fear is extreme and occurs in an older child, teen, or adult, and it impairs normal life or family function, it may be a more severe *separation anxiety disorder.*

Children with separation anxiety may cling to the parent and be unable to go or stay in a room by themselves. They may have trouble sleeping alone at bedtime and want a parent to stay with them until they fall asleep. They also may refuse to go to school for fear of being away from their parent.

Teens and adults with the disorder may have fears of harm that might endanger their family or themselves while away from each other, such as being robbed, being kidnapped, or being in car or plane crashes. They may feel great discomfort if they travel alone. Some with separation anxiety also become homesick and filled with grief when away from home. Some young adults may choose not to attend college because of their anxiety. Adults with the disorder may have constant concern for their children's welfare and check in on them throughout the day. This disrupts their workday and the daily life of their children.

Separation anxiety affects about 4% of boys and girls younger than age 12 in the United States. It is less common in teens and occurs in only about 1.6%. Between 1% and 2% of adults also have the disorder.

Children with separation anxiety disorder are more likely to also have *generalized anxiety disorder* and *specific phobia.* Adults with the disorder can also have other disorders. such as other *anxiety disorders, obsessive-compulsive disorder, posttraumatic stress disorder,* and *depressive, bipolar,* and *personality disorders.*

---

 **Separation Anxiety Disorder**

The disorder is diagnosed when at least three of the following symptoms occur, beyond what is normal for the person's age:

- Frequent and extreme distress when separated, or expecting separation, from home or a loved one (parent or other caregiver).

- Frequent and extreme worry about losing a loved one or possible harm to the loved one, such as illness or death.
- Frequent and extreme worry about a harmful or traumatic event that will cause separation from a loved one, such as getting lost or being kidnapped.
- Firm refusal or being unwilling to go away from home because of fear of separation, such as going to school or work.
- Frequent and extreme fear of being alone without the loved one at home or other settings.
- Firm refusal or being unwilling to sleep away from home or go to sleep without being near the loved one.
- Frequent nightmares about being separated.
- Frequent complaints of physical symptoms because of fear of separation, such as headaches and stomachaches.

The fear, anxiety, or avoidance must persist, lasting at least 4 weeks in children and teens and at least 6 months in adults, before a diagnosis is made. The symptoms cause major distress and impair social, school, work, or other key aspects of function. The symptoms are not due to another mental disorder, such as *autism spectrum, psychotic, generalized anxiety*, or *illness anxiety disorders*, or *agoraphobia*.

## Risk Factors

The causes of separation anxiety disorder are unknown. The following may increase risk for the disorder:

- **Environment.** Separation anxiety disorder often occurs after stressful life events that involve separation from a loved one. This includes the death of a relative or pet, a change in schools, a parents' divorce, a natural disaster, or a move to a new neighborhood or country. In young adults, the life stress may involve leaving the parents' home or becoming a parent. Overprotective or intrusive parenting styles may also increase risk for the disorder.
- **Genetics.** The disorder runs in families. Those with relatives with anxiety disorders may be at higher risk.

### Joey's Story

Joey was a 12-year-old boy who was referred to mental health care for long-standing anxiety about losing his parents. He had begun to have anxieties as a young child and had great trouble starting kindergarten. He had been scared of being away from home for school. He was also briefly bullied in third grade, which made his anxieties worse.

Joey's parents noted that he "always seemed to have a new worry." His most constant fear revolved around his parents' safety. He often was fine when both were at work or home, but when they were in transit or elsewhere, he was afraid that they would die in an accident. When the parents were late from work or when they tried to go out together, Joey became frantic, constantly calling and texting them. Joey was mostly concerned about his mother's safety, and she had gradually reduced her solo activities to a minimum. She said, it felt like "he would like to follow me into the toilet." Joey was less demanding toward his father, who said, "When we comfort him all the time or stay at home, he'll never become independent." He believed his wife had been too soft and overprotective.

Joey's grades were good. His teachers agreed that he was quiet but had a number of friends and worked well with other children. They noted that he seemed sensitive to any hint that he was being picked on.

Joey and his family underwent several months of psychotherapy when Joey was 10 years old. The father said therapy helped his wife become less overprotective, and Joey's anxiety seemed to improve. Joey's mother had a history of *panic disorder, agoraphobia,* and *social anxiety disorder.* His grandmother was described as being as anxious as Joey's mother.

Joey was diagnosed with *separation anxiety disorder.* He has at least four of the eight symptoms: long-standing, extreme fears of anticipated separations, harm to his parents, events that could lead to separations, and being left alone. His mother has panic disorder, agoraphobia, and social anxiety disorder, and both parents agree that her own worries have affected her parenting style. Joey's fears appear to be rewarded: the parents stay home, rarely leave Joey alone, and respond quickly to all his calls and text messages.

## Key Points

- *Anxiety disorders* differ from normal feelings of being worried, ill at ease, or afraid at certain brief times. People with anxiety disorders have extreme fear or worry that impairs their life function and goes beyond what is normal for their age or the setting. Unlike brief times of stress and worry, the symptoms of anxiety disorders often last for 6 months or more.

- Most anxiety disorders respond well to treatment. Often treatment for anxiety disorders involves a mix of psychotherapy ("talk therapy") and medications. Treatment can provide great relief from symptoms and teach healthy coping skills, but it may not always provide a complete cure.

- Cognitive-behavior therapy (CBT) involves helping to change unhealthy thinking and behavior patterns. The mental health care provider may work with the person to develop a plan of action to help reduce fears and improve habits of thinking.

- Medicines that treat depression also can help anxiety disorders. These medications include antidepressants, such as selective serotonin reuptake inhibitors (SSRIs) and serotonin-norepinephrine reuptake inhibitors (SNRIs). Benzodiazepines calm fear, panic, and anxiety. These medications also can be used for a short time.
- People with anxiety disorders also benefit from healthy lifestyle habits. Exercise, limiting caffeine, and joining a support group can boost efforts to cope and reduce symptoms.

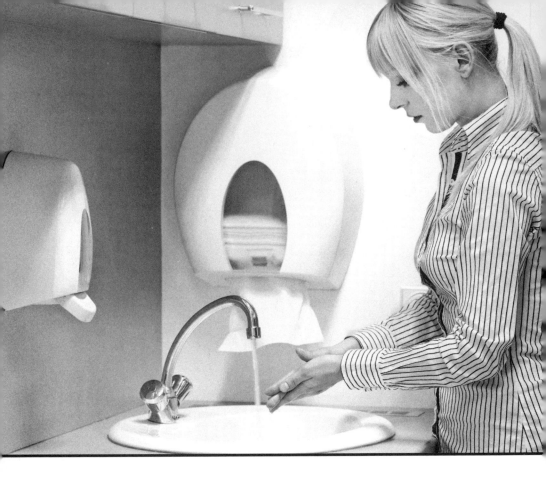

Obsessive-Compulsive Disorder

Body Dysmorphic Disorder

Hoarding Disorder

Other Obsessive-Compulsive Disorders

    Hair-Pulling Disorder

    Skin-Picking Disorder

*For a complete list of DSM-5 disorders, see Appendix A.*

# CHAPTER 6

# Obsessive-Compulsive Disorders

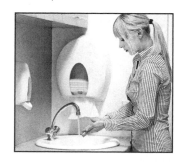

**O**bsessive-compulsive disorders involve frequent fears, worries, urges, or thoughts *(obsessions)* that distract and distress the people who have them. These obsessions often are combined with ritualistic behaviors *(compulsions)* that are repeated in an intense attempt to deal with the unwanted obsessions. Other related disorders in this group involve repeated body-focused behaviors (such as hair pulling or skin picking) despite attempts to decrease or stop them.

These disorders make up a new chapter or grouping of disorders in DSM-5. They include *obsessive-compulsive disorder* (OCD), *body dysmorphic disorder, hoarding disorder, hair-pulling disorder,* and *skin-picking disorder.* Although anxiety is a frequent symptom of these disorders, the obsessions and compulsions are unique features that cause these disorders to be grouped in their own chapter.

At times, people may double-check a locked door, dislike a new facial wrinkle, save a few special items, pull out a stray gray hair, or pick at a blemish. This normal behavior is part of life from time to time, and people resume their daily tasks without much further thought to these concerns. In contrast, people with obsessive-compulsive and related disorders often are held captive by their obsessions and compulsions. Their repeated behaviors and extreme concerns can take over their daily lives, cause health problems, and impair their social ties and school or work functions.

Similar treatments apply to all of these disorders. Treatment can help relieve and control obsessions and compulsions and prevent disorders from getting worse. Treatment often involves a mix of antidepressant medications and a type of psychotherapy ("talk therapy") called *cognitive-behavior therapy* (CBT). CBT teaches people with these disorders to cope with their stress, lessen their fears and worries, and manage their compulsions. Most people with these disorders can go on to live full and satisfying lives with treatment.

## A Healthy Mind and Body

Keeping a healthy lifestyle is important in coping with obsessive-compulsive and related disorders. In addition to following the treatment set by the mental health care provider, these tips can help:

- **Learn basic relaxation techniques.** Relaxation helps ease the stress and anxiety caused by these disorders. Several types of relaxation techniques help relieve stress and worry. These include meditation, visualization, yoga, and massage.
- **Be aware of warning signs.** Learn what triggers the obsessive-compulsive symptoms and what to do if they return.
- **Avoid drugs and alcohol.** Using these substances can make obsessive symptoms worse and can delay the success of treatment.

# Obsessive-Compulsive Disorder

Most people with OCD have both obsessions and compulsions throughout their day. These disrupt their daily routine, making it hard to go to school, work, or have a normal social life. Many people with OCD know or suspect that their obsessions are likely not true. This knowledge is called *insight*. Others with OCD may think that their beliefs could be true (poor insight), or they may be strongly convinced that their beliefs are in fact true (absent insight). Despite the level of insight, people with OCD have a hard time keeping their focus off their strong obsessions and stopping their compulsions.

The worry or stress caused by the obsession (a thought, urge, or image that causes distress) leads to an attempt to ignore or suppress it by another thought or action (that is, by doing a compulsion). Common obsessions include concerns about harm to self or others, fear of getting sick from dirt or germs, and having forbidden or taboo thoughts about topics such as sex or religion. Compulsions can include constant checking (such as locks on doors), frequent hand washing until skin is raw, and counting, praying, or saying words silently over and over.

The compulsions also can be done in an attempt to prevent a feared event. (Children with OCD may not be able to explain the purpose for their compulsions.) The acts cannot prevent the feared event in real life (such as placing objects on a shelf in a certain order to prevent parents from being in a car accident). Or the acts are clearly extreme (for instance, checking that the door is locked 30 times before leaving for work). These acts are performed in the belief that they will counter or render harmless the thought, urge, or fear. Although compulsions may bring some brief relief to the worry and stress of an obsession, the obsession returns, and the cycle of obsessions and compulsions repeats again and again. People with OCD feel driven to perform their compulsions.

While most people will at times have concerned thoughts or repeated behaviors ("Did I check that lock?"), these tend not to disrupt living and only cause concern for a brief time. For many people, minor routines add needed structure to their day and make certain tasks easy. These routines are helpful and are easy to change with new events, such as a guest's visit. For people with OCD, their routines are rigid, and they have great distress if they try not to do them. Their compulsions can become a way of life.

OCD affects 1.2% of Americans. In childhood, it affects more boys, but more women are affected than men in adult years. The average age when symptoms first appear is 19 years. It is rare for the disorder to first appear after age 35. Onset in childhood or teen years can lead to a lifetime of OCD symptoms that can be managed with treatment. In 40% of those with onset in childhood or teen years, there may be no symptoms by early adult years.

People with OCD also may have a *tic disorder, anxiety disorder,* or *major depressive disorder.* Any other mental disorder that occurs with OCD will need to be taken into account when planning treatment.

---

 ## Obsessive-Compulsive Disorder

OCD is diagnosed when the following symptoms occur:

- Obsessions, compulsions, or both.
- Obsessions or compulsions that are time-consuming (take more than 1 hour per day), cause major distress, or impair social, work, or other key aspects of function.

The symptoms are not due to another medical condition, the use of a drug or medication, or another mental disorder, such as an *anxiety disorder,* another *obsessive-compulsive disorder,* an *eating disorder,* or *major depressive disorder.*

---

# Risk Factors

Certain factors may increase a person's risk for OCD:

- **Temperament.** People who often keep their feelings inside, tend to worry or have downbeat thinking styles, or tended to withdraw from unknown settings as a child.
- **Environment.** Some children have a sudden onset of OCD after they have been exposed to a strep infection, such as strep throat or scarlet fever. Being exposed to physical or sexual abuse or other stressful events in childhood also increases the risk of OCD.
- **Genetics.** People with a first-degree blood relative (parent, sibling) with OCD are two to five times at greater risk for the disorder than are people who have no close relative with OCD. The risk is even higher in relatives of those who had OCD in childhood or teen years.

## Allen's Story

Allen, a 22-year-old gay man, came to a mental health clinic for treatment of anxiety. He worked full-time as a janitor and engaged in very few activities outside of work. When asked about anxiety, Allen said he was worried about contracting diseases such as HIV.

Aware of a strong disinfectant smell, the mental health care provider asked Allen if he had any special cleaning behaviors linked to his concern about getting HIV. Allen said that he avoided touching almost anything outside of his home. He said that if he even came close to things that he thought might have been in contact with the virus, he had to wash his hands many times with bleach. He often washed his hands up to 30 times a day, spending hours on this routine. Physical contact was quite difficult. Shopping for groceries and taking the subway were big problems, and he had almost given up trying to go to social events or engage in romantic relationships.

When asked if he had other worries, Allen said that he was bothered by sudden images of hitting someone, fears that he would say things that might be offensive or wrong, and concerns about upsetting his neighbors. To ease the anxiety caused by these thoughts, he often replayed prior conversations in his mind, kept diaries to record what he said, and often apologized for fear he might have sounded offensive. When he showered, he made sure the water in the tub only reached a certain level. He was afraid that if he was not careful, he would flood his neighbors.

Allen used gloves at work and performed well. He spent most of his free time at home. Although he enjoyed the company of others, the fear of having to touch something if he was invited to a meal or to another person's home was too much for him to handle. He knew that his fears and urges were "kinda crazy," but he felt they were out of his control.

Allen was diagnosed with *OCD*. He had many obsessions, including ones related to contamination (fear of contracting HIV), aggression (intrusive images of hitting someone), and symmetry (exactness in the level of water). These caused Allen to spend hours on his OCD routines and to avoid leaving his apartment, engage in social relationships, and perform basic errands.

He also has many compulsions: excessive hand washing, checking (keeping diaries), repeating (often clarifying what he said), and mental compulsions (replaying prior conversations in his mind).

The symptoms also get in the way of Allen's normal daily tasks. Even though he is able to work, his job choice may have been swayed by his symptoms (few other jobs would allow him to always wear gloves and use bleach). Not only do his symptoms consume much of his time, but he appears to be a lonely, isolated man whose quality of life has been greatly affected by his OCD.

## Treatment

Treatments for OCD have improved from the past. Most people with OCD benefit from medication, psychotherapy, or a mix of the two.

The medications most often prescribed to treat OCD are the *selective serotonin reuptake inhibitors* (SSRIs). These antidepressant medications are widely used to treat depression, anxiety, and other conditions, and work well in the treatment of OCD. SSRIs that are approved for the treatment of OCD include clomipramine, fluoxetine, fluvoxamine, paroxetine, and sertraline. The choice of which one to use will depend on the doctor's preference. Although all give medications work well, some people have a better response to one but not another. If one medication is not working, talking with the doctor is key to finding another medication that can improve symptoms. Response to the medication often takes at least 6 to 12 weeks. People with OCD will note that the obsessions are not as bothersome, they spend less time on compulsions, and they are better able to exert control over the disorder, though some symptoms will often remain.

CBT also is an effective treatment for people with OCD. With CBT, the mental health care provider will teach the patient to fight the obsessions more effectively, and to challenge the ritualistic behaviors. During treatment sessions, people may be exposed to the obsessions that create anxiety and provoke the compulsions. They may write a "script" in which the obsessions are described, and then read the script over and over. This technique works well for people whose compulsions cause great problems. For instance, with extreme hand washing, the mental health care provider might have the person touch a "dirty" object such as a doorknob, and then not allow the person to wash his or her hands. This *exposure and response prevention therapy* has been proved useful. It briefly exposes the person to what is feared, in greater amounts of time, and the person's urge to do a compulsion in response to the fear is delayed or blocked. With very anxious people, the mental health care provider might begin with a simpler task, such as thinking of touching a doorknob, and then not washing. The exposure and response prevention methods teach people with OCD to decrease and then stop the rituals that affect their lives.

CBT can help many people with OCD greatly reduce their symptoms. However, treatment only works if they adhere to the treatment methods. Some people may not agree to take part in CBT because of the anxiety it involves, and others have depression that must be treated at the same time.

People with OCD who receive proper treatment function better and improve their quality of life. Treatment does more than just ease symptoms. It may improve people's ability to attend school, work, build and enjoy relationships, and pursue leisure activities. The OCD symptoms cease to control their lives.

# Body Dysmorphic Disorder

People with *body dysmorphic disorder* are obsessed with what they think are flaws or defects in how they look. They think these flaws make them ugly, unattractive, or deformed. However, other people do not see these defects or see them as only being minor.

People with the disorder find it hard to stop or control their negative thoughts. They don't believe people who tell them they look fine. Their extreme concerns can focus on one or many body parts, often the skin, hair, or nose. Any body part can be the focus: the eyes, eyebrows, teeth, weight, stomach, face size or shape, and so on. If they can afford plastic surgery, they may have repeated surgery to correct the perceived flaw— but are rarely pleased with the results.

The obsessions about their appearance can cause people with body dysmorphic disorder severe distress that can last for hours, or even all day. They feel driven to repeat certain behaviors to try to hide or improve the flaws. These frequent behaviors only add to their stress and anxiety. Examples of repetitive behaviors are as follows:

- Constant checking in a mirror
- Constant grooming
- Hiding or covering certain body parts or perceived flaws (frequent use of makeup or choosing certain types of clothing, hairstyles, hats, etc.)
- Comparing their body part to that of others

Body dysmorphic disorder affects almost 2.5% of U.S. adults and affects women and men at about the same rate. For most people with the disorder, the first symptoms appear before age 18. The most common age for the disorder to begin is 12–13 years.

The disorder can cause low self-esteem. People with the disorder may avoid social settings. Some may drop out of school because of their extreme concerns. Thoughts of suicide and suicide attempts are high in those with the disorder, based on distress about their appearance. Teens are at the highest risk for suicide.

Although the disorder can last for many years, proven treatments for the disorder can relieve symptoms (see the "Treatment" section). People with body dysmorphic disorder also may have *major depressive disorder, social anxiety disorder, OCD,* or an *addictive disorder.*

---

 **Body Dysmorphic Disorder**

Body dysmorphic disorder is diagnosed when the following symptoms occur:

- Frequent and intense focus on one or more perceived or slight defects in appearance that are not seen by others or are seen as minor.
- Repeats behavior to try to hide or improve the "flaws" or performs mental acts (for instance, compares self to others) in response to intense concerns.

The symptoms cause major distress or impair social, work, or other key aspects of function. They are not due to concerns about body weight or body fat that come with an *eating disorder.*

---

## Risk Factors

People who have a first-degree blood relative (parent or sibling) with OCD have a higher risk of body dysmorphic disorder. People with the disorder often have had childhood neglect or abuse.

## Treatment

As with OCD, treatment for body dysmorphic disorder relies on CBT, SSRI antidepressants, or a mix of the two. With treatment, the symptoms have less power over time. Those with the disorder also can benefit from the "Healthy Mind and Body" lifestyle tips noted near the start of this chapter.

# Hoarding Disorder

*Hoarding disorder* is marked by long-standing problems throwing away or giving up possessions, regardless of whether the objects have any value ("hoarding"). People who hoard often save items because they believe they will need these items in the future or the items will have value in the future. They also may be strongly attached to the items.

The most common items that people save are newspapers, magazines, clothing, bags, books, junk mail, and paperwork. But any item can be hoarded. Items of value may be mixed with items of little value.

Hoarding is not the same as collecting. Collectors look for specific items of clear, known value, such as stamps or coins. These items are neatly ordered and sometimes displayed. Hoarders often save random items and store them without any sense of order.

People with hoarding disorder have homes where the countertops, desks, tabletops, hallways, stairways, and most of the floor space cannot be used because of the clutter. *Clutter* refers to large piles of mixed objects filling spaces designed for other use. Clutter can be so great that the living spaces of the home cannot be used. For instance, the person may not be able to cook in the kitchen, sleep in his or her bed, or sit in a chair. As the clutter grows, so does the stress and impaired function. People with the disorder may not report their distress, but it is clear to those who know them or see their living spaces.

People who hoard have great distress when an item is thrown out or given away. The feeling shown is either anxiety or grief at the loss. They may tend to give human traits to their belongings, feeling that the item is "part of me." The large mass of clutter also may provide a sense of comfort and safety. The thought of losing the item appears to disturb those feelings.

When severe, the disorder can threaten the safety of those who live in the home. Fires, falling, uncleaned spaces, and rotting food are some of the health risks that can occur. It can disrupt family ties and cause discord with neighbors and local authorities.

Hoarding disorder occurs in about 2% to 6% of the U.S. population and affects both men and women. Hoarding habits may begin early in life—between ages 11–15 years. It then starts to disrupt daily function by the mid-20s and causes impaired function by the mid-30s. It often becomes more severe as a person grows older. The disorder is almost three times more common in adults over age 55.

About 75% of people with hoarding disorder also have depressive or anxiety disorders. The most common are *major depressive, social anxiety,* and *generalized anxiety disorder*. And about 20% of hoarders also have *OCD*.

**Hoarding Disorder**

Hoarding disorder is diagnosed when the following symptoms occur:

- Lasting problems with throwing out or giving away possessions, regardless of their actual value.
- The problems are due to a perceived need to save the items and to distress linked to parting with them.
- Items fill, block, and clutter active living spaces so they cannot be used or use is hampered by the large amount of items (if living spaces are clear, it is due to help from others).

The symptoms cause major distress or impair social, work, or other key aspects of function. They are not due to another medical condition (such as brain injury) or another mental disorder (such as *OCD, major depressive disorder, schizophrenia,* or *autism spectrum disorder*).

## Risk Factors

The cause of hoarding disorder is unknown, but a number of factors increase risk:

- **Temperament.** People who have trouble making decisions are prone to hoarding.
- **Environment.** A stressful or traumatic life event can trigger hoarding, such as the death of a loved one, divorce, or eviction.
- **Genetics.** About half of the people who hoard have a family member who also hoards.

---

### Animal Hoarding

Nearly 40% of people who hoard objects also hoard animals. Animal hoarding is the compulsive need to collect and own animals with the intent to care for them. People who hoard animals follow animal-adoption Web sites, visit shelters, or search alleys for stray animals. These habits lead to a home or yard full of too many pets. Soon the living spaces of people hoarding animals become very messy with animal waste and clutter. The animals are often neglected or abused.

People who hoard animals often ignore their own health and social life as they spend time and money caring for their animals. They rarely seek treatment on their own and need family and friends to get involved and notify authorities.

---

## Lainie's Story

Lainie was a 47-year-old single woman referred to a community mental health team for treatment of *depression* and *anxiety*. She had never taken any psychiatric medication but had undergone CBT for depression 5 years earlier.

Lainie had a college degree and worked as a part-time sales assistant in a charity thrift shop. She said she had dated in college but had "somehow been too busy" in recent years. She was clearly in a down mood. She complained about poor concentration and problems getting organized. She said she hadn't abused any substance.

The mental health care provider noticed that Lainie's purse was filled with bills and other papers. When asked, she first shrugged it off, saying that she "carried around my office." But when asked again, Lainie admitted she had a hard time throwing away business papers, newspapers, and magazines for as long as she could remember. She felt that it all started when her mother got rid of her old toys when she was 12 years old. Now, many years later, Lainie's apartment had become filled with books, stationery, crafts, plastic packages, cardboard boxes, and all sorts of other things. She said she knew it was a little crazy, but these items could be handy one day. She also stated that many of her possessions were beautiful, unique, and irreplaceable, or had strong sentimental value. The thought of throwing out any of these items caused her great distress.

Over a series of interviews, the mental health care provider learned that rooms in Lainie's apartment had begun to fill when she was in her early 30s, and by the time of the interview, she had little room to live. Her kitchen was almost entirely full, so she used a mini-fridge and a toaster oven that she had wedged between piles of paper in the hallway. She ate her meals in the only open chair. At night, she moved a pile of papers from the bed onto that chair so she could sleep. Lainie kept buying items from the charity thrift store where she worked and also picked up daily free newspapers that she planned to read in the future.

Ashamed by the state of her apartment, she had told no one about her behavior and had invited no one into her apartment for at least 15 years. She also avoided social functions and dating, because—despite being friendly and very lonely—she knew she could not invite anyone to her home. She did not want the mental health care provider to visit her home but showed some photographs from her phone's camera. The pictures showed furniture, papers, boxes, and clothes piled from floor to ceiling.

Lainie was diagnosed with *hoarding disorder*. She has had problems throwing away possessions for as long as she can recall, which have resulted in a living space that she can barely live in.

# Treatment

Treatment can help people with hoarding disorder decrease their saving and collecting of items and live safer, more enjoyable lives. Severe hoarding is very hard for people to fully stop and may last despite treatment. Symptoms can be reduced with regular help. Those with the disorder also can benefit from the "Healthy Mind and Body" lifestyle tips noted near the start of this chapter.

The two main types of treatment that help people with hoarding disorder are CBT and SSRI antidepressants, such as paroxetine. With treatment, people learn to throw away unneeded items with less stress, easing their need or desire to save them. They also learn to improve skills such as organization, decision making, and relaxation.

Some people can benefit from hiring a professional organizer to help "declutter" their homes. Because people who hoard tend to have great problems parting with saved items, they must trust the organizer. Because hoarding can last even after the cleanup, the organizer should return from time to time to help keep the person's home tidy.

# Other Obsessive-Compulsive Disorders

People with these disorders have great distress or impaired social, work, or other key aspects of function. People with *hair-pulling disorder* or *skin-picking disorder* often feel shame and a loss of control about their extreme acts of hair pulling or skin picking. They may avoid social and other public settings where the results of these acts may be noticed. They cover the body regions where hair has been lost due to pulling or skin is damaged from picking. Hair pulling and skin picking often are not done in front of other people, except family members. These disorders are not diagnosed if the symptoms are due to another medical condition or another mental disorder. These disorders can come and go for weeks, months, or years if untreated. They are more common in teen girls and women: hair pulling is 10 times more common in females than males, and 75% of those with skin-picking disorder are female.

## Hair-Pulling Disorder

People with *hair-pulling disorder* often pull out the hair from their scalp, eyelashes, eyebrows, or other parts of the body—that is, any region where hair grows. The places where hair is pulled from can change over time. Most people with hair-pulling disorder pull enough scalp hair that they have bald spots, which they may try to cover with hairstyles, scarves, wigs, or makeup.

Often the behavior is a reflex, done without purpose or thought. At other times, it is on purpose or planned. The disorder is diagnosed when the following symptoms occur:

- Frequently pulling out of one's hair, causing hair loss
- Repeated attempts to decrease or stop hair pulling

The hair pulling can lead to lasting damage to hair growth and hair quality. Swallowed hair may collect in the stomach, which can lead to anemia (low iron), stomach pain, nausea, vomiting, bowel blockage, and even bowel tears in the most severe cases.

Treatment often consists of a mix of medication and CBT. SSRI antidepressants are often used and can help curb the urge to pull hair. In therapy, people learn to become more aware of their hair pulling. They also may learn helpful techniques of *habit reversal*. This includes learning to replace hair pulling with less harmful acts, such as squeezing a ball. Some also improve by learning to prevent hair pulling by wearing gloves or a hat.

## Skin-Picking Disorder

People with *skin-picking disorder* often pick, rub, and scratch their skin. They might pick at healthy skin, pimples, calluses, or scabs. Many people with the disorder spend at least 1 hour per day picking their skin, thinking about it, or trying to resist the urge.

The face is the most common site of picking, but the hands, fingers, torso, arms, and legs are also common targets. Fingernails, knives, tweezers, or pins may be used in the process. Picking may result in scars, major tissue damage, and medical problems, such as skin or blood infections.

Skin picking most often begins during teen years, and acne may be a trigger for the symptoms. The picking may occur when a person feels anxious or bored. The picking can lead to a sense of relief or pleasure. It can last for several hours each day. The disorder is diagnosed when the following occurs:

- Frequent skin picking that results in skin lesions or sores
- Repeated attempts to stop or lessen skin picking

Because of the amount of time spent picking, people report missing or being late for work, school, or social functions. The problem also can distract people from their work or school tasks.

Treatment for skin-picking disorder is similar to that for hair-pulling disorder. SSRI antidepressants may help reduce urges and increase control over the picking. Through therapy, people can learn to become more aware of their picking behavior and learn how to stop.

# Key Points

- People with *obsessive-compulsive disorders* have disturbing fears, worries, urges, or thoughts (obsessions) that fill their mind. These are often combined with behaviors (compulsions) that are repeated in an intense attempt to deal with the unwanted obsessions.
- Obsessions and compulsions often rule people with these disorders. Their repeated behaviors and extreme concerns take over their lives and impair their social ties and school or work functions.
- People with these disorders often receive similar treatments. This involves a mix of antidepressant medications and a type of psychotherapy ("talk therapy") called *cognitive-behavior therapy* (CBT). Most people with these disorders can go on to live full and satisfying lives with treatment.
- CBT teaches how to cope with stress, manage fears and worries, and change ways of responding to obsessions. The medications most often prescribed to treat these disorders are antidepressants known as selective serotonin reuptake inhibitors (SSRIs). These include clomipramine, fluoxetine, fluvoxamine, paroxetine, and sertraline.
- Keeping a healthy lifestyle is important in coping with these disorders. The following tips can help: learn basic relaxation techniques to ease stress and anxiety, be aware of warning signs, and avoid drugs and alcohol, which can worsen symptoms.

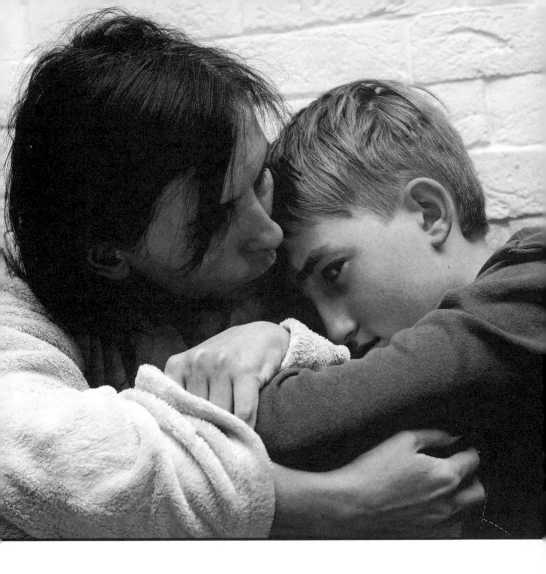

Posttraumatic Stress Disorder

Acute Stress Disorder

Adjustment Disorder

Other Trauma and Stress Disorders

Reactive Attachment Disorder

Disinhibited Social Engagement Disorder

*For a complete list of DSM-5 disorders, see Appendix A.*

# CHAPTER 7

# Trauma and Stress Disorders

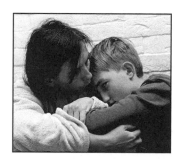

A *traumatic event* is something horrible that people have lived through or seen. It upsets, scares, and disturbs those who survive or learn about the event. *Stress* is a common experience and involves feeling tense or pressured. For some, major stress can lead to feeling overwhelmed and unable to cope.

About 60% of men and 50% of women live through at least one traumatic event in their lives, such as accidents, physical assault, sexual abuse, natural disasters, and war combat. People of all ages react to trauma in many different ways. They often have strong emotions, such as feeling very sad, frightened, guilty, ashamed, or angry. Such feelings can subside with time.

For some people, more lasting problems may occur for weeks, months, or years. About 30% of disaster survivors have some psychiatric symptoms. Nearly 1 in 5 women (18%) have reported rape and sexual abuse, and of these, about 30% have psychiatric symptoms.

*Trauma and stress disorders* are a new group of disorders in DSM-5. These disorders are all caused by events or circumstances that overwhelm the person, often threatening or causing serious injury, neglect, or death. *Posttraumatic stress disorder* and *acute stress disorder* are triggered by traumatic events that lead to distressing symptoms such as nightmares, flashbacks, and vivid upsetting memories. An *adjustment disorder* is a response to a stressful life event that is not life threatening, such as divorce, bankruptcy, or a spouse having an affair.

Two disorders in this chapter are diagnosed in children only. *Reactive attachment disorder* and *disinhibited social engagement disorder* can occur in children who have been subject to abuse or neglect, and both disorders can have lifelong effects.

# Posttraumatic Stress Disorder

People with *posttraumatic stress disorder* (PTSD) have a range of symptoms as a result of trauma. PTSD symptoms vary from person to person. A person may not appear sad or afraid, but may be angry, reckless, moody, withdrawn, jumpy, forgetful, or hard to talk to and get along with. PTSD is diagnosed when the person has had symptoms for longer than 1 month.

DSM-5 makes clear that the trauma must involve real or threatened death, severe injury, or sexual assault (such as rape). Learning that a family member has died from natural causes or watching a terrorist attack on the evening news does not meet the standards for the diagnosis. It can affect soldiers who have returned from combat, as well as men, women, and children who have lived through other traumatic events.

People with PTSD often relive the experience through sudden disturbing memories that repeat and involve what they saw, felt, heard, or smelled, as if the event were happening again. They may have distressing dreams, intense fear, helplessness, horror, nightmares, and problems sleeping, and feel detached or distant. Sights, sounds, and other settings may trigger symptoms, and these triggers are often avoided. Up to 30% of disaster victims develop PTSD.

Others with the disorder may have changes in thinking and mood. They may make vague and extreme negative statements about themselves or others, such as "I always had bad judgment" or "People in authority can't be trusted." They may blame themselves or others for the trauma.

PTSD can occur at any age. Symptoms often begin within the first 3 months after the trauma, but they may appear even later. Those with PTSD often have a first response to trauma that meets the guidelines for *acute stress disorder*, which lasts no longer than 1 month. About one-half of adults who have PTSD will fully recover within 3 months, while some have symptoms longer than a year and sometimes for more than 50 years.

Children can also develop PTSD and at first may be restless or confused after the traumatic event. They also may show intense fear and sadness. Their play often reflects the trauma they lived through or witnessed. DSM-5 has set forth guidelines for children age 6 and younger who have this disorder to detect their unique symptoms.

Most people with PTSD have at least one other mental disorder. The most common are *depressive, bipolar, anxiety,* and *substance use disorders.* PTSD and mild traumatic brain injury have been diagnosed in nearly one-half of U.S. combat veterans from the Iraq and Afghanistan wars.

---

 ## Posttraumatic Stress Disorder

PTSD is diagnosed when the following symptoms occur in adults, teens, and children older than age 6 years (see the symptom list for children age 6 years and younger on later pages):

- Being exposed to threatened or real death, severe injury, or sexual assault in at least one of the following ways:
  - Living through the traumatic event.
  - Seeing the event in person as it happens to others.
  - Learning the traumatic event happened to a family member or close friend. In the threatened or real death of a family member or friend, the event must be violent or due to accident.
  - Being exposed to horrible details of trauma again and again (such as medics collecting body parts or police officers exposed to details of child abuse cases). Watching events via computers, TV, movies, or pictures does not apply unless it is work related.
- Having at least one of the following symptoms of *intrusion* for 1 month or more after the traumatic event:
  - Memories of the trauma recur without warning and cause distress ("intrude" into current life). In children older than age 6, play may repeat with themes or aspects of the trauma expressed.
  - Nightmares that reflect details or feelings during the trauma. (In children, scary dreams may not have content that is clearly tied to the trauma.)
  - Flashbacks that cause the person to feel or act as though the trauma is happening again. (In children, this may be expressed in play.)
  - Intense or lasting distress when exposed to thoughts, memories, or other reminders that reflect aspects of the trauma, such as objects, sounds, and sights.
  - Physical responses (such as rapid heartbeat, feeling dizzy, sweating) to thoughts, memories, or other reminders that reflect aspects of the trauma, such as objects, sounds, and sights.

- Frequent *avoidance* of any reminder of the event for 1 month or more, shown by one or both of the following:
  - Avoids or tries to avoid memories, thoughts, or feelings about the event.
  - Avoids or tries to avoid settings or tasks that are reminders of the event (such as people, places, objects, or conversations).
- Showing at least two of the following negative changes in beliefs and feelings for 1 month or more, which began or became worse after the trauma:
  - Cannot recall key parts of the event (not due to head injury, alcohol, or drugs).
  - Frequent and extreme negative beliefs about self, others, or the world ("I am bad," "No one can be trusted").
  - Lasting malformed thoughts about the cause or results of the trauma that lead to blaming self or others.
  - Frequent and lasting fear, horror, anger, guilt, or shame.
  - Greatly decreased interest or not taking part in activities once enjoyed.
  - Feeling detached or distant from others.
  - Often cannot have positive, happy, pleased, or loving feelings.
- Showing at least two major changes in *arousal* (being keyed up) and response for 1 month or more, which began or became worse after the trauma:
  - Irritable or angry outbursts (even when not provoked) often shown as verbal or physical anger toward people or objects.
  - Reckless or self-destructive behavior.
  - Hypervigilance (being on high alert for threats or danger, constant scanning of surroundings).
  - Greatly startled by loud noise or surprise.
  - Problems staying focused in thoughts or attention.
  - Trouble sleeping (such as problems falling asleep or staying asleep; having restless sleep).

These symptoms cause major distress and impair social, work, or other key aspects of function. They are not due to a drug, alcohol, medication, or another medical condition. Some people with PTSD may have *dissociative symptoms*: They feel like an outside observer to their own thoughts or body, as if in a dream. They also may feel as if the world around them is unreal, dreamlike, or distant. Dissociative symptoms also include flashbacks and not being able to recall key parts of the traumatic event (as described in the guidelines above).

## Posttraumatic Stress Disorder for Children 6 Years and Younger

A PTSD diagnosis for young children age 6 years and under includes the following features:

- Being exposed to threatened or real death, severe injury, or sexual assault in at least one of the following ways:
  - Living through the traumatic event.
  - Seeing the event in person as it happens to others, such as parents or key caregivers (doesn't include events seen via computers, TV, movies, or pictures).
  - Learning the traumatic event happened to a parent or caregiver.
- Having at least one of the following symptoms of *intrusion* for 1 month or more after the traumatic event:
  - Memories of the trauma recur without warning and cause distress ("intrude" into current life). (Sudden memories may not cause distress in some children and may be expressed in play.)
  - Nightmares that reflect details or feelings during the trauma. (In children, scary dreams may not have content that is clearly tied to the trauma.)
  - Flashbacks that cause the child to feel or act as though the trauma is happening again. This may be expressed in play.
  - Intense or lasting distress when exposed to thoughts, memories, or other reminders that reflect aspects of the trauma, such as objects, sounds, and sights.
  - Physical symptoms (such as rapid heartbeat, feeling dizzy, sweating) in response to reminders of the trauma.
- At least one of the following symptoms is present and reflects frequent efforts to avoid reminders of the trauma or negative changes in thinking and mood. These symptoms began or became worse after the trauma and have lasted for 1 month or more:
  - Avoids or tries to avoid activities, places, or objects that bring back memories of the event.
  - Avoids or tries to avoid people, conversations, or settings that are reminders of the event.
  - More frequent feelings of fear, guilt, sadness, shame, or confusion.
  - Greatly reduced interest or not taking part in activities once enjoyed, such as less play.
  - Withdraws from others.
  - Seldom shows happy, positive, or loving feelings.

- Showing at least two major changes in *arousal* (being keyed up) and response for 1 month or more, which began or became worse after the trauma:
  - Irritable or angry outbursts (even when not provoked) often shown as verbal or physical anger toward people or objects (such as in extreme temper tantrums).
  - Hypervigilance (being on high alert for threats or danger, constant scanning of surroundings).
  - Greatly startled by loud noise or surprise.
  - Problems staying focused in thoughts or attention.
  - Trouble sleeping (such as problems falling asleep or staying asleep; having restless sleep).

These symptoms cause major distress; impair ties with parents, siblings, friends, or other caregivers; or impact school behavior. They are not due to a drug, alcohol, medication, or another medical condition. Some children with PTSD may have *dissociative symptoms*: They feel like an outside observer to their own thoughts or body, as if in a dream. They also may feel as if the world around them is unreal, dreamlike, or distant. Dissociative symptoms in children also include flashbacks (as described in the guidelines above).

## Risk Factors

The risk factors for PTSD are divided into three categories: pretraumatic (before the trauma), peritraumatic (at the time of the trauma), and posttraumatic (after the trauma). Social support and a stable family for children help to protect from or lessen risk of the disorder.

### Pretraumatic Factors

- *Temperament.* People who had childhood emotional problems before age 6. These can include a traumatic event or mental disorder, such as *panic disorder, major depressive disorder,* or *obsessive-compulsive disorder*.
- *Environment.* A background of lower socioeconomic status, lower education, past history of trauma, divorce, death in the family, and a family history of mental health problems.
- *Genetics.* Women and younger persons are at higher risk.

### Peritraumatic Factors

- *Temperament.* People who have dissociative symptoms during and after the trauma may be at increased risk.
- *Environment.* The chances of developing PTSD are higher based on how severe the event was, perceived life threat, harm to self, or vio-

lence between persons. For instance, a child being harmed by a parent or a soldier seeing the death of a fellow soldier is at increased risk.

### Posttraumatic Factors

- *Temperament.* Those without healthy coping skills or who develop acute stress disorder.
- *Environment.* Being around constant reminders of the event, further life crises, and financial or other losses from the trauma.

## Jared's Story

Jared was a 36-year-old married veteran who had returned from Afghanistan, where he had served as an officer. He went to the Veterans Affairs outpatient mental health clinic complaining of having "a short fuse" and being "easily triggered."

Jared's symptoms involved out-of-control rage when startled, constant thoughts and memories of death-related events, weekly vivid nightmares of combat that caused trouble sleeping, anxiety, and a loss of interest in hobbies he once enjoyed with friends.

Although all of these symptoms were very distressing, Jared was most worried about his extreme anger. His "hair-trigger temper" caused fights with drivers who cut him off, cursing at strangers who stood too close in checkout lines, and shifts into "attack mode" when coworkers startled him by accident. In a recent visit to the doctor, he was drifting off to sleep on the exam table. A nurse brushed by his foot, and he leapt up, cursing and threatening her—scaring both the nurse and himself.

He kept a handgun in his car for self-protection, but Jared had no intent to harm others. He had deep remorse after a threatening incident and worried that he might accidently hurt someone.

These moments reminded him of a time in the military when he was on guard at the front gate. While he was dozing, an enemy mortar round stunned him into action.

Jared was raised in a loving family that struggled to make ends meet as Midwestern farmers. At age 20, he joined the U.S. Army and deployed to Afghanistan. He described himself as having been upbeat and happy before his army service. He said he enjoyed basic training and his first few weeks in Afghanistan, until one of his comrades got killed. At that point, all he cared about was getting his best friend and himself home alive, even if it meant killing others. His personality changed, he said, from that of a happy-go-lucky farm boy to a frightened, overprotective soldier.

When he returned to civilian life, he got a college degree and a graduate business degree. He chose to work as a self-employed plumber because of his need to stay alone in his work. He had been married for 7 years and was the father of two young daughters. In his retirement, he looked forward to woodworking, reading, and getting some "peace and quiet."

Jared was diagnosed with *posttraumatic stress disorder.* His main concerns were due to his symptoms of fear, and his aggression when startled by someone. Jared was jittery and always on the lookout for danger. He also had intrusive memories, nightmares, and flashbacks.

Jared's attempts to reduce the risk of conflict has reduced his social and career opportunities. For instance, his decision to work as a plumber rather than to use his M.B.A. seemed based largely on his effort to control his personal space.

## Treatment

People with PTSD may require different types of help at different stages. Some recover with the help of family, friends, or clergy. But many do need mental health treatment to get better. Psychiatrists and other mental health care providers have good success in treating the painful effects of PTSD. A range of treatment methods are used to help people with this disorder work through their trauma and pain (see Chapter 20, "Treatment Essentials," for more detail):

- **Medication.** The selective serotonin reuptake inhibitor (SSRI) antidepressants, such as paroxetine and sertraline, can help in treating the symptoms of PTSD, such as nightmares and flashbacks. Tranquilizers in the benzodiazepine class, such as clonazepam or lorazepam, can help reduce anxiety on a short-term basis. Alpha-adrenergic antagonists, such as prazosin (Minipress), have been shown to help reduce nightmares and improve sleep.
- **Cognitive-behavior therapy (CBT).** This form of psychotherapy focuses on changing painful patterns of behavior and intrusive thoughts by teaching relaxation techniques. CBT also pinpoints, reviews, and challenges the thoughts that are causing problems.
- **Hypnosis.** Helping to enhance control over dissociative states and experiences can be of great benefit to those with PTSD. The power of the trauma and the state of focused attention in hypnosis can be used to retrieve traumatic memories, face them, and view them in a clearer or broader perspective.
- **Exposure therapy.** This behavior therapy uses careful, repeated, detailed reliving of the trauma (exposure) to "trigger" symptoms in a safe, controlled context. This helps the survivor face and gain control of the extreme fear and distress from the trauma. In some cases, trauma memories can be faced all at once (known as "flooding"). In others, it is better to work up to the most severe trauma slowly or by taking the trauma one piece at a time (known as "desensitization").

**Talk about it**
- Seek support from family members.
- Speak to other service members who have been through similar situations.
- Speak to a mental health care provider (either one-on-one or as a family). See Appendix C, "Helpful Resources," for support services, such as **Give an Hour.**
- Get advice from people you trust or respect.

**Strive for balance**
- Avoid extremes in personal behavior, such as drinking too much alcohol.
- Seek out people who are supportive and positive.

**Take care of yourself**
- Engage in healthy behaviors, such as getting exercise, adequate rest, and a balanced diet.
- Avoid alcohol and drugs. They won't improve your symptoms, but only mask them for a short time.

**Take care of your loved ones**
- Spend more time with your romantic partner, children, or other family members.
- Focus some of your energy on helping your family cope with their problems.

**Give yourself a break**
- Limit your exposure to distressing news reports and violent movies or games.
- Focus more time on what you enjoy.

**Help others**
- Provide aid to other service members or families who are coping with trauma.
- Helping others will also help you to cope. Find and get engaged in volunteer activities you enjoy.

## Helping a Child Cope With Trauma

When children experience a trauma or stressful event, they are often afraid it will happen again. Getting early treatment and help is essential. Support from parents or caregivers, school, and peers is key. Psychotherapy sessions alone or with other family members can also help children to speak, play, draw, or write about the event and work through their fears. It's important to assure children they are safe and their feelings are normal. Just knowing a parent is there to listen and give attention, love, and time is helpful to the child. The **American Academy of Child and Adolescent Psychiatry** (www.aacap.org) offers resources for families about coping with life crises, as well as how to find a local child and adolescent psychiatrist. The Web site contains helpful tips such as avoiding violent or upsetting TV images and setting routines to help the child feel safe.

## A Healthy Mind and Body

Taking care of your body and emotions can go a long way in helping to ease the stress and anxiety caused by a traumatic event. A few lifestyle changes can help:

- **Stay connected with family and friends.** Try to keep close contact through talking and being with loved ones who can offer emotional support as you work through PTSD.
- **Join a support group of trauma survivors.** Group therapy or discussion groups encourage survivors of similar events to share their experiences and reactions to them. Group members help one another realize that many people would have done the same thing and felt the same emotions. (See Appendix C, "Helpful Resources," for groups that can help.)
- **Exercise.** Almost any type of physical activity, such as walking, jogging, biking, and weight lifting can boost mood, reduce tension, and improve self-esteem.
- **Avoid drugs and alcohol.** Many who suffer from PTSD symptoms turn to alcohol and drugs for relief. These only make the symptoms worse and delay the success of treatment.

# Acute Stress Disorder

*Acute stress disorder* occurs in some people after traumatic events. Traumatic events that can cause acute stress disorder are the same as those that can cause PTSD. These include threatened or real death, serious accidents, violent personal attack, sexual assault or abuse, disasters, and war combat. The symptoms for acute stress disorder last for a shorter time than for PTSD.

Traumatic events cause strong feelings of anxiety, fear, helplessness, or horror. People with acute stress disorder often may relive the trauma. Some may have *dissociative symptoms*: They feel numb, dazed, or detached from themselves. They may see things happen in slow motion.

The disorder cannot be diagnosed until 3 days after the traumatic event. When symptoms last longer than 1 month, the disorder may progress to PTSD. The stress response also may end shortly after 1 month. About 50% of people with acute stress disorder may go on to have PTSD.

The number of people who have acute stress disorder varies for different types of trauma. Survivors of car accidents have rates of 13% to 21%. Those who survive assault, rape, or mass shootings have higher rates, between 20% and 50%. Women are diagnosed with acute stress disorder more often than men. The higher numbers may be due to higher rates of personal violence against women.

---

##  Acute Stress Disorder

The following must occur for a diagnosis of acute stress disorder:

- Being exposed to threatened or real death, severe injury, or sexual assault in at least one of the following ways:
  - Living through the traumatic event.
  - Seeing the event in person as it happens to others.
  - Learning the traumatic event happened to a family member or close friend. In the threatened or real death of a family member or friend, the event must be violent or due to accident.
  - Being exposed to horrible details of trauma again and again (such as medics collecting body parts or police officers exposed to details of child abuse cases). Watching events via computers, TV, movies, or pictures does not apply unless it is work related.
- Having at least nine of the following symptoms from any of the five categories below. Symptoms begin or become worse after the traumatic event. They last for at least 3 days and up to 1 month after the trauma:

### Intrusion Symptoms

- Memories of the trauma recur without warning and cause distress. In children, play may repeat with themes or aspects of the trauma expressed.
- Nightmares that reflect details or feelings during the trauma. (In children, scary dreams may not have content that is clearly tied to the trauma.)
- Flashbacks that cause the person to feel or act as though the trauma is happening again. (In children, this may be expressed in play.)
- Intense or lasting distress when exposed to thoughts, memories, or other reminders that reflect aspects of the trauma, such as objects, sounds, and sights.

### Negative Mood

- Often cannot have positive, happy, pleased, or loving feelings.

### Dissociative Symptoms

- An altered sense of what is real in one's surroundings or self (such as seeing oneself as if watching from the other side of the room, being in a daze).

- Cannot recall key aspects of the trauma (not because of head injury, alcohol, or drugs).

### Avoidance Symptoms

- Tries to avoid memories, thoughts, or feelings about the event.
- Tries to avoid reminders (such as people, places, objects, tasks, or conversations) that raise memories, thoughts, or feelings about the event.

### Arousal Symptoms

- Trouble sleeping (such as problems falling asleep or staying asleep; having restless sleep).
- Irritable or angry outbursts (even when not provoked) often shown as verbal or physical anger toward people or objects.
- Hypervigilance (being on high alert for threats or danger, constant scanning of surroundings).
- Problems staying focused in thoughts or attention.
- Greatly startled by loud noise or surprise.

These symptoms cause major distress or impair social, work, or other key aspects of function. They are not due to a drug, alcohol, medication, another medical condition, or *brief psychotic disorder.*

## Risk Factors

Several factors can increase a person's risk of developing acute stress disorder:

- **Temperament.** A history of another mental disorder, frequent downbeat thinking, feeling guilty or hopeless, greater sense of threat from the event, and a coping style based on avoiding thoughts and feelings.
- **Environment.** Being exposed to other traumas.
- **Genetics.** Women (and girls) are at higher risk.

## Mary's and Robert's Stories

### Traumatic Event

Mary went to a theater to see a movie premiere. As she settled into her seat, a young man in a ski mask suddenly appeared in front of the screen. Holding an assault rifle, he fired into the crowd. She saw many people get shot, including the woman sitting next to her. People all around began screaming, and there was a confused stampede for the exit door. Terrified, she somehow fought her way to the exit. She escaped, uninjured, to the parking lot, just as police cars arrived.

Robert was in the same movie theater at the same time. He too feared for his life. Hiding behind a row of seats, he was able to crawl to the aisle and quickly sprint to the exit. Although covered in blood, he escaped without physical injury.

Two days later, both Mary and Robert considered themselves "nervous wrecks." Grateful that they were alive and uninjured, they still found themselves very anxious and on edge. They jumped at the slightest noise. They kept watching TV for the latest news about the shooting. Every time there was real video of the event, they had panic attacks, broke out into a sweat, were unable to calm down, and could not stop thinking about the trauma. They could not sleep at night because of nightmares, and during the day they had constant intrusive and unwelcome memories of gunshots, screams, and their own personal terror during the event.

### Mary—Two Weeks Later

Mary was feeling and behaving like her normal self within 2 weeks. Although reminders of the shooting sometimes led to a brief panic or physical reaction, they did not dominate her waking hours. She no longer had nightmares. She knew that she would never forget what happened in that movie theater, but for the most part, her life was returning to normal.

### Robert—Two Weeks Later

Robert had not recovered 2 weeks later. He felt unable to express his feelings and to have pleasant or positive feelings. He jumped at the slightest sound and was unable to focus on his work, and he had nightmares. He tried to avoid any reminders of the shootings but still remembered the sound of gunfire, the screams, and the sticky feel of the blood pouring out of his neighbor's chest and onto him as he hid behind the seats. He felt disconnected from his surroundings and from himself. He viewed his life as having been changed by this trauma.

### Diagnosis

Mary had a normal reaction to the trauma and was not diagnosed. Robert, however, was diagnosed with *acute stress disorder*. Right after a traumatic event, almost everyone is upset. They often feel better within 2–3 days and normal recovery is expected. Mary's response after the shooting was normal for the trauma: shock, fear, grief, confusion, trouble staying focused, fatigue, trouble sleeping, easily startled, racing pulse, nausea, and loss of appetite. These symptoms had gone away after about 2 weeks.

Robert developed acute stress disorder. This involved more intense symptoms during the month after the shooting. He had at least 9 of 14 possible symptoms, including nightmares, flashbacks, trouble sleeping, and hypervigilance.

# Treatment

CBT (described in "Posttraumatic Stress Disorder") has shown the most success for treating people with acute stress disorder. It can help stop symptoms from getting worse and growing into PTSD.

Other therapies also can help. Supportive psychotherapy works through emotional responses to trauma or stress. Training in self-hypnosis can induce a pleasant sense of floating lightness to replace distress. Relaxation techniques, such as progressive muscle relaxation and biofeedback, also can help. *Biofeedback* is a technique that helps a person gain control over his or her body functions. A desired response is learned when instruments record information such as muscle tone, skin temperature, and breathing rate. This feedback helps the person to make certain changes (such as in breathing rate) to create a desired response (such as breathing more deeply to reduce tension). Some of the same healthy lifestyle changes recommended for people with PTSD also can be of benefit.

Medication may be prescribed to ease symptoms of anxiety on a short-term basis. These include the SSRI antidepressants and the benzodiazepine tranquilizers.

# Adjustment Disorders

Changes in life often cause stress—whether it's a single event, such as a new job or going away to school, or a series of events, such as marital problems, financial troubles, or a death in the family. Stressful change also can be an ongoing problem, such as a serious illness or a child being near parents who have constant fights. Some people adjust to such changes in a couple of months.

When people feel distressed and down for a longer time, these symptoms can lead to an adjustment disorder. Those with the disorder have a hard time with the changes in their life. They may have a range of symptoms. These include depressed moods, thoughts of suicide, anxiety, and impaired work function. These "walking wounded" may have symptoms that are severe enough to require treatment or care.

After the stressful event or circumstance occurs, signs of adjustment disorder often begin within 3 months and go away after 6 months. Between 5% and 20% of people in the United States seeking mental health treatment have symptoms of the disorder.

If the person's symptoms lead to a more specific disorder, such as *major depressive disorder* or *panic disorder*, that diagnosis will be given. Adjustment disorder would not be diagnosed, even when a stressor appears to have caused the symptoms.

---

 **Adjustment Disorders**

The disorder is diagnosed when one or both of the following symptoms occur within 3 months after the stressful event began:

- Extreme and lasting distress that exceeds the type of stressor. This includes depressed mood, anxiety, or a mix of anxiety with depressed mood.
- Major problems in social, work, or other key aspects of function.

These symptoms are not due to another mental disorder. They do not reflect normal grieving over a loved one's death. Once the stressful event has passed, symptoms do not last for more than another 6 months.

## Risk Factors

People who may have a higher risk for adjustment disorders are those from disadvantaged surroundings (such as being poor, having been in foster care, or having less education). They are faced with many stressful life events that may increase risk.

## Treatment

Most people with adjustment disorder do well with treatment and often need treatment for only a short time. There are two main types of treatment for adjustment disorder—psychotherapy (counseling or "talk therapy") and medications.

Brief psychotherapy, either alone or in a group, helps people learn why the stressful event had such a great impact on them. Putting painful feelings and fears into words lessens the pressure caused by the stressor and helps people with the disorder to cope better. As they see this connection, they also learn coping skills to help deal with any future stressful events.

Group therapy involves people with similar problems. In the group, people can learn more about their problem, gain a fresh view on it, face emotional issues, release pent-up feelings, and feel less alone.

Medications also may reduce symptoms and can be used for a short time. Most often prescribed and shown to be of help are antidepressant and anti-anxiety medications. Most people may need medications for only a few months.

# Other Trauma and Stress Disorders

Two disorders describe how some children respond to the distress of severe neglect (that is, not receiving enough needed love and care when they were infants or very young children). Even though these disorders share the same cause, they reflect whether the child's response is inward (*reactive attachment disorder*) or outward (*disinhibited social engagement disorder*). These disorders are diagnosed when symptoms have occurred in a child older than 9 months for more than 1 year.

These disorders also can occur along with malnutrition and delays in language and thinking skills. They have one key feature in common—the child has had an extreme lack of needed care as shown by at least one of the following:

- Social neglect (lack of comfort, relating, and affection from parents or caregivers).
- Frequent changes of main caregivers, such as in foster care. This limits being able to form stable attachments (connections) with known caregivers.
- Being raised in a setting that greatly limits chances to closely attach to certain caregivers (such as institutions with many children and few caregivers).

Family therapy and parenting skills can help parents and caregivers give more frequent, stable, and loving care, such as holding the child often. A healthy, caring bond with the child and a mental health care provider can also help.

## Reactive Attachment Disorder

*Reactive attachment disorder* affects infants and very young children. The key feature is absent or very little attachment between the child and key adults who provide care. When distressed, children with the disorder rarely turn to these adults for comfort, support, nurture, or protection. When given comfort, the child does not seem to respond or responds very little. The child shows few happy feelings, withdrawn behavior, and depressive symptoms. Without normal comfort, holding, and relating with the child, signs of the disorder may last for years. The disorder occurs in less than 10% of children in foster care or institutions. It must be diagnosed with caution in children older than 5 years. The behavior is not due to *autism spectrum disorder,* and the following symptoms appear before age 5:

- A frequent pattern of withdrawn and restrained behavior toward parents or other adult caregivers, as shown by the following:
  - Rare or little effort to seek comfort when distressed.
  - Rare or little response to comfort when distressed.
- Frequent social and emotional problems shown by at least two of the following:
  - Little social and emotional response to others.
  - Little positive emotion (such as smiling).
  - Sudden moments of irritable, sad, or fearful behavior when no threat or harm exists with adult caregivers.

# Disinhibited Social Engagement Disorder

Children with *disinhibited social engagement disorder* relate to strangers in the same way they relate with their parents or other adult caregivers. They aren't shy or hesitant—and are too friendly—around strange adults. The disorder occurs in about 20% of children in foster care or institutions. When the disorder lasts into teen years, social ties may be on a surface level, with more risk for peer conflicts. The disorder has not been reported in adults. Symptoms include the following:

- A frequent pattern in which the child approaches and interacts with strangers, showing at least two of the following:
  - Little or no shyness in approaching and interacting with unknown adults.
  - Very talkative or physical (cuddly) with strangers.
  - Little or no checking back with the parent or caregiver after venturing off, even in unknown settings.
  - Willing to go off with an unknown adult with little or no caution.

## Key Points

- A *traumatic event* is something horrible that people have lived through or seen. It upsets, scares, and disturbs those who survive or learn about the event. Stress is a common experience and involves feeling tense or pressured. For some, major stress can lead to feeling overwhelmed and unable to cope.
- People of all ages react to trauma in many different ways. They often have strong emotions, such as feeling very sad, frightened, guilty, ashamed, or angry. Such feelings can subside with time. More lasting problems also can occur. *Trauma and stress disorders* are all caused by events or circumstances that overwhelm the person, often threatening or causing serious injury, neglect, or death.
- A number of treatment options can help those with trauma and stress disorders. These include cognitive-behavior therapy (CBT), hypnosis, exposure therapy, and medications, such as antidepressants, anti-anxiety medications, and medications to help reduce nightmares.
- Those healing from *posttraumatic stress disorder* (PTSD) can take steps to improve their symptoms and relieve stress while seeking treatment. These include staying connected with family and friends, joining a support group of trauma survivors, getting exercise, and avoiding drugs and alcohol, which worsen symptoms.

- When children go through a trauma or stressful event, they are often afraid it will happen again. Getting early treatment and help is key to prevent lasting effects throughout their lives. Assure children they are safe and their feelings are normal. The American Academy of Child and Adolescent Psychiatry (www.aacap.org) offers resources for families who are coping with life crises, as well as information on how to find a local child and adolescent psychiatrist.

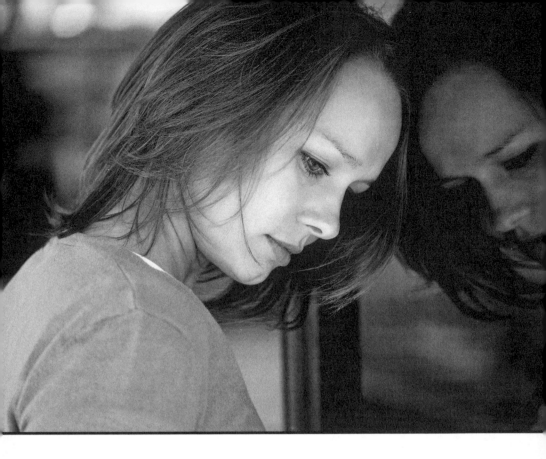

Dissociative Identity Disorder

Dissociative Amnesia

Depersonalization/Derealization Disorder

*For a complete list of DSM-5 disorders, see Appendix A.*

# CHAPTER 8

# Dissociative Disorders

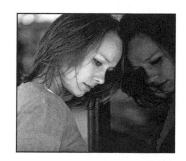

**D**issociative disorders cause problems in people's normal sense of awareness and affect their sense of identity, memory, or consciousness. *Dissociation* is a change in awareness that alters a person's sense of identity or self. It affects the person's ability to connect memories and perceptions. In dissociative disorders, events that would be linked in normal memory are separated from one another. A normal part of people's lives may include mild dissociative behavior. For example, it is normal for a person to occasionally get lost in thought or to drive somewhere and not recall the details of the trip. Dissociative disorders, however, involve severe changes in a person's mental state, and some can cause big gaps in memory. They can become an unhealthy way for the person to avoid reality.

There are three types of dissociative disorders discussed in this chapter: *dissociative identity disorder, dissociative amnesia*, and *depersonalization/derealization disorder*. People may keep the symptoms of these disorders secret because they feel embarrassed or confused. Trauma (such as constant or extreme abuse or violence, whether recent or in the past) is a risk factor for all of these disorders. People with dissociative identity disorder or dissociative amnesia are at increased risk for suicide.

Several different types of treatment are available for dissociative disorders. There is not a single, standard treatment, and treatment is tailored to each person. Treatment should always be guided by a mental

**127**

health care provider who understands the life events and stresses that the person has endured, as well as his or her environment and personality. These treatments include psychotherapy, hypnosis, and medications to relieve anxiety symptoms. Anxiety or mood problems may occur at the same time as the dissociative symptoms. Particularly helpful medications may include the selective serotonin reuptake inhibitors (SSRIs) that are commonly prescribed for depression.

# Dissociative Identity Disorder

In the past, this disorder was known as "multiple personality disorder." People with *dissociative identity disorder* behave and feel as if they have more than one "identity." At times, they may relate to others as if they have more than one type of personality. People with the disorder may say they feel the presence of one or more different identities. These identities may feel like different people within them that influence the way they think and interact with others.

Some people with dissociative identity disorder may feel they have suddenly become outside observers of their own speech and actions, which they may feel powerless to stop. In some cultures, this is thought of as "being possessed"—as if a spirit or supernatural being has taken control of a person in a distressing way.

More women than men are diagnosed with dissociative identity disorder. Men with the disorder may deny their symptoms and history of abuse. About 70% of people with the disorder have attempted suicide. Frequent abuse, severe medical illness, and other mental disorders may worsen symptoms.

---

 **Dissociative Identity Disorder**

Dissociative identity disorder is diagnosed when:

- There is a presence of at least two distinct identities (or "personality states") that control the person's behavior.
- Ongoing gaps occur in recall of daily events, personal information, or traumatic events that is beyond normal forgetting.
- The symptoms cause distress or impair social, work, school, or other key aspects of function.

Dissociative identity disorder cannot be diagnosed when the behavior is part of a widely accepted practice in someone's culture or religion, and when the practice does not cause distress or disrupt daily life. (For instance, some faiths have an accepted practice to feel that a spiritual presence is guiding a person's thoughts and behaviors.) The disorder is also not diagnosed when gaps in memory are due to medications, medical conditions, or use of drugs, such as alcohol.

It is normal to have different personality states that change based on the setting (such as being at home or being at a party) and to daydream at times. But when these shifts in personality and awareness cause problems with school, work, or relationships, then it is vital to seek help. Meeting with a mental health care provider to discuss the symptoms can be helpful. For some people, special therapy may be needed to help them think about how they managed stressful events in the past and how they now think about those events. Along with therapy, antidepressants may relieve depressive symptoms and block panic attacks, if these occur.

# Dissociative Amnesia

*Dissociative amnesia* is memory loss in which the person cannot remember personal information that is normal to know or recall. The *amnesia*, or memory loss, can be so extreme that a person is not able to recall his or her own name. It is often short-term and exceeds normal forgetting. With dissociative amnesia, the person is often confused and perplexed. He or she may not know, or be only slightly aware, of the memory problems. It can occur in children, teens, or adults. This disorder disrupts the person's ability to form and keep relationships.

There are different types of dissociative amnesia:

- *Localized amnesia* is most common and prevents people from recalling events that happened during a certain time frame.
- *Selective amnesia* blocks memory of some but not all of the events during a certain time. Or the person may recall only parts of the event.
- *Generalized amnesia* causes people to have a complete loss of memory of their entire life.
- *Systematized amnesia* is memory loss for a certain type of information (such as all events linked to a single person).
- *Continuous amnesia* involves forgetting each new event as it occurs.

**Dissociative Amnesia**

Dissociative amnesia is diagnosed when:

- A person cannot recall personal information, often of a traumatic or stressful nature. This lack of recall is beyond normal forgetting.
- The symptoms cause distress or impair social, work, school, or other key aspects of function.

The disorder is not diagnosed when the amnesia is caused by an injury or illness that causes damage to the brain. Medications or drug use, other medical conditions, or another mental disorder, such as *acute stress disorder* or *posttraumatic stress disorder,* can also cause amnesia. Dissociative amnesia is not diagnosed if the amnesia results from any of these causes.

Extreme mental stress may bring on the disorder (it occurs in 5%–14% of military members who have been diagnosed with a mental disorder from combat). The amnesia may end on its own, and safe settings may foster recovery. A return of memories may bring great distress or *posttraumatic stress disorder*. When memories return, mental health care providers can help people to manage any stressful symptoms, understand the reason for their memory loss, and learn healthy ways of coping.

# Depersonalization/Derealization Disorder

People with *depersonalization/derealization disorder* feel detached or separated from themselves or their surroundings, as though they were an outside observer to their lives. This feeling persists and causes much distress.

*Depersonalization* is a sense of being cut off from one's whole self ("I am no one"), thoughts, feelings, body, or actions. Some people experience a dreamlike state. Others may feel like robots. They may appear stiff and without feeling to others, despite having great inner pain.

Depersonalization may occur with *derealization,* which is a sense of detachment from the outside world. Time may seem to slow down and the outside world may seem unreal.

People with depersonalization/derealization symptoms may feel that they go through their daily lives as if they are someone watching a movie. They can see people and events happening around them, but they are not part of the movie.

Episodes of depersonalization/derealization can be brief (a few hours or days) or may come and go for weeks, months, or years. The disorder tends not to occur after age 40. It can be triggered by stress, mood or anxiety symptoms that worsen, new settings, or lack of sleep.

 ## Depersonalization/Derealization Disorder

Depersonalization/derealization disorder is diagnosed when:

- There are ongoing episodes of depersonalization, derealization, or both:
  - *Depersonalization*: experiences of unreality, detachment, or being an outside observer to one's own thoughts, feelings, body, or actions.
  - *Derealization*: experiences of unreality or detachment from one's surroundings (people or objects seem unreal, dreamlike, or lifeless).
- During such episodes, the person can tell what is occurring in his or her mind and what is occurring in the outside world.
- The symptoms cause distress or impair social, work, school, or other key aspects of function.

People can feel detached at times in daily life from events around them, and this is normal. Depersonalization/derealization disorder is diagnosed if the feelings of unreality or detachment greatly disrupt daily living or cause severe distress or anxiety for the person having them. Some medications or drugs can cause feelings of depersonalization and derealization, such as anesthesia used for medical procedures or surgeries. Thus, the disorder is not diagnosed if there are medications or drug use, other medical conditions (such as seizures), or another mental disorder, such as *acute stress disorder* or *posttraumatic stress disorder,* causing these symptoms.

For some people, special therapy may be needed to help them think about how they perceive the world around them. It can help them to pinpoint and possibly avoid settings that tend to bring on symptoms. These treatment options are as follows:

- *Cognitive-behavior therapy* can help to confront distorted thoughts and challenge feelings of unreality.
- *Self-hypnosis* may help to replace distressing feelings with a pleasant sense of floating lightness.

- *Relaxation techniques,* such as progressive muscle relaxation and biofeedback, also can help. *Biofeedback* is a technique that helps a person gain control over his or her body functions. A desired response is learned when instruments record information such as muscle tone, skin temperature, and breathing rate. This feedback helps the person to make certain changes (such as in breathing rate) to create a desired response (such as breathing more deeply to reduce tension).
- *SSRI medications* may be helpful but also pose a risk. Depersonalization and derealization can be side effects of these medications.

## Key Points

- *Dissociation* is a change in awareness that alters a person's sense of self. It disrupts the person's ability to connect memories and perceptions.
- It is normal for people to have mild dissociative behavior from time to time. For instance, a person can get lost in thought or drive somewhere and not recall the details of the trip. This does not signal a dissociative disorder.
- *Dissociative disorders* cause severe changes in a person's mental state. Large gaps in memory about events may also occur. When dissociative symptoms and behaviors persist or are frequent; impair social, work, school, or other functions; or trigger distress, then the person or his or her loved one should seek help.
- People may keep the symptoms of these disorders secret because they feel embarrassed or confused. Trauma (such as constant or extreme abuse or violence, whether recent or in the past) is a risk factor for these disorders.
- Several different types of treatment are available for dissociative disorders. Treatment should always be decided on by a mental health care provider who understands the life events and stresses that the person has endured, as well as his or her environment and personality. These treatments include psychotherapy, hypnosis, and medications such as selective serotonin reuptake inhibitors (SSRIs) to relieve anxiety symptoms. Medications should be used with care for some of these disorders because certain side effects mimic symptoms for the disorder.

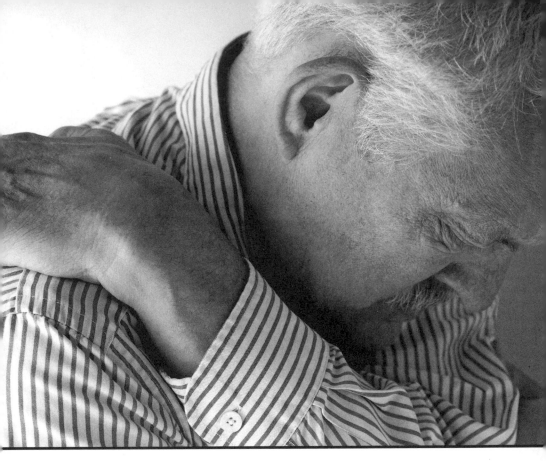

Somatic Symptom Disorder

Conversion Disorder

Other Somatic Symptom Disorders

    Illness Anxiety Disorder

    Factitious Disorder

*For a complete list of DSM-5 disorders, see Appendix A.*

# CHAPTER 9

# Somatic (Physical) Symptom Disorders

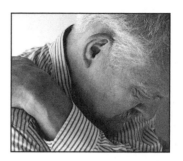

**S**omatic (or physical) symptom disorders involve pronounced physical problems and a high level of health concern that disrupts or impairs work and home life. These disorders involve abnormal thoughts, feelings, and behaviors about real, perceived, or feigned health problems. For instance, when health problems occur, the extreme concern about them is often greater than the actual physical problem itself.

People with these disorders describe physical pain and discomfort. They see these symptoms as real health problems, not a mental health issue. These concerns can lead to tests, surgery, or medication that may not be needed and can be a source of stress and frustration.

A person can have both a medical disorder and a somatic symptom disorder at the same time. People with strong health concerns are not diagnosed as having a somatic symptom disorder only because a medical cause cannot be found. For some somatic symptom disorders, the lack of a medical cause for the symptoms is still a key factor of the diagnosis. Risk factors for somatic symptom disorders include increased sensitivity to pain and early trauma or neglect.

Four somatic symptom disorders are included in a new chapter in DSM-5—*somatic symptom disorder, conversion disorder, illness anxiety dis-*

*order,* and *factitious disorder.* Each of these disorders shares some common features: People who have them are more likely to go to a medical clinic or hospital instead of seeking mental health care. Each disorder is marked by a great concern for physical health:

- In *somatic symptom disorder,* the person mainly seeks help to try to explain physical discomfort.
- In *illness anxiety disorder,* some physical discomfort may exist but the main problem is a constant worry about being sick (or about becoming sick). These mental worries impair daily life more so than any mild physical symptoms, if they exist.
- In *conversion disorder,* one sudden, major physical problem occurs and involves a loss of ability (such as sudden paralysis or seizures) that leads to an urgent visit to an emergency room or hospital.
- In *factious disorder,* a person seeks help for a physical complaint while aware that no physical problem exists—or hides the fact that he or she caused the physical problem on purpose.

# Treatment

As a group, somatic symptom disorders can sometimes get better or be managed without mental health care. For some people, the anxiety and stress may go away after medical tests prove no sign of a medical illness. The tests are enough to resolve the cause of concern. Others with a disorder may struggle for some time and need mental health care to return to normal function. Treatment works best for those who seek care for their symptoms early.

A major goal of treating somatic symptom disorders is to build a relationship of trust (what is known as a *therapeutic alliance*) between the doctor and patient. When this happens, the doctor admits that the person's discomfort is real and takes seriously his or her medical complaints. The doctor and patient also work toward a return to healthy daily activities.

Education is key in helping people to understand that somatic symptom disorders are complex medical illnesses. Some treatment options have been found useful. Cognitive-behavior therapy can address beliefs and behaviors about having an illness. It may help people learn to think positively about coping with daily life even if a medical cause is not found to be the source of their physical ailments. Therapy also teaches ways to cope with pain and learn what seems to make the pain worse. Group therapy may be helpful if group members can go beyond talking about their symptoms and deal with the stress that may be causing or worsening their physical symptoms. Antidepressant medications can also help reduce the pain, anxiety, irritable mood, and panic that often occur with somatic symptom disorders.

# Somatic Symptom Disorder

*Somatic symptom disorder,* once known as "somatization disorder," is a mental disorder that causes multiple physical symptoms. These include chronic pain, nausea, dizziness, fatigue, and weakness. People with the disorder have these symptoms for a long time, but doctors may not find any health condition or disease that might explain them.

People with somatic symptom disorder have constant worry about their health. Their health concerns play a central role in their life and relationships. They see their symptoms as harmful and think the worst about their health, even when test results show no reason for concern.

Although a medical condition may not be diagnosed, they are not faking their symptoms and really believe they are sick. The symptoms and pain are real and can linger for months or years. People with the disorder often have intense worry and anxiety that there is a cancer or infection causing their physical problems—but that their doctors are not finding it. Because of this fear, persons with somatic symptom disorder will often seek out many different doctors, hoping to find someone who will solve their physical complaints by finding the source of them.

The disorder occurs more often in women. Many with the disorder also have other medical conditions, as well as *anxiety disorders, depressive disorders,* and *personality disorders.* The disorder is common in people who have a diagnosed medical condition, but with symptoms that persist or go beyond what is normal. For instance, a person may have a medical problem such as a stomach ulcer that needs treatment. The person with somatic symptom disorder will feel distress about his or her stomach and bowels that persists, consumes his or her life, and goes far beyond what would be normal for a stomach ulcer. More problems also may occur in day-to-day life (such as more missed days of work) than is normal for the medical issue.

---

 ## Somatic Symptom Disorder

The disorder occurs when a person has the following:

- One or more physical symptoms that cause distress or much trouble with daily tasks.

- Excessive thoughts, feelings, or behaviors related to the symptoms or concerns about personal health, as shown by at least one of the following:
  - Constant thoughts about the seriousness of the symptoms.
  - Constant high level of anxiety or stress about health or symptoms.
  - Great amounts of time or energy spent thinking or worrying about these symptoms or health concerns.
- Although physical symptoms may come and go, at least one other symptom is present for more than 6 months before the diagnosis is made.

## Risk Factors

The following factors are believed to raise the risk of developing somatic symptom disorder:

- **Temperament.** People who have a downbeat outlook on life, who are often angry, or who often complain. Having anxiety or depression is also common and can make physical symptoms worse.
- **Environment.** The disorder is more common in people with few years of education and low socioeconomic status, as well as those who have recently gone through a stressful or traumatic event. It also runs in families.

# Conversion Disorder

*Conversion disorder* is a condition in which one or more symptoms emerge quickly and affect awareness, perception, sensation, or movement without any apparent physical cause.

People with conversion disorder may have multiple symptoms that affect their body movements and senses. Trouble with walking, weakness or paralysis, deafness or hearing loss, blindness, difficulty in swallowing, seizures, inability to speak, loss of consciousness, and numbness are all common symptoms of the disorder. The body shaking and loss of consciousness that happen during an epileptic seizure can also occur in conversion disorder, except that an actual seizure is not happening in the brain. Symptoms of conversion disorder tend to come on quickly, such as a sudden paralysis or weakness on one side or in one limb. Because of its sudden onset, conversion disorder can result in an urgent visit to a clinic or emergency room. Sometimes conversion symptoms can come and go or last for a longer time. It has been thought that because conversion symptoms may come on quickly, they might be a response to mental stress, but many times there is no sign of a source for emotional distress.

In the United States, conversion disorder is two to three times more common in women than in men. Conversion symptoms often first occur in the teen or early adult years, but may start at any age. For many people, symptoms of conversion disorder start quickly, last for only a short time, and get better without treatment, often after gentle reassurance and support from the doctor that their symptoms aren't caused by a serious problem. The symptoms can come on quickly and stop fairly quickly, and the person can return to normal daily life.

People with conversion disorder also often have *anxiety disorders* (such as *panic disorder*) and *depressive disorders*. People with *depersonalization/derealization disorder* may also have sudden physical symptoms, such as a sudden paralysis, that may be a sign of conversion disorder. Both of these disorders can occur at the same time.

 **Conversion Disorder**

Conversion disorder is diagnosed when:

- At least one symptom affects the function of the senses or body movement.
- Medical tests or a physical exam cannot find a neurological (brain-based) or other medical cause for the symptom.

The symptom is not caused by another medical condition or mental disorder. It causes great distress or problems in social, work, or other daily functions.

## Risk Factors

The following factors may increase the risk of conversion disorder:

- **Temperament.** People who often don't deal with problems or situations in a healthy way.
- **Environment.** Victims of childhood abuse and neglect. A stressful life event may also increase the risk.
- **Genetics.** Having a neurological (brain) disease that causes similar symptoms. For instance, nonepileptic seizures are more common in people who also have epilepsy.

Conversion disorder often develops during the course of other mental disorders, especially *major depressive* or *panic disorder*.

# Other Somatic Symptom Disorders

## Illness Anxiety Disorder

People with *illness anxiety disorder* are obsessed with having an illness or believing they may possibly get sick. The term "hypochondriasis" was used in the past to describe this disorder, which causes constant anxiety and stress. People with illness anxiety disorder spend a lot of time and energy worrying about their health. They may also organize their life around trying to avoid settings that may expose them to health risks or ill people, such as traveling. They may be greatly focused on health behaviors, such as taking vitamins and other supplements, and they may devote a lot of time and money to these behaviors. Although the results of physical exams and tests may prove negative, they are not reassured or relieved that they are healthy. If they do have a medical condition, the symptoms are often mild when compared with the stress imposed.

The disorder is diagnosed when the following occur:

- Extreme concern about having or getting a serious illness.
- Physical symptoms are not present or are only mild. If the person has a medical condition or a high risk of getting one, he or she often is preoccupied by it.
- A high level of anxiety and frequent worries about his or her own health.
- The person obsesses over health-related behaviors, such as frequent and repeated checking of his or her body for signs of illness. The person avoids hospitals and doctors who could confirm or dismiss the presence of health problem.
- The preoccupation with illness has lasted for at least 6 months and is not due to another mental condition, such as *panic, generalized anxiety,* or *body dysmorphic disorders*.

## Factitious Disorder

People with *factitious disorder* produce or feign a physical or mental illness when they are not really sick. They might lie about symptoms, hurt themselves to cause symptoms, or change test results to make it look like they have an illness. For instance, people with the disorder may claim to be depressed or suicidal over a loved one's death that never happened. Sometimes people with factitious disorder do have a real illness or injury, such as a wound or sore, but they make it worse on purpose. For instance, they may expose their wounds to germs or do other things that prevent healing. Because of these behaviors, they may make a minor illness into a more severe problem by preventing their own recovery. They will not reveal their own actions to worsen the wound or illness.

There are two types of factitious disorders that can be diagnosed:

### Factitious Disorder Imposed on Self

- Fakes physical or mental symptoms or hurts oneself to cause symptoms.
- Claims to be ill or injured.

### Factitious Disorder Imposed on Another

- Fakes physical or mental symptoms in another (children, adults, or pets) or hurts others to create symptoms.
- Tells others that someone in their care is ill or injured.
- The person who causes these symptoms is diagnosed with the disorder, not the person or animal who received the illness or injury symptoms.

In either type of factitious disorder, there is not a clear reason why the person pretends to have an illness. The person may or may not stand to benefit from faking the illness or injury, such as gaining money by blaming someone else for the problem. There may be complex reasons that the person feels better when getting care and attention as if he or she were a sick person or were caring for a sick person. To have factitious disorder, the person must not have another mental disorder, such as *delusional disorder,* in which the person truly believes that he or she is sick.

People with factitious disorder often do not seek mental health treatment on their own. There are no research studies showing which types of treatment are best. There is no evidence that psychiatric medications help. Supportive psychotherapy or biofeedback has been reported to help some people with the disorder. *Biofeedback* is a technique that helps a person gain control over his or her body functions. A desired response is learned when instruments record information such as muscle tone, skin temperature, and breathing rate. This feedback helps the person to make certain changes (such as in breathing rate) to create a desired response (such as breathing more deeply to reduce tension).

## Key Points

- *Somatic (or physical) symptom disorders* involve abnormal thoughts, feelings, and behaviors about real, perceived, or feigned health problems. Each of these disorders shares some common features:

People who have them are more likely to go to a medical clinic or hospital instead of seeking mental health care. Each disorder is marked by a great concern for physical health.

- As a group, somatic symptom disorders can sometimes get better or be managed without mental health treatment. For some people, the high anxiety and stress about their health may go away after medical tests prove no sign of a medical illness. The tests are enough to resolve the cause of concern.
- Other people with these disorders may struggle for some time and need mental health treatment to return to normal function. Treatment includes trust between the doctor and patient. The doctor agrees that the person's discomfort is real and takes seriously his or her medical complaints. The doctor and patient also work toward a return to healthy daily function.
- Education is key in helping people to understand that somatic symptom disorders are complex medical illnesses. Cognitive-behavior therapy may be helpful to address beliefs and behaviors about having an illness. It may help people learn to think positively about coping with daily life even if a medical cause is not found to be the source of their physical ailments. Therapy also teaches ways to cope with pain and learn what seems to make the pain worse.
- Antidepressant medications can help reduce the pain, anxiety, irritable mood, and panic that often occur with somatic symptom disorders.

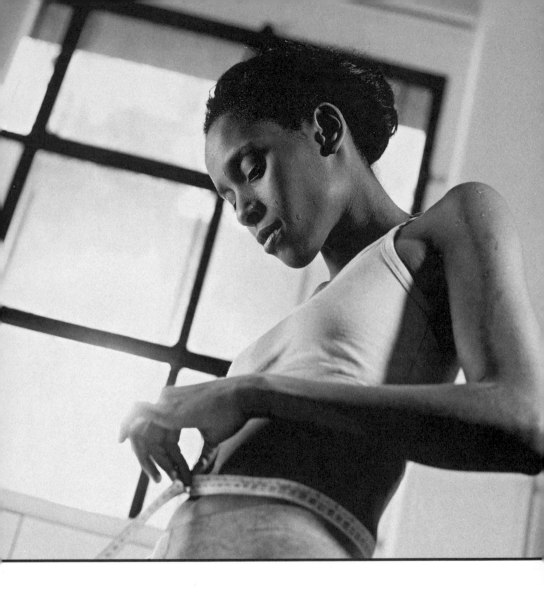

Anorexia Nervosa

Bulimia Nervosa

Binge-Eating Disorder

Other Eating Disorders

    Pica

    Rumination Disorder

    Avoidant/Restrictive Food Intake Disorder

*For a complete list of DSM-5 disorders, see Appendix A.*

# CHAPTER 10

# Eating Disorders

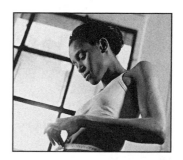

**E**ating disorders involve chronic eating problems that disrupt how someone eats food and absorbs nutrients. These disorders greatly impair physical health and how the person thinks, feels, and relates to others. People with these disorders may be intensely concerned about their body weight and shape. Eating disorders affect millions of people each year in the United States—most often girls and women between ages 12–35.

There are three main types of eating disorders: *anorexia nervosa, bulimia nervosa,* and *binge-eating disorder.* Many people believe eating disorders are somewhat new and reflect the culture's obsession with youth and beauty—yet these disorders have been seen for centuries.

In many cases, eating disorders occur with other mental disorders, such as *anxiety, depressive, panic, obsessive-compulsive,* and *substance use disorders.* Heredity may play a part in why certain people develop eating disorders, but these disorders also appear in many people who have no family history.

Besides anorexia nervosa, bulimia nervosa, and binge-eating disorder, three other disorders are discussed in this chapter: *pica, rumination disorder,* and *avoidant/restrictive food intake disorder.* These are feeding disorders that often first occur in childhood and involve disturbed eating behaviors.

# Treatment

Eating disorders reveal the close link between emotional and physical health. Eating disorders can lead to serious health trouble, such as malnutrition and heart problems. Proper medical and mental health care are lifesaving for people with these disorders. They can learn healthy eating habits, restore their weight to a normal range, and control binge episodes (eating large amounts of food in a short period of time) and purge episodes (vomiting or using laxatives, diuretics, or enemas to counteract the effect of the binge).

Because of the serious health problems caused by eating disorders, any plan for treating anorexia nervosa, bulimia nervosa, or binge-eating disorder must include a thorough assessment of the person's medical condition. This involves a physical exam, lab tests, and often X-rays to check for osteoporosis (thinning of bones common in eating disorder patients).

While the main goals of treating the various eating disorders differ slightly, the treatments are similar. With anorexia nervosa, the first step is to restore a healthy weight. For people with bulimia nervosa, stopping the binge-purge cycle is key. And for people with binge-eating disorder, it is vital that binge episodes stop.

Restoring weight, curbing binge and purge episodes, and psychotherapy are the mainstays of treatment. Cognitive-behavior therapy is often used to help address the disturbed thoughts, feelings, and behaviors related to the eating disorder. Group and family-based therapy may help the person resolve any relationship problems or conflicts that may have caused the unhealthy eating behavior.

Medications such as antidepressants, antipsychotics, and mood stabilizers are sometimes used. These can help relieve depression, psychotic symptoms, or unstable moods that can impede treatment.

Nutritional counseling can help manage diet and eating habits. With nutritional counseling, a dietitian and other health care providers can explain how nutrition affects the body and how to return to healthy eating patterns of three meals each day. These measures help rebuild physical well-being and healthy eating habits.

# A Healthy Mind and Body

Getting healthy again, both mentally and physically, is the number one goal of overcoming an eating disorder. Along with the treatment plan set by the mental health care provider and treatment team, following these steps can help:

- **Set and conquer small goals.** Whether it's eating three meals a day that include all food groups or trying a new activity, changing behavior is a good start.
- **Build a support network.** Join a support group with others who are trying to heal. The National Association of Anorexia Nervosa and Associated Disorders (www.anad.org) and the National Eating Disorders Association (www.nationaleatingdisorders.org) provide a directory of groups around the country, as well as online forums. The organizations also offer telephone, instant message, and e-mail help lines.
- **Practice embracing a positive body image.** People with eating disorders find that a top-ten list of things they like about themselves—that aren't related to weight or looks—helps. They read the list often. Looking at themselves as a whole person, not just as a body or only one body part, is key to recovery.

## What Is a Healthy Weight?

Our culture can seem obsessed with appearance. It often promotes a thin ideal that may not reflect normal, good health. Knowing what a healthy weight looks like can become confused by the pictures seen on TV and in magazines. The answer used by many health care providers is based on *body mass index* (BMI). BMI is a number based on age, height, and weight (see Figure 1 for an adult BMI chart). This is a trusted measure to define what is underweight, normal, overweight, or obese. The **Centers for Disease Control and Prevention** (CDC) Web site contains an easy tool in which height and weight can be entered for adults or children to find BMI: www.cdc.gov/healthyweight/assessing/bmi/index.html. The site also provides tips for healthy eating and healthy weight.

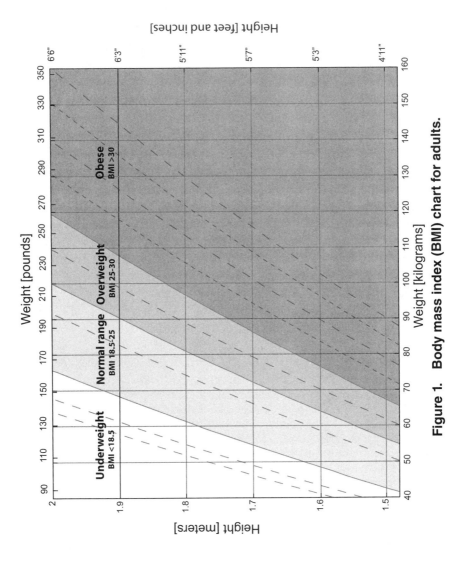

**Figure 1.  Body mass index (BMI) chart for adults.**

Understanding Mental Disorders

# Anorexia Nervosa

People with *anorexia nervosa* severely restrict their food intake. They have an intense fear of gaining weight or of becoming fat, even when they are starved and appear thin and gaunt to others. They see themselves as fat or overweight, and their fear is not relieved by weight loss. In fact, concern about weight gain may increase as their weight falls. They may weigh themselves often and eat very small amounts of only certain foods. People with the disorder may not accept or admit to others their fear of weight gain. Their self-esteem is based on their view of their body shape and weight.

Anorexia nervosa affects about 0.4% of girls and young women per year. The disorder is 10 times more common in girls and women than in boys and men. Body mass index (BMI) is a useful measure to assess body weight for height (see Figure 1 for a BMI chart for adults). The DSM-5 diagnosis of anorexia nervosa uses BMI levels for thinness derived from the World Health Organization to show how severe the disorder is.

Instead of weight loss in children and teens with the disorder, there may be a failure to gain normal weight or to maintain normal development (such as growth). As with adults, weight history, body build, and physical health also are reviewed for a diagnosis.

There are two types of anorexia nervosa. The first is called the *restricting type,* in which people maintain weight loss by dieting, fasting, or exercising in excess. They might consume only a few hundred calories a day or just water. The second type is the *binge-eating/purging type,* in which people have *binge episodes* (eating large amounts of food in a short period of time) and then *purge* (vomit or use laxatives, diuretics, or enemas) to counteract the effect of the binge.

Anorexia nervosa rarely begins before puberty or after age 40 years. It often starts after a stressful life event, such as leaving home for college. Some people who have anorexia nervosa recover with treatment after only one episode, but others may improve only to relapse and fall back into unhealthy eating behaviors. Those with the more chronic form of anorexia nervosa may struggle with the illness for years and have severe health problems. In very severe cases, people can die from the medical effects of self-starvation.

Often, a person with anorexia nervosa is brought to a doctor by concerned family members after a marked weight loss. It is rare for someone with anorexia nervosa to complain of weight loss. People with anorexia nervosa often deny the problem. Family members can help provide the history of weight loss and other features of the illness to the doctor.

##  Anorexia Nervosa

Anorexia nervosa is diagnosed when a person has:

- Limited food intake that leads to marked, low body weight below the normal minimum for his or her age and height.
- Intense fear of gaining weight or being fat, even though underweight; or frequent behavior that obstructs weight gain.
- Body image problems or a denial that his or her low body weight is serious.

How thin a person is suggests how severe the disorder is. The following ratings are derived from the World Health Organization levels of thinness for adults. The level of thinness for children and teens is based on the BMI of others their same age and sex. Problems with work, school, family, or friendships can increase the rating:

- Mild: BMI$\geq$17
- Moderate: BMI=16–16.99
- Severe: BMI=15–15.99
- Extreme: BMI<15

## Risk Factors

Studies have shown certain factors may increase a person's risk for anorexia nervosa:

- **Temperament.** People who have *anxiety disorders* or show obsessive traits in childhood.
- **Environment.** Living in a culture in which being thin is valued. People who work in fields that promote thinness, such as models, dancers, and athletes, are at higher risk.
- **Genetics.** People with a first-degree blood relative (parent, sibling) who had anorexia nervosa.

### Helena's Story

Helena was a 16-year-old girl who lived at home with her parents and younger sister. Throughout her teenage years, she had been a normal weight, but she worried a great deal about her body weight and shape. She often compared her body weight with that of other girls and women she met or saw—and then judged herself as too heavy.

Often, Helena checked her body weight by looking in the mirror. She would pinch the skin on her sides and notice that her thighs touched each other. At about age 14 she began to diet, first off and on, and then all the time. At 15, she decided to become a vegetarian and began to cut out many foods from her diet. She was 5'6" and weighed 125 pounds at age 15, but by her 16th birthday she had dropped to 110 pounds.

Rather than being relieved by this weight loss, she kept seeing herself as too heavy. She weighed herself throughout the day. She spent most of her time worrying about her weight. Time spent on her weight concerns took the place of other activities she used to enjoy, such as school work and having fun with friends. She became more alone. And she kept losing weight.

Her parents became more alarmed about her weight loss and behavior. They talked about this between themselves and started watching and checking her eating behavior at meals. They urged her to eat more often, without success. She kept losing weight, and 6 months later she weighed 98 pounds.

Helena appeared very thin. She often was withdrawn, hard to talk to, and distracted. She seemed weak—but did heavy exercise twice each day. She preferred to stand or pace rather than to sit and relax. Because of their concerns, her parents took Helena to see the family doctor for an evaluation.

Helena was diagnosed with *anorexia nervosa, restricting type*. Her low food intake, low weight (BMI of 15.8), frequent exercise, and constant concern about her body weight despite being very thin are hallmarks of the diagnosis.

# Bulimia Nervosa

People with *bulimia nervosa* binge eat often. At these times, they may consume a shocking amount of food, often eating thousands of calories that are high in sugars, carbohydrates, and fat. They can eat very quickly, sometimes gulping down food without even tasting it. Their binges often end only when another person disrupts them, they fall asleep, or they have stomach pain from the stomach being stretched beyond capacity.

People with bulimia nervosa can be slightly underweight, normal weight, overweight, or even obese. They often diet and do intense exercise to keep their weight down but are never as underweight as people with anorexia nervosa.

During an eating binge, the person feels out of control. After a binge, people with bulimia purge by throwing up or using a laxative, often because of stomach pains and the fear of weight gain. This cycle is repeated at least several times a week, or in extreme cases, several times a day. The constant bingeing and purging can damage the digestive system. Frequent vomiting can also cause swelling of the cheeks and jaws, as well as tooth decay and staining from stomach acids.

People with this disorder manage to almost always hide their binges and purges. Because they don't become severely thin, family members and friends may not notice these behaviors. The chance of getting better increases the sooner bulimia nervosa is detected and treated.

Bulimia nervosa affects 1%–2% of teenage girls and young adult women in the United States. About 80% of people with the disorder are female.

---

 **Bulimia Nervosa**

Bulimia nervosa is diagnosed when a person has:

- Repeated episodes of binge eating with both of the following:
  - Eating in a discrete period of time (such as within 2 hours) a larger amount of food than what most people would eat in that same time.
  - A lack of control over eating during this episode (feeling unable to stop eating or control how much to eat).
- Frequent use of unhealthy purge behaviors to prevent gaining weight, such as self-induced vomiting, laxative or diuretic abuse, fasting, or extreme exercise.
- Both binge eating and purging behaviors that occur at least once a week for 3 months.
- Extreme concern with body weight and shape.

These symptoms need to occur outside an episode of *anorexia nervosa* for a diagnosis. The number of episodes per week of unhealthy purge behavior suggests how severe the disorder is. Problems with work, school, family, or friendships can increase the rating:

- Mild: 1–3 purging episodes per week
- Moderate: 4–7 purging episodes per week
- Severe: 8–13 purging episodes per week
- Extreme: 14 or more purging episodes per week

---

## Risk Factors

A few factors may play a role in the development of bulimia nervosa:

- **Temperament.** People who worry about weight; who have low self-esteem, depressive symptoms, or *social anxiety disorder*; or as children had *generalized anxiety disorder*.

- **Environment.** People who are made to believe that being thin is ideal are more likely to have concerns about their weight. Those who were victims of sexual or physical abuse as children have a higher chance of bulimia nervosa. A series of stressful life events can also increase risk.
- **Genetics.** Childhood obesity and early puberty raise the risk. People with a first-degree blood relative (parent or sibling) with an eating disorder may also be at higher risk.

# Binge-Eating Disorder

People with *binge-eating disorder* often eat unusually large amounts of food. This overeating is often done in secret. People with the disorder can't resist the urge to eat and feel shame and guilt once they stop. Unlike bulimia nervosa, the binge episodes are not paired with purging through vomiting or other means.

A person of any weight size—from normal weight to obese—can have binge-eating disorder. Studies have shown that people with the disorder consume more calories and have more problems in daily function and overall quality of life than those who are obese.

Compared to the other eating disorders, binge eating affects a closer ratio of men to women. Each year in the United States, about 1.6% of women and 0.8% of men engage in binge eating. It strikes women of all races and ethnic groups equally.

People with binge-eating disorder may also be diagnosed with *bipolar, depressive,* and *anxiety disorders. Substance use disorders* may also be present.

---

 **Binge-Eating Disorder**

Binge-eating disorder is diagnosed when a person binge eats at least once a week for 3 months and has the following symptoms:

- Repeated episodes of binge eating that is characterized by both of the following:
  - Eating in a discrete period of time (such as within 2 hours) a larger amount of food than what most people would eat in that same time.
  - A lack of control over eating during this episode (unable to stop eating or control how much to eat).
- Binge-eating episodes that involve at least three of the following:
  - Eating much faster than normal.
  - Eating until feeling uncomfortably full.

- Eating large amounts of food although not feeling hungry.
- Eating alone because of being ashamed by the amount consumed.
- Feeling disgusted, depressed, or very guilty afterward.

The binge eating must occur outside periods of *bulimia nervosa* or *anorexia nervosa* and be a source of distress. The number of episodes per week of binge eating suggests how severe the disorder is. Problems with work, school, family, or friendships because of the disorder can increase the rating:

- Mild: 1–3 binge-eating episodes per week
- Moderate: 4–7 binge-eating episodes per week
- Severe: 8–13 binge-eating episodes per week
- Extreme: 14 or more binge-eating episodes per week

## Risk Factors

Binge-eating disorder appears to run in families, which signals a possible genetic link or learned behavior.

# Other Eating Disorders

These disorders often first occur in childhood and involve disturbed eating behaviors. They also can occur in teens and adults. They include *pica, rumination disorder,* and *avoidant/restrictive food intake disorder.*

## Pica

*Pica* is the eating of nonfood items on a regular basis. Objects that people with pica eat include paint chips, paper, chalk, hair, talcum powder, starch, dirt, and ice. These items have no nutrients. They can be harmful if they are toxic or cause cuts in the person's stomach or bowels. The disorder can occur in children, teens, and adults. Pregnant women may also crave these nonfood items. In some cases, a lack of certain nutrients during pregnancy, such as iron deficiency anemia, can trigger the cravings. The disorder is diagnosed by the presence of the following:

- Constant eating of nonfood items with no nutritional value for at least 1 month.
- Eating nonfood items does not fit the person's stage in life (for instance, young children under 3 may attempt to eat or put in their mouths a variety of nonfood objects, but this is not standard for teens or adults).
- The eating behavior is not part of the person's cultural practice.

The eating behavior can occur with other conditions, such as *intellectual disability, autism spectrum disorder,* or pregnancy.

## Rumination Disorder

*Rumination disorder* occurs when a person *regurgitates* often (brings food up from the stomach into the mouth) and rechews the food. This occurs without gagging or disgust. It is frequent and occurs at least several times per week, often daily.

Rumination disorder can occur in people of all ages. Risk factors include lack of social contact, neglect, stressful life events, and problems in the parent-child relationship. People who have *intellectual disability* may be more at risk. When it occurs in infants, it tends to start after age 3 months. Teens and adults may attempt to disguise the regurgitation behavior by placing a hand over their mouth or coughing. The regurgitation and rumination behavior appears to have a self-soothing function. It can lead to problems with growth, learning, and severe malnutrition if it persists. The disorder is diagnosed when the following occur:

- Repeatedly regurgitate food to rechew, re-swallow, or spit out several times per week, often daily, for at least 1 month.
- The repeated regurgitation is not due to a gastrointestinal or other medical condition.

The behavior does not occur as a symptom of another eating disorder. The symptoms can occur as part of another mental disorder, such as *intellectual disability* or another childhood disorder.

## Avoidant/Restrictive Food Intake Disorder

*Avoidant/restrictive food intake disorder* is a condition in which people avoid or restrict food intake and fail to meet needs for proper nutrition and energy. It is more common in children than adults. People with the disorder do not seem to like eating or food. They may have problems digesting certain food, avoid foods of certain colors and textures, or not tolerate the smell of other people's food. The disorder is diagnosed when the:

- Eating or feeding problem, such as a lack of interest in eating, causes a failure to take in proper calories or nutrition, signaled by at least one of the following:
  - Marked weight loss (or in children, failure to reach height or growth for age).
  - Marked nutritional deficits.

- Dependence on a feeding tube or oral nutrition supplements.
- A disruption of social function (such as avoiding work lunches or seeing friends or family at social events where food is present).

The problem is not due to lack of food or because of cultural practice. The symptoms do not occur as part of another *eating disorder*. It is also not due to another mental disorder or medical condition.

## Key Points

- *Eating disorders* reveal the close link between emotional and physical health. They can lead to major health trouble, such as malnutrition and heart problems. Proper medical and mental health care are lifesaving for people with these disorders.
- Nutritional counseling can help manage diet and eating habits. A dietitian and other health care providers can explain how nutrition affects the body and how to return to healthy eating patterns of three meals each day. These measures help rebuild physical well-being and healthy eating habits.
- Restoring weight, curbing binge and purge episodes, and psychotherapy are the mainstays of treatment. Cognitive-behavior therapy is often used to help address the disturbed thoughts, feelings, and behaviors related to the eating disorder. Group and family-based therapy may help the person resolve any relationship problems or conflicts that may have caused the unhealthy eating behavior.
- Medications such as antidepressants, antipsychotics, and mood stabilizers are sometimes used. These can help relieve depression, psychotic symptoms, or unstable moods that can impede treatment.
- Along with the treatment plan set by the mental health care provider and treatment team, the following steps can help combat eating disorders: setting and meeting small goals, building a support network, and embracing a positive body image and self-image.

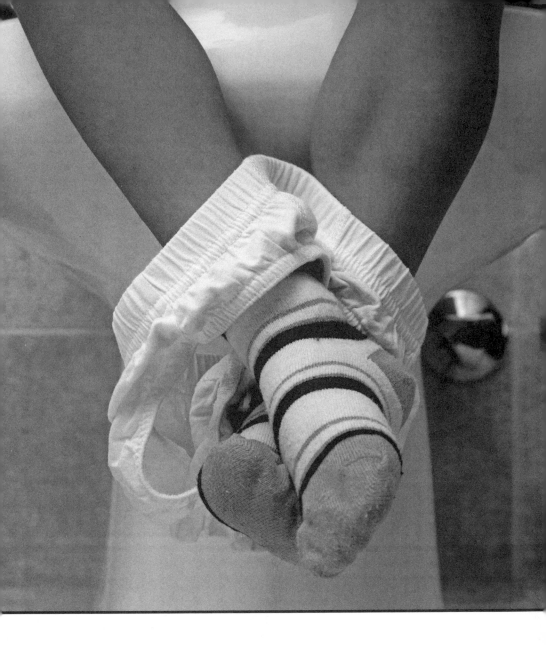

Enuresis

Encopresis

---

*For a complete list of DSM-5 disorders, see Appendix A.*

# CHAPTER 11

# Elimination Disorders

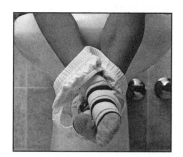

People with *elimination disorders* have problems urinating (passing urine from the bladder), called *enuresis*, or defecating (passing stools from the bowels), called *encopresis*. They pass their urine or stools into bedding, clothing, or other inappropriate places. Both disorders can occur during the day or at night. A person can have one or both disorders at the same time. These disorders are most often first diagnosed in children, after the age when a child is expected to be toilet trained. The disorders occur less often in teens and adults.

The causes of these disorders are not always known. Medical conditions or medications can affect bowel or bladder function and cause these problems. Thus, seeing a doctor is key to rule out medical causes. When the medical issue is resolved, often so is the elimination disorder.

These disorders are included in DSM-5 because they also can result from problems with toilet training or stress, such as the start of school or the birth of a sibling. They are diagnosed after the age a child is expected to be toilet trained. Although most often these behaviors are not done on purpose, sometimes they are. This points to an emotional or psychological reason for the behavior. No matter the reason, these disorders cause great distress to children and parents.

These disorders often resolve on their own without treatment as the child grows. If people with these disorders feel shame, embarrassment, or guilt from the disorder or are dealing with other stresses and worries in their life that could be making it worse, psychotherapy ("talk therapy") can help. Psychotherapy can also address emotional reasons for the behavior if it is done on purpose. One form of psychotherapy is *behavior therapy*, which works with parents and child to teach methods to change behaviors and learn new skills. Parents and the child can learn new habits that they can work on together. Parents' support, love, and calm attitude as new skills are practiced will greatly help a child learn to control his or her bladder or bowel and use the toilet.

# Enuresis

*Enuresis* involves urinating into bedding, clothing, and other inappropriate places. Enuresis may be caused or worsened by heavy fluid intake (drinking), particularly before bedtime.

Children who have never been able to control urination during the day or night have *primary enuresis.* Those who begin to wet their beds after at least 1 year of bladder control have *secondary enuresis.* The most common type of enuresis involves urinating in the bed during the night (bed-wetting). The second type occurs during the day (urinary incontinence). Most often the urinating is by accident and out of the child's control. However, in rare cases it is done on purpose.

Enuresis is common in children. About 3% of girls and 7% of boys at age 5 years have the condition, and 2% of girls and 3% of boys at age 10. Bed-wetting at night is more common in boys, and urinary incontinence is more common in girls. The disorder is most common among children ages 5–8 years. There is an increased risk for the disorder if either parent also had this problem when younger. The disorder tends to resolve in most children by the time they are teens.

In 1% of cases, the disorder lasts into adulthood. The rate of incontinence tends to increase when the condition persists.

The condition is diagnosed only in those age 5 years and up. In younger children it is not considered a disorder because it can be part of normal development.

---

 **Enuresis**

Enuresis is diagnosed when the person:

- Urinates repeatedly into bed or clothes, whether by accident or on purpose.

- Does so for at least twice a week for 3 months in a row.
- Has trouble with daily life in going to work or school or taking part in social activities because of the behavior.

Enuresis is not diagnosed if the problem is caused by a medication (such as a diuretic) or another medical condition, such as a problem with bladder anatomy or a bladder infection.

## Treatment

Children with nighttime enuresis often outgrow the problem on their own. After a doctor has ruled out any physical cause of the bed-wetting, parents are counseled on changing bedtime habits to reduce the amount of fluid the child drinks at night and to make sure he or she uses the bathroom regularly during the day and evening.

If the problem lasts, bed-wetting alarms that wake the child or parent when the child starts to urinate also can train the child to get up and use the bathroom during the night. The child will need a parent's help. It may take 2–12 weeks to see gradual results, from fewer accidents, to smaller accidents, to complete dryness. Use of the alarm (often referred to as the *bell-and-pad method*) can be stopped after 14 days in a row of dryness. (For more tips, see box at the end of this chapter.)

Adults with urinary incontinence also are treated with bladder retraining exercises. They are asked to keep a "bladder diary" to record how much and how often during the day they urinate. The doctor then uses the diary to find a pattern and to suggest specific times for the person to control his or her bladder and use the bathroom. For women with urinary incontinence, *Kegel exercises* strengthen certain muscles in the vagina that control the flow of urine and can also help improve bladder control.

Children and adults who have enuresis may be prescribed medication to help calm the bladder. For children, behavior therapy (such as the bell-and-pad method) is just as useful and leads to less risk of relapse and side effects.

# Encopresis

*Encopresis* involves repeatedly defecating (passing stools) in inappropriate places (such as in underwear or on the floor) after the age when bowel control is normally expected. It is also called "fecal incontinence."

The most common reason for encopresis is chronic constipation, which can be caused by stress, not drinking enough water (stools become too hard to pass), and pain caused by a sore near the anus. Poor diet (such as too much sugar or fatty, fried foods) and lack of exercise can also worsen constipation. If a person is not fully passing stool, overflow incontinence can occur and result in leakage.

About 1% of children age 5 years have encopresis, and it is more common in boys than in girls. In most cases, encopresis is not done on purpose, but is out of the person's control, usually because of constipation. It may result from anxiety that leads the person to avoid defecating. When encopresis is clearly done on purpose, it may be related to *oppositional defiant disorder* or *conduct disorder* (see Chapter 15, "Disruptive and Conduct Disorders").

The condition is diagnosed only in those age 4 years and up. In younger children, it is not considered a disorder because it can be part of normal development.

---

 ## Encopresis

Encopresis is diagnosed when the person:

- Repeatedly passes stools in inappropriate places whether by accident or on purpose.
- Does so for at least once a month for 3 months in a row.
- Has trouble with daily life in going to work or school or taking part in social activities because of the behavior.

Encopresis is not diagnosed if the problem is caused by a medication (such as a laxative) or another medical condition.

---

## Treatment

Because encopresis is often due to constipation, treating the medical cause may resolve the problem. Preventing any constipation and teaching good toilet-training habits are the goals of treating encopresis (for more tips, see box).

Changing the child's diet to include foods high in fiber (fruits, vegetables, and whole grain foods) and making sure the child is drinking enough water during the day can help. If this doesn't relieve the constipation, stool softeners or suppositories can help. These also may be used under the guidance of a doctor or mental health care provider to build a regular pattern of bowel habits. A mental health care provider also may help to address any emotional issues that may be causing the problem.

These basic techniques from behavior therapy can help parents whose children have enuresis or encopresis.

- When accidents happen, maintain a neutral and matter-of-fact, problem-solving attitude. This helps the child not to be afraid of reporting accidents—or not to try hiding the accident until it is discovered.
- The child who had the accident can help with the cleanup of soiled bedding and clothing in age-appropriate ways, such as putting soiled clothes in the washing machine, cleaning himself or herself as best he or she can, or helping to put clean sheets on the bed. These tasks are performed by the child to help him or her take part in getting better, not to punish the child.
- Parents need to be supportive and patient. Reward small steps taken to improve and slight progress made (such as fewer accidents or smaller accidents).
- Solving the problem together can help the parent and child learn new skills and increase their bond.

Young or physically small children will often sit on the toilet with their feet dangling. This position makes it hard for them to relax enough or to use the muscles needed for a bowel movement. A footstool can be placed under their feet while they are sitting on the toilet. This solid support for their feet can help the child have the seating position needed to have a bowel movement.

## Key Points

- *Elimination disorders* can occur during the day or at night. They often are not done on purpose and are accidents. These disorders are more common in children, and they are diagnosed after the age when a child is to be toilet trained.
- These disorders can be very upsetting to both children and their parents. Keeping a neutral, supportive attitude when accidents happen lowers the child's stress about the accident. Solving the problem together includes the child's help in cleaning up accidents in ways that suit his or her age.
- Medical conditions or medications can affect bowel or bladder function and cause these disorders. When these conditions are treated (or certain medications stopped or replaced under a doctor's guidance), the elimination disorder can resolve. Seeing a doctor to rule out medical causes for the problem is key. If not caused by medical conditions or medications, these disorders often end on their own without treatment as the child grows.

- Treatments for *enuresis* include drinking less fluid at night, regular bathroom use during the day and evening, bed-wetting alarms if the problem lasts, and medications. Adults can take medication, learn bladder retraining exercises, keep a bladder diary, and strengthen muscles to help bladder control.
- Treatments for *encopresis* include cutting out sugar and fatty foods, eating more fiber (vegetables, fruit, whole grains), drinking water during the day, getting more exercise, using stool softeners or suppositories, and placing a footstool under the child's feet while he or she is sitting on the toilet to achieve the posture needed.

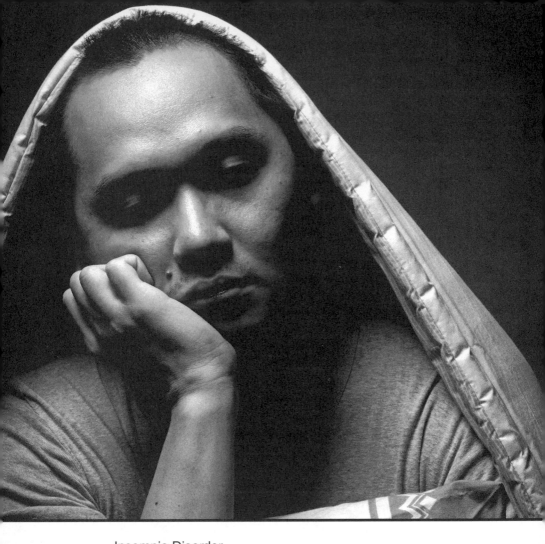

Insomnia Disorder
Narcolepsy
Breathing-Related Sleep Disorders
    Obstructive Sleep Apnea Hypopnea
    Central Sleep Apnea
    Sleep-Related Hypoventilation
Parasomnias
    Non–Rapid Eye Movement Sleep Arousal Disorders
    Nightmare Disorder
    Rapid Eye Movement Sleep Behavior Disorder
Other Sleep-Wake Disorders
    Hypersomnolence Disorder
    Circadian Rhythm Sleep-Wake Disorders
    Restless Legs Syndrome

*For a complete list of DSM-5 disorders, see Appendix A.*

# CHAPTER 12

# Sleep-Wake Disorders

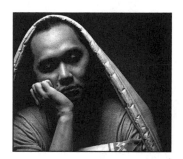

**T**he purpose of sleep is a mystery, yet it fills about one-third of our lives. Regular and consistent sleep can make a big difference in quality of life, day-to-day function, and mood. It is no wonder that sleep complaints are among the most common that people report to their doctors.

To feel fully rested and refreshed, most healthy adults need from 7.5 to 8.5 hours of uninterrupted sleep each night, although some people need more and some less to feel rested. Teens need about 9.5 hours. Without these needed hours of sleep, the body doesn't have enough hours to repair and restore itself for the next day. The longer a person has been awake, the more quickly he or she tends to fall asleep.

*Sleep-wake disorders* disrupt the quality, timing, and amount of sleep. These disorders can cause a wide range of physical and emotional problems, such as fatigue, depression, concentration problems, irritability, and obesity. On any given night, one in three people has a problem falling or staying asleep.

This chapter details the sleep-wake disorders of *insomnia disorder, narcolepsy, breathing-related sleep disorders* (*obstructive sleep apnea hypopnea, central sleep apnea,* and *sleep-related hypoventilation*), and *parasomnias* (*non–rapid eye movement sleep arousal disorders, nightmare disorder,* and *rapid eye movement sleep behavior disorder*). Also described briefly are *hypersomnolence disorder, circadian rhythm sleep-wake disorders,* and *restless legs syndrome.*

## How Are Sleep Disorders Diagnosed?

To diagnose sleep problems, the doctor will review medical history and use of medications. Certain medical conditions and medications are known to affect sleep. People with sleep problems should keep a sleep log to track the following items:

- Bedtime
- Amount of time (best guess) before they fall asleep
- Wake time(s)
- Number of awakenings
- Daytime naps
- Any use of drugs or medications

The person's bed partner may be able to describe the person's snoring, breathing difficulties, leg jerks, or other body movements that might help diagnose a sleep disorder.

If the sleep disorder is severe or greatly impairs home and work function, getting a sleep study at a sleep disorders clinic is needed. Several tests can help identify the problem, but the most common is *polysomnography.* This test traces electrical activity in the brain and eye muscles during sleep, as well as other major body functions. The results can help to diagnose a range of sleep-wake disorders, such as *narcolepsy, breathing-related sleep disorders,* and *rapid eye movement sleep behavior disorder.*

Knowing about the normal stages of sleep can explain how different disorders cause problems in the night. Sleep stages in adults are divided into *rapid eye movement* (REM) and *non-REM* (NREM) sleep. These sleep stages switch back and forth in a cycle that lasts 70–120 minutes. In normal sleep, three to six NREM/REM cycles occur nightly.

- When people fall asleep, they enter NREM sleep that takes up most (75%) of the night. During this stage, body functions are restored, breathing becomes slower, muscles are relaxed, body temperature drops, and tissue growth occurs. The deepest level of sleep occurs during NREM sleep.
- The first stage of REM sleep occurs about 90 minutes after falling asleep and lasts 5–10 minutes. During REM sleep, the brain is active and the eyes dart back and forth. REM sleep repeats about every 90 minutes, with each REM period getting longer later in the night. During the night, REM periods become closer together.

Without the full cycle of both REM and NREM sleep stages, the body may not feel fully restored. These changes from sleep to wakefulness are controlled by messages from the brain. Seeking a diagnosis and treatment, changing sleep habits and settings, and making lifestyle changes can return these sleep stages to more normal patterns. See the box at the end of this chapter for tips on building good sleep and lifestyle habits that can improve and prevent sleep disorders.

# Insomnia Disorder

People with *insomnia disorder* are often unable to fall asleep or stay asleep. They do not get enough sleep or do not feel restored (with energy) or refreshed when they wake. As a result, they may have low energy and feel tired, worried, or depressed. It is the most common sleep problem of all the sleep disorders. About 30% of adults report insomnia symptoms in any given year. Sometimes insomnia can happen during stressful events, such as loss of a loved one, loss of a job, or relationship problems. Looking forward to a happy event such as a wedding or vacation also can disrupt a person's sleep.

Insomnia can be situational (also known as acute), episodic, persistent, or recurrent (chronic).

- *Situational insomnia* lasts a few days or weeks and is often brought on by life events or changes to sleep schedules or settings.
- *Episodic insomnia* occurs for at least 1 month but less than 3 months.
- *Persistent insomnia* occurs when the sleep problems last 3 months or longer after the life event or changes to sleep schedules or settings.
- *Recurrent insomnia* is when two or more insomnia episodes recur at least twice within 1 year. People with chronic insomnia often have trouble sleeping for a few nights, followed by a few nights of good sleep, before the trouble returns.

Insomnia is more common in women, people in middle age, and older adults. Women often have symptoms during pregnancy, as well as menopause. Insomnia is also often linked to some other medical conditions, such as diabetes, heart disease, arthritis, and other chronic pain conditions. Sleep schedules that vary can cause insomnia in children and teens, as well as adults.

Persistent insomnia is a risk factor of *bipolar, depressive,* and *anxiety disorders.* People with the condition often begin to rely on medications to help with sleep or use caffeine to stay awake during the day. This practice also can lead to a *substance use disorder.*

**Insomnia Disorder**

The disorder is diagnosed when:

- A person does not get enough sleep or good sleep because of at least one of the following symptoms:
    - Problems falling asleep (children may have trouble falling asleep without the help of parent or caregiver).
    - Problems staying asleep (waking up often or problems going back to sleep after being awake).
    - Waking early in the morning and unable to go back to sleep.
- The sleep problem causes much distress or hinders social, work, school, behavior, or other major functions.
- The problem occurs at least 3 nights a week.
- The problem lasts for at least 3 months.

The insomnia is not due to another sleep-wake disorder, such as *narcolepsy* or a *parasomnia*. It is not due to a drug, alcohol, or medication. Another mental disorder or medical condition is not the main cause of the insomnia.

## Risk Factors

The following factors may make people more prone to insomnia. A life event, such as illness, separation, or chronic stress, can trigger a sleep problem in people with these traits:

- **Temperament.** People who tend to be anxious or worried are more prone to insomnia, as well as people who tend to repress their emotions.
- **Environment.** Noise, light, a room that is too warm or cold, and a high altitude can increase insomnia.
- **Genetics.** Having a first-degree blood relative (parent or sibling) with the condition.

 ### Warren's Story

Warren, a 30-year-old graduate student, saw a doctor to discuss his problems staying asleep. The trouble began 4 months prior when he started to wake up at 3:00 A.M. every morning, no matter when he went to bed, and he was unable to fall back to sleep. As a result he felt "out of it" during the day. This led him to feel more worried about how he was going to finish his thesis when he was unable to focus due to extreme fatigue. At first, he did not recall waking up with any concern on his mind. As the problem lasted, he found himself dreading the next day and wondering how he would teach his classes or focus on his writing if he was only getting a few hours of sleep. Some mornings he lay awake in the dark next to his fiancée, who was sleeping soundly. On other mornings he would cut his losses, rise from bed, and go very early to his office on campus.

After a month of poor sleep, Warren went to the student health services clinic, where he received his medical care. (He had asthma, for which he sometimes used an inhaler.) The physician assistant prescribed a sleep medication, which did not help. Falling asleep was never his problem, Warren explained. Meanwhile, he followed some of the advice he read online. Although he often relied on coffee during the day, he never drank it after 2:00 P.M. An avid tennis player, he chose to play only in the early morning. He did have a glass or two of wine every night at dinner with his fiancée, however. "By dinner, I start to worry about whether I'll be able to sleep," he said, "and to be honest, the wine helps."

Warren did not appear tired but told the doctor, "I made a point to see you in the morning, before I hit the wall." He did not look sad or on edge and was not sure if he had ever felt depressed. But he was certain of nagging, low-level anxiety. "This sleep problem has taken over," he explained. "I'm stressed about my work, and my fiancée and I have been arguing. But it's all because I'm so tired."

Warren was diagnosed with *insomnia disorder.* His sleep problem began during a period of high stress. His worries about not sleeping may have made the problem worse. Warren may also be self-medicating with caffeine to stay alert during the day and with wine to slow down during the evening.

Also noted is a past medical history of asthma, for which Warren sometimes uses an inhaler. Because the inhaler medication may be stimulating, knowing when and how much of them he uses would be helpful.

## Treatment

There are many methods used to treat insomnia and most people find relief—although it may take a bit of time for some. Treatment often combines both behavior therapy and medication.

With behavior therapy, one of the first steps may be to create a sleep environment that promotes sleep, as well as practicing good sleep hygiene (see box at the end of this chapter). Relaxation techniques, such as yoga and meditation, can also be very helpful in getting the body to sleep.

Sleeping pills, such as one of the benzodiazepines, or sedating antidepressants, are helpful in many cases. Which medication is prescribed and at what dose depends on the specific symptoms of insomnia. Sleeping pills should only be used on a short-term basis.

# Narcolepsy

People with *narcolepsy* have an extreme need to sleep during the day, with frequent daytime naps or sleep attacks that are hard to stop. They also may have *cataplexy*—a sudden loss of muscle tone triggered by emotions such as laughter or surprise. Cataplexy can affect the neck, jaw, arms, legs, or whole body, resulting in falls.

Narcolepsy can make people fall asleep while talking, while at work or school, while driving, or at other inappropriate times. The sleep attacks can last from seconds to minutes. People with the disorder often wake up through the night, for brief or long amounts of time. Right before falling asleep or just before waking up, they may also have *hallucinations* (seeing, smelling, or hearing things that are not there) or *sleep paralysis* (a brief loss of muscle tone, being unable to move or speak). Vivid dreams and nightmares are also common, as is *REM sleep behavior disorder* (described later in this chapter).

Social life can suffer as people with the disorder try to control their emotions to prevent symptoms. They may avoid social contact because they are embarrassed by their symptoms. When treated, people with the disorder can drive for short distances, but they should not drive or operate machines for a living because of safety concerns. There is not a complete cure for the disorder, but treatment helps people to manage and cope with symptoms.

Narcolepsy with cataplexy affects about 1 in every 3,000 Americans. There are likely more people who have narcolepsy without cataplexy. The condition may affect slightly more men than women, and research suggests it may be caused by a shortage of *hypocretin* (a protein made by the brain).

Symptoms of narcolepsy often start in childhood and teen years. The symptoms may go unnoticed because they progress slowly over time. The disorder often first appears at ages 15–25 years and 30–35 years. It rarely first appears in older adults. The disorder is also linked to obesity. Young children who suddenly develop the symptoms often have rapid weight gain. People with *bipolar, depressive,* and *anxiety disorders* may also suffer from narcolepsy.

---

 **Narcolepsy**

Narcolepsy is diagnosed when people have:

- Periods of a strong urge to sleep, followed by a short nap (sleep attack). These naps happen at least three times per week over the past 3 months.

- The presence of at least one of the following:
  - Episodes of cataplexy (either one of the following) that occur at least a few times per month:
    - In people whose symptoms have lasted for a long time, a brief and sudden loss of muscle tone while awake that makes them unable to move and is triggered by emotions such as laughter or joking.
    - In children or people whose symptoms have lasted for 6 months or less, sudden grimaces or episodes with an open jaw and thrusting tongue, without any emotional triggers.
  - Lab tests showing a low amount of hypocretin in the brain.
  - Nighttime sleep study results showing that REM sleep occurs at abnormal times.

## Risk Factors

The following factors may make people more prone to narcolepsy:

- **Temperament.** *Parasomnias* (such as *sleepwalking* or *REM sleep behavior disorder*), teeth grinding, and bed-wetting may be more common in people who develop narcolepsy. Those with narcolepsy often notice that they need more sleep than other family members.
- **Environment.** Certain types of flu or strep throat, immune system problems, head trauma, and sudden changes in sleep-wake patterns, such as job changes or stress, may be triggers.
- **Genetics.** People with a first-degree blood relative (parent or sibling) with narcolepsy are at a higher risk of also developing the condition.

## Treatment

Treatment of narcolepsy often combines both behavior therapy and medication. These may relieve the symptoms enough for many people with the condition to once again have almost-normal sleep habits.

Behavior therapy may include making lifestyle changes, such as taking several short naps (10–15 minutes) during the day and sticking to a regular schedule for sleep, exercise, and meals. Avoiding heavy meals and alcohol, which can disturb or induce sleep, is also suggested.

Stimulants, such as methylphenidate (Ritalin), are often used to treat sleep attacks and can help with staying alert. Modafinil (Provigil) is an effective alternative to the stimulants and is well tolerated. Tricyclic antidepressants are sometimes used to treat cataplexy or sleep paralysis but have little impact on sleep attacks. Sodium oxybate can be used to treat cataplexy.

# Breathing-Related Sleep Disorders

*Breathing-related sleep disorders* cause problems in a person's normal breathing that disturb sleep. These often lead to more serious health and social concerns. Seeking treatment quickly for these disorders can prevent serious health problems. This group of disorders includes *obstructive sleep apnea hypopnea, central sleep apnea,* and *sleep-related hypoventilation.*

## Obstructive Sleep Apnea Hypopnea

*Obstructive sleep apnea hypopnea*—or sleep apnea—causes breathing to briefly stop during sleep. *Apnea* refers to a total pause in breathing, and *hypopnea* refers to reduced breathing for at least 10 seconds (in children, two missed breaths). The pause or reduction in breathing occurs when the muscles in the back of the throat do not keep the airway open. This can happen hundreds of times throughout the night.

Sleep apnea is the most common breathing-related sleep disorder, affecting more than 18 million American adults. Most people who have sleep apnea, however, don't know it because it only happens while they are asleep. A family member or other person sharing the bedroom might be the first to notice the symptoms. It is more common in men, people ages 40–60, older adults, and people who are overweight. Weight loss can resolve the problem.

At least 1% to 2% of children also suffer from sleep apnea, and the numbers may be as high as 10% to 20% in children who snore. Children who have enlarged tonsil tissues in their throats may also have the problem. The disorder tends to peak in children ages 3–8 years. It can resolve as the child grows, but if the problem exists, getting help is key for the child's health. In children, delayed growth and behavior and learning problems can result. Children with the disorder may have problems breathing while asleep, a dry mouth, morning headaches, problems swallowing, bed-wetting, and problems forming words.

For all people with the condition, sleep apnea can cause disturbed sleep and low oxygen levels. The most common symptoms in adults include snoring, dry mouth, sleepiness during the day, heartburn, morning headaches, and loss of sex drive. More than 60% of people with sleep apnea develop high blood pressure.

# Obstructive Sleep Apnea Hypopnea

The condition is diagnosed when a person has either one of the following:

- A sleep study shows at least five obstructive apneas or hypopneas per hour of sleep and either of the following sleep symptoms:
  - Snoring, snorting/gasping, or breathing pauses during nighttime sleep.
  - Daytime sleepiness, fatigue, or unrefreshing sleep, despite enough time to sleep, that is not due to another mental disorder or medical condition.
- A sleep study shows at least 15 obstructive apneas and/or hypopneas per hour of sleep regardless of other symptoms.

 ## Carlos's Story

Carlos, a 57-year-old man, came in for reevaluation of his antidepressant medication. He described several months of worsening fatigue, daytime sleepiness, and generally "not feeling good." He lacked the energy to do his usual activities, but he still enjoyed them when he took part in them. He had some trouble staying focused on his work in computers and was worried that he would lose his job. A selective serotonin reuptake inhibitor (SSRI) antidepressant had been prescribed 2 years earlier, and symptoms improved somewhat. Carlos insisted he was still taking the medication.

He said he didn't feel stressed. Along with *depression*, he also had high blood pressure, diabetes, and heart disease. He complained of heartburn as well as erectile dysfunction, for which he had not seen a doctor.

Carlos was born in Venezuela. He was married and had two grown children. He did not smoke or drink alcohol but did drink several servings of coffee each day to help stay alert.

The exam showed he was 5 feet 10 inches tall, weighed 235 pounds, and had a body mass index (BMI) of 34. His neck width was 20 inches.

More questions revealed that Carlos not only had trouble staying awake at work, but sometimes nodded off while driving. He slept 8–10 hours nightly but woke up often, made nightly trips to the bathroom (nocturia), and often woke with a choking sensation and sometimes with a headache. He had snored since childhood, but he added, "All the men in my family are snorers." Before his wife chose to sleep in their guest bedroom, she said he snored very loudly and sometimes stopped breathing and gasped for air.

Carlos was sent for a sleep study, which showed he had 25 events of apnea per hour. He was diagnosed with *obstructive sleep apnea hypopnea*. His history of loud snoring and episodes of choking and gasping suggested that apnea was likely the problem.

Carlos has many of the risk factors for obstructive sleep apnea hypopnea. For example, he is over age 50 and obese, and has a family history of "all the men" being snorers. Snoring is a specific sign of sleep apnea, especially when the snoring is very loud, occurs more than 3 days per week, and is accompanied by episodes of choking and gasping.

## Risk Factors

Many genetic and physical factors increase the risk of sleep apnea, such as having a first-degree blood relative (parent or sibling) with the condition, obesity, a recessed chin, a small jaw, a large overbite, a large neck size (17 inches or greater in a man or 16 inches or greater in a woman), smoking, and alcohol use. Men are at higher risk than women because of the design of their airway structure. Menopause can increase risk in women.

## Treatment

Treatment for sleep apnea helps people breathe normally during sleep and relieves symptoms such as loud snoring and daytime sleepiness.

- Lifestyle changes are a major part of treating apnea. Because many people with sleep apnea are obese, weight loss can help in many cases.
- People also find that sleeping on their side instead of their back helps keep the throat open, and can reduce the symptoms of sleep apnea.
- Seeing a doctor for any medical or medication problems that might be causing the sleep apnea can also resolve the sleep problem.
- A custom-made mouthpiece can be used to adjust the lower jaw and tongue to keep the airways open during sleep.
- For those with moderate to severe apnea, a *continuous positive airway pressure (CPAP)* device is prescribed. A CPAP machine consists of a face mask that gently blows air into the person's throat to keep airways open during sleep.
- In rare and severe cases, surgery can help to keep the airway open during sleep.

# Central Sleep Apnea

*Central sleep apnea* is a disorder in which the brain fails to correctly control breathing during sleep. This causes people to make no effort to breathe for brief periods. The condition is a rare type of sleep apnea.

Central sleep apnea is more common in people with certain medical conditions, such as heart failure, stroke, or kidney failure. People with these health problems usually develop a type of disturbed breathing pattern known as *Cheyne-Stokes breathing.* Breathing increases and decreases, sometimes quickly, like a tidal wave, with periods of sleep apnea and waking. Hyperventilation (fast, deep, rapid breaths) and hypoventilation (shallow and few breaths) occur.

Central sleep apnea is more common in people over age 60. It is also more common in people who use opioids, with as much as 30% of opioid users having the condition.

---

 **Central Sleep Apnea**

The condition is diagnosed when:

- A sleep study shows at least five central apneas per hour of sleep.
- The disorder is not due to another current sleep disorder.

---

## Risk Factors

Many genetic and health factors increase the risk of central sleep apnea, such as heart failure, older age, and male gender. Kidney failure, stroke, and taking long-acting opioid medication (painkillers) also increase risk.

## Treatment

Treating the underlying condition that is causing central sleep apnea can help relieve and manage symptoms. If opioid medications are causing the apnea, the doctor may lower the dose or change the medicine. Devices used during sleep to aid breathing also may be used. These include CPAP (described above for obstructive sleep apnea hypopnea), bilevel positive airway pressure (BiPAP), and adaptive servo-ventilation (ASV). These devices provide pressured air in different ways. BiPAP and ASV can deliver a breath if one hasn't been taken for a certain number of seconds. Some types of central sleep apnea are treated with medicines that promote breathing. Oxygen treatment may help ensure the lungs get enough oxygen while sleeping.

# Sleep-Related Hypoventilation

*Sleep-related hypoventilation* is a rare condition marked by shallow breathing with either high carbon dioxide or low oxygen levels only during sleep. It can occur on its own or with medical conditions, medication use, or *substance use disorders*. Daytime sleepiness, frequent waking during sleep, morning headaches, and complaints of insomnia are common. The disorder is slow to progress and can occur at any age, even in infants. It can result in heart failure and problems in brain, blood, and heart function.

**Sleep-Related Hypoventilation**

The condition is diagnosed when:

- A sleep study shows decreased breathing with high carbon dioxide or low oxygen levels.
- The disorder is not due to another current sleep disorder.

## Risk Factors

The following factors increase the risk of developing the condition:

- **Environment.** People who take central nervous system depressants to treat anxiety or insomnia, such as benzodiazepines, opiates, or alcohol.
- **Genetics and biology.** Other medical conditions, such as obesity, breathing disorders (for instance, asthma, lung diseases), hypothyroidism, neuromuscular or chest wall disorders, or spinal cord injury.

## Treatment

Treating the underlying condition that is causing sleep-related hypoventilation can help relieve and manage symptoms. When the other condition improves or worsens, it can likewise improve or worsen sleep-related hypoventilation. Treatments also can include oxygen treatment and CPAP.

# Parasomnias

*Parasomnias* are disorders that involve abnormal dreams and behaviors that happen during sleep or as someone begins to awake. *Non–rapid eye movement (NREM) sleep arousal disorders* and *rapid eye movement (REM) sleep behavior disorder* are the most common. They reveal that being asleep and being awake are not always distinct states.

When episodes of parasomnias are frequent and cause much distress, medications are usually prescribed for treatment. In most cases, benzodiazapine tranquilizers or antidepressant medications can be very helpful in stopping the episodes.

## Non–Rapid Eye Movement Sleep Arousal Disorders

The most common type of *non-REM sleep arousal disorders* are *sleepwalking* and *sleep terrors.* These disorders involve partial waking during the night, and the person's eyes may be open when these occur. The person is confused when wakened or can be hard to wake. Many people have both sleepwalking and sleep terrors.

While sleepwalking, people may just sit up in bed, look about, or pick at the blanket or sheet. Or they may do such things as leave the room, use the bathroom, and talk with someone. Most episodes last from 1–10 minutes to a half hour or full hour.

During a sleep terror, people have an extreme sense of dread and danger, and an urge to escape. There may be several episodes of terrors throughout the night.

It is common for non-REM sleep arousal disorders to occur just once or rarely (after a long while if it happened before). Between 10% and 30% of children have sleepwalked at least once, and 2%–3% sleepwalk often. Nearly 30% of adults sleepwalk in their lifetime and almost 4% sleepwalk in any given year. Sleep terror episodes are more common in young children under age 3 (20%–40%) than in adults (2%).

---

 ## Non–REM Sleep Arousal Disorders

The disorder is diagnosed when the following occur:

- Regular episodes of incomplete awakening from sleep, usually during the first third of the sleep hours, along with one of the following:
  - **Sleepwalking:** Repeated episodes of rising from bed during sleep and walking about. While sleepwalking, the person has a blank, staring face; does not respond to others trying to talk to him or her; and can be hard to wake.
  - **Sleep terrors:** Extreme nightmares that wake a person from sleep, most often with a panicked scream. There may be intense fear, rapid breathing, and sweating during each episode. The person does not respond to others who try to give comfort during the episode.
- None or little of the dream is recalled.
- The person does not recall that sleepwalking or sleep terrors occurred.
- The episodes cause much distress or disrupt social life, work, or daily functions.

The problem is not due to the effects of a substance such as drugs or medication. It is not due to another mental disorder or medical condition.

---

## Risk Factors

These factors increase the risk of sleepwalking or sleep terrors:

- **Environment.** Use of sedatives (medicines that cause sleep or rest), lack of sleep, change of sleep schedule, fatigue, fever, and physical or emotional stress.
- **Genetics.** Up to 80% of people who sleepwalk have a family history of sleepwalking or sleep terrors. Children whose mother and father both sleepwalk are 60% more likely to also have the problem. And those with a first-degree blood relative (parent or sibling) who sleepwalks or has sleep terrors are up to 10 times more likely to have sleep terrors as well.

# Nightmare Disorder

*Nightmares* are vivid, detailed dreams that cause worry or fear. Attempts to avoid danger are a common theme, and feelings of worry or fear may persist after waking. Nightmares occur during REM sleep. They involve quick waking after the dream and good recall of the dream content.

Episodes of nightmares increase through childhood into teenage years. Between 1% and 4% of parents report that their preschool-age children "often" or "always" have nightmares. Nightmares often begin between ages 3–6 years but become more frequent and severe in the teens and early adult years. Women ages 20–29 are twice as likely to have nightmares than men of their age. About 6% of adults have nightmares at least once a month, and 1% to 2% have them frequently. Parents who soothe their children after nightmares may protect them against chronic nightmares.

---

 **Nightmare Disorder**

The disorder is diagnosed when:

- Repeated instances of long, very restless, and well-remembered dreams occur that often involve trying to avoid physical harm and safety threats. These happen during the second half of sleep hours.
- The person wakes from a dream and quickly is alert.
- The episodes cause much distress or interfere with social life, work, or other major daily functions.

The problem is not due to the effects of a substance such as drugs or medication. It is not due to another mental disorder or medical condition. The nightmares can occur less than once a week, more than once a week, or each night. They can happen for 1 month or less, more than 1 month, or 6 months or more.

## Risk Factors

These factors increase the risk of nightmares:

- **Temperament.** Harmful or stressful life events, such as trauma. Having a mental disorder may increase risk.
- **Environment.** Lack of sleep, jet lag, and changing the times for sleeping and waking can upset REM sleep stages.
- **Genetics.** A family history of nightmares.

# Rapid Eye Movement Sleep Behavior Disorder

People with *REM sleep behavior disorder* act out their dreams during sleep. They may perform strong and violent acts in dreams of being attacked or escaping harm. The violent behavior includes loud, profane screams or movement that harms the person and the bed partner, such as falling, jumping, punching, thrusting, hitting, or kicking. The person's eyes may be closed during these episodes. When awakened, the person is quickly alert and may be able to recall the upsetting dream.

The disorder is much more common in men over age 50, but it can occur in women and younger people. It may be more common in people who take medications for a mental disorder.

---

 **REM Sleep Behavior Disorder**

The disorder is diagnosed when:

- Repeated episodes of waking during sleep occur, with talking and/ or complex movement.
- These behaviors arise during REM sleep and often happen more than 90 minutes after sleep begins, tend to occur later in the sleep cycle, and rarely happen during daytime naps.
- The person wakes fully alert, and not confused or disoriented.
- Either of the following exists:
  - REM sleep without relaxed muscles on sleep study recording.
  - A history of possible REM sleep behavior disorder and a diagnosis of a disease with abnormal levels of synuclein protein (a type of protein in the brain), such as *Parkinson's disease* or *Lewy body disease.*

- The behaviors cause much distress or interfere with social life, work, or other major daily functions.

The problem is not due to the effects of a substance such as drugs or medication. It is not due to another mental disorder or medical condition. Special regard is given to how often symptoms occur, the potential for harm, and the degree of distress in other household members.

### Risk Factors

REM sleep behavior disorder is often a side effect of many antidepressant medications and beta-blockers commonly prescribed to treat high blood pressure.

# Other Sleep-Wake Disorders

These other sleep-wake disorders also cause distress and disrupt social, work, or other major daily functions. They require treatment and are discussed briefly below: *hypersomnolence disorder, circadian rhythm sleep-wake disorders,* and *restless legs syndrome.*

## Hypersomnolence Disorder

*Hypersomnolence* is a condition that causes people to sleep for long periods during the day or night. Most people with the condition sleep about 9.5 hours each night but do not feel refreshed or energized when they awake. About 5% to 10% of people who complain of being sleepy during the day and get examined at a sleep clinic are later diagnosed with *hypersomnolence disorder*. The same treatments for *narcolepsy* also improve symptoms of this disorder.

The condition is diagnosed when:

- Extreme sleepiness occurs with 7 or more hours of sleep, with at least one of the following symptoms:
  - Frequent periods of sleep or sleep attacks within the same day.
  - Sleeping for more than 9 hours per day without feeling refreshed.
  - Trouble fully waking up.
- The problem happens at least three times per week for at least 3 months.

The problem is not due to the effects of drugs or medication. It is not due to another sleep disorder, mental disorder, or medical condition, although these can also be present. Hypersomnolence disorder may require a special evaluation, and a number of medical disorders may need to be ruled out as the cause.

# Circadian Rhythm Sleep-Wake Disorders

*Circadian rhythm sleep-wake disorders* occur with changes to the normal sleep-wake routine, such as with shift work. *Circadian rhythm* is a 24-hour cycle often referred to as the "body clock." This internal body clock is affected by factors such as sunrise and time zones. When the body's circadian rhythm is disrupted (for instance, by jet lag), sleeping patterns can be affected. Treatment involves resetting the sleep-wake schedule by fixing environmental cues and the use of light therapy. Behavior approaches also help (see the box at the end of this chapter).

These disorders are diagnosed when:

- A constant or frequent pattern of disturbed sleep occurs when a person's normal sleep-wake schedule is changed.
- The disturbed sleep leads to extreme sleepiness, insomnia, or both.

# Restless Legs Syndrome

*Restless legs syndrome* causes uncomfortable feelings in the legs, often in the evenings, while sitting or lying down. It makes people feel like getting up and moving around, which eases the discomfort. The uncomfortable feelings are often described as creeping, crawling, tingling, or burning. As with the other sleep disorders, this condition can interrupt the sleep of the person's bed partner. The treatment for restless legs syndrome involves medications. These include benzodiazepines and medicines that increase levels of dopamine (a chemical in the brain)—for instance, pramipexole.

The condition is diagnosed when:

- A person has an urge to move the legs in response to uncomfortable sensations, characterized by all of the following happening at least three times a week for at least 3 months:
  - The urge to move the legs begins or worsens during periods of rest or inactivity.
  - The urge to move the legs is partly or totally relieved by movement.
  - The urge to move the legs is worse at night or only happens at night.

The problem is not due to the effects of a substance such as drugs or medication. It is not due to another mental disorder or medical condition, such as arthritis or leg swelling.

While many factors can disrupt sleep, these steps can help provide a better night's rest:

- **Make your bedroom comfortable.** Have a quiet setting that is dark and cool and a bed with cozy bedding and pillows. Remove the distractions of computers, televisions, and electronic devices. Use the bed for sleeping and sex only. Paying bills or going over work issues will link sleep with stress.
- **Get regular exercise.** Brisk exercise, such as cycling or swimming, at least three times a week is best. Any form of exercise can help as long as it does not occur close to sleep time.
- **Maintain sleep times.** Get as much sleep as you need, not too much or too little.
- **Limit worry.** Schedule a regular worry time earlier in the day to think about issues in your life. Write down concerns and possible solutions so they don't prevent you from sleeping.
- **Set a routine.** Stick to a regular pattern of sleep and wake hours—wake up and go to bed every day at the same time and avoid daytime naps even on weekends.
- **Stay away from stimulants.** Cut off substances such as caffeine, nicotine, and alcohol, at least a few hours before bedtime.
- **Find a relaxing bedtime routine.** A regular ritual of a warm bath or listening to soft music can mentally prepare the body and mind for sleep.
- **Create a soothing sleep environment.** Keep the lights turned down. Use earplugs or a sound machine that produces soothing sounds.

## Key Points

- *Sleep-wake disorders* disrupt the quality, timing, and amount of sleep. These disorders can cause a wide range of physical and emotional problems, such as fatigue, depression, concentration problems, irritability, and obesity. On any given night, one in three people has a problem falling or staying asleep.
- Certain medical conditions and medications are known to affect sleep. To diagnose sleep problems, the doctor will review medical history and use of medications.
- People with sleep problems should keep a sleep log to track the following items for their doctor: bedtime, amount of time (best guess) before they fall asleep, wake time(s), number of awakenings, daytime naps, and any use of drugs or medications. The person's bed partner may be able to describe the person's snoring, breathing difficulties, leg jerks, or other body movements that might help diagnose a sleep disorder.
- If the sleep disorder is severe or greatly impairs home and work function, getting a sleep study at a sleep disorders clinic is needed.

Several tests can help identify the problem, but the most common is polysomnography. This test traces electrical activity in the brain and eye muscles during sleep, as well as other major body functions.

- Seeking a diagnosis and treatment, changing sleep habits and settings if needed, and making lifestyle changes can greatly improve sleep. The following tips can help: make your bedroom comfortable and use it only for sleep and sex; get regular exercise as long as it does not occur close to sleep time; limit worry; stick to a regular pattern of sleep and wake hours; stay away from caffeine, nicotine, and alcohol at least a few hours before bedtime; find a relaxing bedtime routine; and create a soothing sleep environment.

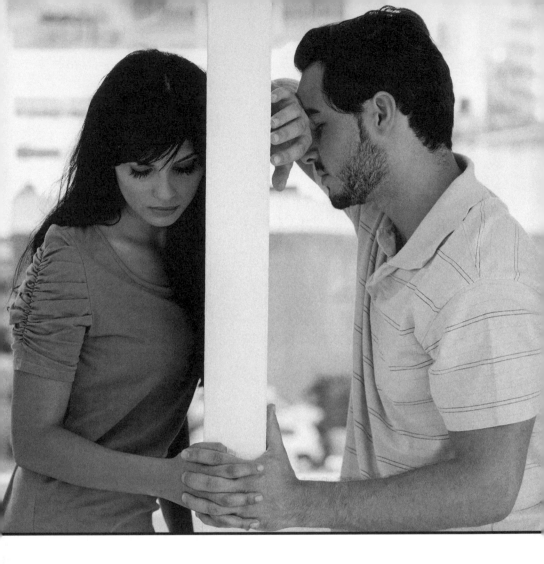

Substance/Medication-Induced Sexual Dysfunction
Erectile Disorder
Premature (Early) Ejaculation
Female Orgasmic Disorder
Other Sexual Dysfunctions
    Delayed Ejaculation
    Genito-Pelvic Pain/Penetration Disorder
    Female Sexual Interest/Arousal Disorder
    Male Hypoactive Sexual Desire Disorder

*For a complete list of DSM-5 disorders, see Appendix A.*

# CHAPTER 13

# Sexual Dysfunctions

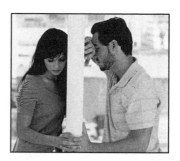

The complete giving of oneself to another person touches the essence of what it means to be human. For this reason, of all our contact with others, sexual intimacy can be the most rewarding. Although it can provide intense joy, it also can produce distress.

*Sexual dysfunctions* disrupt the ability to respond to sexual activity or to enjoy sex. Sexual dysfunctions occur across a range of sexual response stages (see box). Learning the reasons for the problem is key to how these disorders are diagnosed and treated. For instance, aging brings a normal decrease in sexual response. Because the sexual response involves the body, mind, and emotions, quite often more than one factor is involved:

- *Partner factors,* such as a partner's sexual or health problems, lack of desire.
- *Relationship factors,* such as not talking openly about feelings, likes, and dislikes; not feeling close; having levels of desire that differ.
- *Individual factors,* such as aging, poor body image, low self-esteem, inhibitions with sexual activity, past sexual or emotional abuse.
- *Cultural or religious factors,* such as laws or rules against sexual activity or pleasure.
- *Medical factors,* such as injury, diabetes, thyroid problems, and heart disease.

Four stages of human sexual response help describe sexual function:
- **Desire** is the key factor that begins sexual response.
- **Sexual excitement** causes biological changes in the man (erection) and woman (vaginal lubrication).
- **Orgasm** produces ejaculation in men and vaginal contractions in women.
- **Resolution** involves a state of well-being and relaxing as sexual organs return to their normal, nonexcited state.

It is normal for sexual problems to occur from time to time, and a diagnosis of a sexual dysfunction involves problems that last for at least 6 months (except for substance/medication-induced sexual dysfunction, which can occur shortly after a drug, alcohol, or medication is taken). Sexual dysfunctions include the following: *substance/medication-induced sexual dysfunction, erectile disorder, premature (early) ejaculation, female orgasmic disorder, delayed ejaculation, genito-pelvic pain/penetration disorder, female sexual interest/arousal disorder,* and *male hypoactive sexual desire disorder.* They can be mild, moderate, or severe, and are described based on when they begin or occur:

- *Lifelong* sexual problems are present since the first sexual experience.
- *Acquired* problems begin after a time of normal sexual activity.
- *Generalized* problems occur with any partner or sexual act.
- *Situational* problems occur with only certain types of stimulation, situations, or partners.

# Substance/Medication-Induced Sexual Dysfunction

Sexual problems can occur from using certain kinds of substances, such as alcohol, opioids (narcotic painkillers such as codeine and oxycodone), sedatives or hypnotics (sleep medications), amphetamines, cocaine, and other stimulants. Some medications that can cause sexual problems include antidepressants, antipsychotics, estrogens, steroids, and medications for heart, stomach, and high blood pressure problems. Sexual problems can occur when people start or stop taking a medication or substance or when their dosage is increased.

People who use drugs often have problems with sexual desire, keeping erections, and reaching orgasm. About 60% to 70% of heroin users have these problems, but the numbers are lower for those who abuse amphetamines or cocaine. Men who drink and smoke on a frequent basis often have trouble getting or keeping an erection.

Sexual problems caused by antidepressants can start as early as 8 days after the first dose. The most common problems relate to reaching orgasm in women and keeping an erection or ejaculating in men. Some people who take antidepressants also have loss of sexual desire. The side effects vary based on the agent. People taking monoamine oxidase inhibitors, tricyclic antidepressants, and selective serotonin reuptake inhibitors (SSRIs) more often have sexual side effects. Certain antidepressants such as bupropion and mirtazapine are less likely to cause these problems.

About one-half of the people taking antipsychotic medications have sexual side effects. These include problems with sexual desire, erection, dryness (in women), ejaculation, or having orgasm.

## Substance/Medication-Induced Sexual Dysfunction

The condition is diagnosed when there is:

- A major problem in sexual function.
- Based on the person's history, lab tests, and physical exam:
  - The problem began during or soon after starting or stopping the use of a medication.
  - The medication or substance can cause sexual problems.
- Great distress about the problem.

A substance/medication-induced sexual dysfunction is *not* diagnosed when the sexual dysfunction was present before the substance or medication use began or if it lasts more than 1 month after the person stops using the substance or medication.

## Daniel's Story

Daniel, a 55-year-old married accountant, saw a doctor for a second opinion about his ongoing *major depression*. He had not improved after trying two antidepressants (fluoxetine and then sertraline) at high doses for 3 months. He had not taken medications for about a month after the sertraline did not work.

Daniel was severely depressed, with poor concentration, early morning waking, decreased sex drive, and loss of interest in normal activities. He said that he didn't abuse any substance, drank little, and did not smoke. He had started taking propranolol for high blood pressure about 6 months before.

Daniel was treated with the antidepressant clomipramine and anti-anxiety medication buspirone. After 5 weeks, he said he felt much better. He was sleeping and eating well and taking part in activities with greater enthusiasm. For the first time in many months, he felt a return of his sexual interest.

After not having sexual intercourse in months, Daniel tried to have sex several times. He was distressed to find that for the first time in his life, he could not keep an erection during intercourse. He could not ejaculate during masturbation. These problems lasted for a month. He recalled having had slightly delayed ejaculation while taking fluoxetine. He did not recall sexual problems while using sertraline.

Daniel was diagnosed with *medication-induced sexual dysfunction* and *depression*. His erection and ejaculation problems appear to have begun directly after starting clomipramine. The antidepressant is known to cause problems with sexual function, most often erectile dysfunction. Clomipramine's sexual side effects also include delayed or inhibited ejaculation.

If clomipramine caused the problem, then Daniel's sexual dysfunction is a medication-induced sexual dysfunction. The sexual dysfunction started with a new medication or a change in dosage of a medication.

Certain medical illnesses (such as diabetes and heart disease) also are linked with sexual problems. Daniel was diagnosed with high blood pressure and started taking propranolol 6 months before starting clomipramine. Both the high blood pressure and the medication for it can impair sexual function. Daniel did not report sexual dysfunction until after he started taking the clomipramine, months after starting the propranolol. This self-report would seem to rule out both high blood pressure and propranolol as the cause for the sexual problems. It is also possible that Daniel's depression led to sexual inactivity so that the sexual dysfunction simply went unnoticed. However, the most likely culprit for his sexual dysfunction remains the clomipramine, the same medication that has greatly improved the quality of his life.

## Treatment

The first approach to treating substance/medication-induced sexual dysfunction is to know which substance or medication is causing the problem and to see whether it can be stopped. In some cases, the condition being treated also may cause the problem. Checking first with the doctor is key. The dosage for some medications must be slowly reduced to avoid adverse effects or health problems. The doctor can then suggest other medication that can replace the agent causing the problem and provide guidance on switching and starting new medications. SSRI antidepressants often can be replaced with bupropion, which is a different kind of antidepressant. Other medications that do not cause sexual side effects are often available, and a doctor can help based on each person's needs and diagnosis. Alcohol, heroin, and cocaine are some drugs that can cause sexual dysfunctions. If a drug of abuse is involved, learning about the problems caused by the drug and treatment for substance abuse are needed.

# Erectile Disorder

*Erectile disorder* (impotence) involves a man's repeated failure to get or keep an erection during sex with his partner. As many as 20%–40% of men may have an erectile disorder at some point in their lives. Many men with the condition have low self-esteem and low confidence that may lead them to fear or avoid sexual encounters.

Erectile disorder can be *lifelong/acquired* and *generalized/situational*. Lifelong erectile disorder is rare and affects about 1% of men under age 35. Acquired erectile disorder is often caused by many factors, such as diabetes and heart disease, as well as alcohol, smoking, and a number of prescribed medications. Most men with the disorder have the acquired form. Generalized erectile disorder occurs with all types of stimulation, in any setting, and with all partners. Situational erectile disorder only occurs with certain types of stimulation, settings, or partners. Symptoms of erectile disorder increase as a man ages—often after age 50. About 13% to 21% of men between ages 40–80 have occasional problems with erections, and 75% of men over age 80 are impotent.

Erectile disorder occurs in men with other sexual disorders, such as *premature (early) ejaculation,* as well as *anxiety* and *depressive disorders*. It is also common in men with urinary tract problems related to an enlarged prostate gland. Impotence also may reflect problems with the man's partner or occur after a stressful event, such as divorce or the death of a loved one.

---

 **Erectile Disorder**

The disorder is diagnosed when:

- At least one of the following symptoms happens almost every time (at least 75% of the time) during sexual activity:
  - Problems getting an erection during sexual acts.
  - Problems keeping an erection until a sexual act is finished.
  - Erections are much less rigid or hard than in the past.
- Symptoms have lasted for at least 6 months.

The symptoms cause the man much distress. They are not due to a nonsexual mental disorder, stress in the relationship or in other areas of life, another medical condition, or drug, alcohol, or medication use.

---

## Risk Factors

Erectile problems may be more common in men with *depressive disorders, posttraumatic stress disorder,* and diabetes. Smoking, older age, heart disease, and lack of exercise each increase risk. Stress and anxiety also can play a part in erectile problems.

## Treatment

Treatment of erectile disorder should involve a mental health care provider experienced in treating sexual and relationship problems. Therapy focuses on reducing anxiety by taking the focus off intercourse. Couples are taught how to give sexual pleasure without having intercourse. Without the pressure to have an erection, a man often is soon able to have an erection and have intercourse. Brief one-on-one psychotherapy ("talk therapy") and lifestyle changes (see box at end of this chapter) also may help.

Men with erectile disorder may be prescribed medication that helps cause an erection by increasing blood flow to the penis: avanafil, sildenafil, vardenafil, or tadalafil. In some cases, men may benefit from the use of penile implants or vacuum pumps.

Over-the-counter tonics, potions, and gadgets do not work. They are untested in terms of their effects on the body (such as possible harm), side effects, and interactions with other medications.

# Premature (Early) Ejaculation

Men with *premature (early) ejaculation* ejaculate before or within 1 minute after vaginal penetration and before the man wishes it. Those with the disorder often feel a sense of lack of control over ejaculation and concern about being able to delay ejaculation in future attempts.

More than 20%–30% of men ages 18–70 around the world report a concern for ejaculating too quickly. About one-third of men who seek help for sexual dysfunction report premature ejaculation. The disorder affects about 1%–3% of men. The guideline of ejaculation in 1 minute or less may apply to men of all sexual orientations.

---

 **Premature (Early) Ejaculation**

The condition is diagnosed when:

- Ejaculation happens during sexual activity with a partner within about 1 minute after vaginal penetration or before the person wishes it.

- The problem has occurred for at least 6 months and happens during almost all sexual activity (75%–100% of the time).

The symptoms cause the man much distress. They are not due to a non-sexual mental disorder, stress in the relationship or in other areas of life, another medical condition, or drug, alcohol, or medication use.

## Risk Factors

Factors that may increase risk for premature ejaculation include the following:

- **Temperament.** Premature ejaculation is more common in men with anxiety disorders, especially *social anxiety disorder (social phobia)*.
- **Genetics and biology.** Lifelong premature ejaculation may be inherited. Acquired premature ejaculation can occur with thyroid disease or drug withdrawal.

## Treatment

Treatment of premature ejaculation often is highly successful. It includes medications or behavior therapy techniques. The use of medications has been most studied and found helpful. Behavior therapy techniques are popular methods of treatment.

Men may be prescribed an SSRI antidepressant (fluoxetine, paroxetine, or sertraline) or the antidepressant clomipramine. A common side effect of these medications is delayed ejaculation. The dosage prescribed often does not cause any other side effects. For the SSRIs, the doctor should ensure that the man does not have certain prostate or thyroid problems. Another option is a topical anesthetic cream that contains lidocaine. It lessens sensation to the penis and helps delay ejaculation. Because this may also decrease sensation for the man's partner, oral medications often are preferred.

In behavior training, a partner stimulates the man until he signals that ejaculation is near. The partner stops stimulation and then restarts once the man's level of arousal is lowered. Over time, the man gains greater control over ejaculation. Another popular method is the "squeeze technique," in which a man's partner is instructed to squeeze the end of the man's penis for several seconds when he feels the urge to ejaculate, until the urge passes. With practice, the man learns how to delay ejaculation.

# Female Orgasmic Disorder

Women who have *female orgasmic disorder* have trouble reaching orgasm after sexual arousal and stimulation. Women with the disorder also may have problems with sexual interest or arousal. The disorder can be linked to physical causes, such as medications or surgery, or psychological stress, such as marital or family conflict.

About 10%–42% of women report problems with having an orgasm, varying across age, culture, and how long the problem has lasted. These numbers do not reflect whether there is distress due to the problem, however. A women's first time having an orgasm can happen anytime from before puberty until well into adult years. About 10% of women never have an orgasm in their lifetimes.

---

 **Female Orgasmic Disorder**

The condition is diagnosed when:

- One of the following symptoms happens almost all the time during sexual activity (75% to 100% of the time):
  - Delayed, infrequent, or no orgasm.
  - Reduced orgasmic sensations.
- Symptoms have lasted for at least 6 months.

These symptoms cause the woman much distress. They are not due to a nonsexual mental disorder, severe stress in the relationship (such as partner violence), another medical condition, or drug, alcohol, or medication use.

---

## Risk Factors

These factors can increase a woman's risk for female orgasmic disorder:

- **Temperament.** A wide range of emotional factors, such as worry or marital stress, can disrupt a woman's ability to have orgasm.
- **Environment.** Problems with relationships, physical health, and mental health are strongly linked to orgasm problems in women. Cultural beliefs about strict gender roles and religious laws against sexual pleasure or activity also play a role.
- **Genetics and biology.** Medical conditions and medications can cause women's orgasm problems. Medical conditions include multiple sclerosis, pelvic nerve damage, and spinal cord injury. Medications such as the selective serotonin reuptake inhibitors (SSRIs) can delay or prevent orgasm.

## Treatment

Treating female orgasmic disorder may include training a woman how to have an orgasm through masturbation. Other methods include *sen-*

*sate focus* (a method of touching skin, being aware of what is pleasing, and not touching sex organs or genitals until later sessions), clitoral stimulation, and Kegel exercises (these involve tightening and relaxing the muscles around the vagina). Once women have orgasm through self-stimulation, they can teach their partners the most pleasurable ways to stimulate them. Therapy also involves teaching the couple exercises to improve intimacy and communication.

# Other Sexual Dysfunctions

These sexual dysfunctions also cause much distress to the man or woman with the disorder. Symptoms for all of these disorders must last for at least 6 months for a diagnosis. They are not due to severe stress in the relationship (this includes partner violence) or drug or alcohol use. These other disorders are *delayed ejaculation, genito-pelvic pain/penetration disorder, female sexual interest/arousal disorder,* and *male hypoactive sexual desire disorder.* The mental health care provider should ensure that no medications, other mental disorders, or other medical conditions are causing the symptoms.

## Delayed Ejaculation

*Delayed ejaculation* occurs when a man takes a long time to reach sexual climax and ejaculate during sex with his partner. Some men are unable to ejaculate at all, despite a desire to do so.

There is no exact definition of *delayed* and what is a reasonable time for a man to reach climax. Men and their partners may report prolonged thrusting to achieve orgasm, to the point of fatigue or pain, at which point they cease their effort. Some partners may report feeling less sexually attractive because their partner cannot easily ejaculate. Men older than age 50 are at increased risk because of changes due to aging. The condition is diagnosed when a man experiences one of the following during almost every sexual encounter with his partner:

- Long delay in ejaculation.
- No or rare ejaculation.

Treatment can include meditation, relaxation, and psychotherapy ("talk therapy"). Cognitive-behavior therapy may include asking the man to refrain for a time from all sexual acts leading to orgasm. Sexual exercises with a partner that involve masturbation or vibrators may be used.

## Genito-Pelvic Pain/Penetration Disorder

Women with *genito-pelvic pain/penetration disorder* have pain with sexual intercourse or at other times of vaginal penetration, such as during a gynecology exam or when inserting a tampon. The intense pain is often described as "burning," "cutting," "shooting," or "throbbing."

Women who have this type of pain often become fearful of intercourse or penetration. They may begin to avoid sexual or intimate acts. Although the number of women who have genito-pelvic pain/penetration disorder is unknown, about 15% of U.S. women report ongoing pain during intercourse. The disorder is diagnosed when a woman has frequent problems with at least one of the following:

- Vaginal penetration during intercourse.
- Vulvovaginal or pelvic pain during vaginal intercourse or other attempts at penetration.
- Fear of vulvovaginal or pelvic pain before, during, or after penetration.
- Tensing or tightening of the pelvic muscles during attempts at vaginal penetration.

Treatment options include cognitive-behavior therapy (group or one-on-one) and sex therapy (such as sex education, sensate focus, and Kegel exercises that strengthen the pelvic floor). Physical therapies to help dilate the vagina also may be helpful. Surgery to remove sensitive tissue causing painful intercourse has been used with success. Treatment should be tailored to the woman and involve health care providers across different fields (such as mental health and gynecology).

## Female Sexual Interest/Arousal Disorder

Women with *female sexual interest/arousal disorder* have low or absent desire for sex for 6 months or more. Having a level of desire lower than a partner's is not enough for diagnosis. Rather, it is the woman's own distress about the problem that prompts the diagnosis. Short-term changes in arousal or interest because of life events are common and do not represent a dysfunction.

Women with the disorder may no longer get pleasure during sex. They often will describe themselves as feeling numb. Causes may include sexual trauma, fear of pregnancy, performance anxiety, body image problems, and marital discord. Diabetes and thyroid problems may increase risk. The disorder is diagnosed when a woman has low or no interest in sexual activity as shown by at least three of the following:

- No or low interest in sexual activity.
- No or few sexual thoughts or fantasies.
- Stops or reduces initiating sexual activity and often is not open to a partner's attempts to start.
- No or low sexual excitement or pleasure during almost all sexual activity.
- No or low interest in sex in response to any sexual cues (such as written, verbal, visual).
- No or low genital or other body sensations during almost all sexual activity.

Treatment includes a number of options, which can be combined. Although this is a new disorder, problems with desire and arousal have been treated in the past with the following methods: Sex therapy includes sex education, sensate focus, and stopping intercourse for a time. Couples therapy may be helpful to build emotional connection between the couple and address any discord. Cognitive-behavior therapy has proved useful to address any thoughts that are not helpful or true that the woman may have about herself and sex. It has been shown to increase women's sexual pleasure and satisfaction.

## Male Hypoactive Sexual Desire Disorder

*Male hypoactive sexual desire disorder* occurs when a man lacks any interest in sexual fantasies or acts for 6 months or more. Having a level of desire lower than a partner's is not enough for diagnosis. How long the symptoms have lasted is key to the diagnosis. Some men may have low desire in response to short-term life events (such as concern about a partner's pregnancy when thinking of ending the relationship).

Risk factors include mood and anxiety symptoms, alcohol use, and early trauma. About 6% of men ages 18–24 and about 40% of men ages 66–74 have problems with sexual desire. The disorder is diagnosed when a man has low or no interest in or desire for sexual activity for at least 6 months.

Treatment includes one-on-one psychotherapy or couples therapy based on the nature of the problem. If testosterone is below normal levels, testosterone replacement therapy with a daily patch or gel may be prescribed, with careful evaluation and education about side effects. Oral testosterone should not be used because of the risk for liver damage. Weight loss (if needed) and changing sexual activities to increase levels of desire also may help.

## Key Points

- Sexual intimacy involves the whole person and can bring great joy. *Sexual dysfunctions* disrupt the ability to respond to sexual activity or to enjoy sex.
- These problems occur for many reasons, which can impact how the disorder is diagnosed and treated. Quite often, more than one factor causes a sexual dysfunction. These include health problems, medications, poor body image or low self-esteem, and relationship issues (such as lack of trust or communication).
- Treatment for sexual dysfunctions takes into account all the factors that can cause these problems and that are unique to each person and his or her partner. There may be medications that can be taken or changed, medical conditions to be treated, techniques to learn, and behaviors to help build trust and communication.
- Drugs, alcohol, and tobacco can impair sexual response. Alcohol is a depressant that can blunt response to sex. Smoking slows blood flow to the sexual organs, which decreases sexual arousal. Quitting or cutting back on these substances can improve sex.
- Others ways to improve sexual health include getting regular exercise (boosts stamina, mood, and self-esteem), coping with stress (so it won't distract from sex), and sharing feelings and preferences (to build closeness and learn what pleases the other).

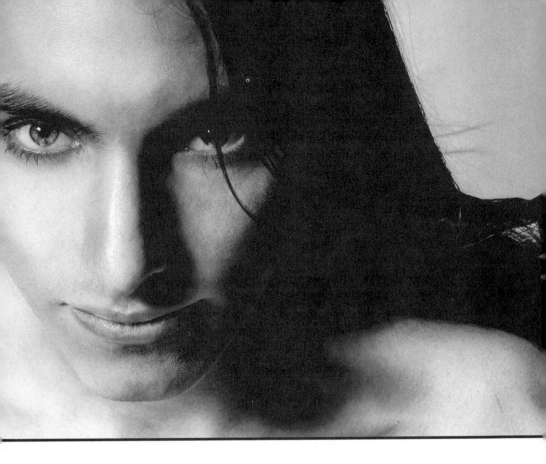

Gender Dysphoria in Children

Gender Dysphoria in Teens and Adults

*For a complete list of DSM-5 disorders, see Appendix A.*

# CHAPTER 14

# Gender Dysphoria

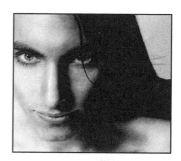

For many people, their gender is never something to question or a source of conflict for their sense of identity. Other people strongly identify themselves as a member of the opposite sex. They have great distress that their physical gender does not match the way they think and feel about themselves. This distress and sense of conflict is described as *gender dysphoria.* The gender that fits with the way they feel is called their *experienced/expressed gender,* and the gender they were born with is called their *assigned/natal gender.*

Gender dysphoria may start in childhood or may start later in the teen or adult years. Symptoms differ by age groups. The dysphoria or distress does not always persist over time, but often the feelings of the mismatch between assigned and experienced gender do last to some degree.

In children, the disorder is defined by the presence of firm statements that they are the opposite sex or desire to be. Their behavior also seems to reflect that wish. The behavior tends to start between ages 2–4 years—the age that children begin to have gender-specific behaviors and interests.

- Young girls may say they wish to be a boy and prefer boys' clothing and hairstyles, boy playmates, and rough-and-tumble play and sports. Many girls who show these signs are labeled "tomboys" at this age. Such behaviors are very common and are not always gender dysphoria. To have a diagnosis of gender dysphoria, the girl must have the firm thought that she is truly a boy and will become upset when told that she must behave as a girl.

- Young boys may wish to be a girl, prefer dressing in girls' clothing, and engage in playing house and playing with dolls. They often avoid rough play and sports. Some boys may pretend not to have a penis and insist on sitting down to urinate. These behaviors are fairly common in boys and do not always mean that the child has gender dysphoria.

In teens and adults, their distress is based more on the conflict between their expressed gender and their assigned gender. Teens and adults may be more upset by their primary and secondary sex features (see box).

- When puberty brings body changes, girls with gender dysphoria may wear baggy clothing or bind their breasts to hide them. Boys may shave their body hair at the first sign of hair growth. These behaviors relieve their distress, which improves when their looks match the way that they feel.
- Adults with gender dysphoria may want to get rid of the sex features of their physical gender and adopt the behavior, clothing, and manners of the opposite sex. They may try to reduce their symptoms of dysphoria by living in the role of their experienced gender as much as possible in their work, looks, and social lives.

It is common for children who have gender dysphoria to also have emotional and behavioral problems—mostly depression, anxiety, and disruptive and impulse-control problems. As children become teens, teasing or conflicts with their peers may increase and lead to more problems. Teens and adults are at increased risk to have *anxiety* and *depressive disorders.*

---

### Sex Features: Growth Brings Changes

People with gender dysphoria may be distressed by one or both types of sex features as they grow from children to adults:
- **Primary sex features** are organs for reproduction present at birth (such as a uterus or penis).
- **Secondary sex features** appear in puberty (such as body hair or breasts).

---

**Gender Dysphoria**

This disorder is diagnosed when the following symptoms have occurred for at least 6 months.

## Gender Dysphoria in Children

- A clear mismatch between one's expressed gender and assigned gender as shown by the first trait on the list and at least five more of the following:
    - Strong desire to be, or insistence that one is, the other gender.
    - In boys, a strong preference for cross-dressing in women's clothing. In girls, a strong preference for wearing only masculine clothing and strong resistance to wearing anything that is feminine.
    - Strong preference for cross-gender roles in make-believe or fantasy play.
    - Strong preference for toys, games, or activities that are often used or done by the other gender.
    - Strong preference for playmates of the other gender.
    - In boys, a strong rejection of masculine toys or games and avoidance of rough-and-tumble play. In girls, a strong rejection of feminine toys, games, or activities.
    - Strong dislike of one's sexual anatomy.
    - Strong desire for the primary sex features (sex organs) and/or secondary sex features (breasts, facial hair) to match one's experienced gender.
- The condition causes much distress and impairs social, school, or other key aspects of function.

## Gender Dysphoria in Teens and Adults

- A clear mismatch between one's expressed gender and assigned gender as shown by at least two of the following:
    - A clear mismatch between one's expressed gender and primary or secondary sex features.
    - Strong desire to be rid of one's primary and/or secondary sex features because of a strong disagreement with one's expressed gender.
    - Strong desire for the primary and/or secondary sex features of the other gender.
    - Strong desire to be the other gender.

- Strong desire to be treated as the other gender.
- Strong conviction that one has the typical feelings and reactions of the other gender.
- The condition causes much distress and impairs social, work, or other key aspects of function.

# Risk Factors

The following factors are believed to play a role in gender dysphoria:

- **Temperament.** Those who behave out of character for their gender at early preschool age may be more likely to develop gender dysphoria.
- **Environment.** Males with gender dysphoria are more likely to have older brothers. Men who develop gender dysphoria in teenage or adult years often have a history of sexual arousal with fantasies of being a woman.
- **Genetics.** Gender dysphoria with a disorder of sexual development (a rare condition that appears at birth when the infant's gender is unclear) is linked to a genetic abnormality.

### Christine's Story

Christopher, a 52-year-old salesperson, has begun a legal process to change her gender to female. Her new name is Christine.

Christopher had been born with male genitals and was raised as a boy. Nothing unusual was noted by Christopher's parents until childhood, at which point Christopher was viewed as a "sissy" by other children. Christopher sought out female friends in school and chose activities and clubs that mainly involved girls. He did not wish to play contact sports, much to the dismay of his father. Christopher did well in tennis and competed in the sport to please his father.

Christopher began to sense that his feelings and thoughts were those of a girl's. He felt he was "Christine" instead of "Christopher." He knew his strict father would never accept such an idea, so he never spoke about it.

Christopher did well in college and became very fond of a longtime girlfriend. Although he did not feel sexually drawn to her, he wanted very much to please his father, so he married her after college. He was fairly content with his married life, but he knew he was living mostly to please his family. The way he was living never matched the way he felt inside. He felt much more at ease when he could think of himself as Christine. When his wife was not at home, he would often wear her clothing.

Over years of marriage, Christopher felt more unhappy and upset with himself that he was not being honest with his own life goals or honest with his wife and family. He sought treatment from a mental health care provider. After he talked about his life at length, he began to talk about his sense that he is "Christine" and his fears of letting down his family. As "Christine," he began to share more private feelings in therapy. He became more secure in describing himself as a woman and began to ask some of his closest friends to refer to him as "she."

Over time, she (Christine) began to realize that she was not going to have the quality of life that she wanted unless she began to live openly as a woman. Over the next several months, she worked with her mental health care provider to gain courage to tell her wife that she wanted to separate. She also sought a referral with a specialist who could inform her about hormone treatments and surgeries. She might someday explore these options if she wanted to change her physical appearance to a female, but she knew this would be a big decision. The first step would be to learn how to discuss her condition with all of her family and friends and decide how to begin changing her life to match the female role. She sought out a specialist who works with people who have *gender dysphoria* to help with this process, as she knew that it would be a very hard transition for her wife. Christine's father also would have trouble accepting the diagnosis and why it was crucial to Christine to be able to live her life as a woman.

# Treatment

Many children go through phases of behavior as they are learning their likes and dislikes. They may at times behave as "tomboys" or "sissies" as part of normal childhood growth. Often it is helpful simply to give support and encourage them to choose activities, toys, and clothes that they enjoy the most. If there are signs of ongoing distress or problems at school, such as refusing to use the restroom for their assigned gender, then it is helpful to seek out a mental health care provider who has treated others with gender dysphoria.

Gender dysphoria requires care not only for the person who has it, but also for the rest of the family to adjust and know how the child is feeling. Family and friends may have a hard time accepting what is happening and what it means to have this condition. Family education can prevent other behavior and emotional problems in the child, such as anxiety.

Treatment also may vary based on how the person handles the dysphoria symptoms. Treatment options differ when the gender dysphoria lasts into adult years. Some people can do well if they can live in relationships that respect their expressed gender and if they can purse activities and lifestyles that feel natural to them. Other people with gender dysphoria will choose to have *sex reassignment surgery*—major surgery that changes their bodies so that their physical sex matches their experienced gender. This may involve breast implants or removing the penis and creating an artificial vagina. In the United States, people wishing to have sex reassignment surgery are asked to live as a member of the opposite sex for more than 1 year before the medical team proceeds with the surgery. When people change their appearance and begin living fully in the role of the opposite sex, this is called being *transsexual*. Someone can live as a transsexual whether or not sex reassignment surgery is chosen.

For a change from male to female, hormones are first prescribed to help alter appearance. Female hormones given to a male cause the breasts to enlarge and other changes in the body to create a female appearance. After the person has adjusted to the hormones, surgery may be done to remove the male genitals. Surgery also may create an artificial vagina. Sometimes other surgeries help adjust facial features to reflect the experienced gender.

For a change from female to male, hormones may be given to increase muscle mass and deepen the voice. Surgery may remove the breasts, uterus, and ovaries. Some people will choose to have an artificial penis made through surgery. Surgery is followed by psychotherapy to help people adjust to their new gender.

Therapy also can help those who do not choose sex reassignment surgery to cope with any issues gender dysphoria may cause. Some people can feel happy with their lives and manage the gender dysphoria by living as a transsexual without having sex reassignment surgery. Some people dress and live at times as the opposite gender but never feel any distress about a mismatch in their identity. These people do not have gender dysphoria. One way to gauge whether seeking treatment is needed is the presence of great distress and frequent unhappiness. In the case of Christine, many years of suffering might have been avoided if she had been able to seek help and talk about her condition much earlier in life.

## Key Points

- People with *gender dysphoria* strongly identify as a member of the opposite sex. They have great distress that their biological gender does not match the way they think and feel about themselves.
- Gender dysphoria may start in childhood or may start later in the teen or adult years. Children may at times behave as "tomboys" or "sissies" as part of normal childhood growth without having the disorder.

- Treatment for gender dysphoria includes therapy for the family to adjust and know how the person is feeling. Family education may also reduce the risk of other mental disorders that may result from gender dysphoria, such as *anxiety* and *depressive disorders*.
- Treatment options differ when the gender dysphoria lasts into adult years. Some people with gender dysphoria will choose to have sex reassignment surgery. Whether or not sex reassignment surgery is chosen, people can change their appearance and begin living fully in the role of the opposite sex. Some people can feel happy with their lives and manage the gender dysphoria by living this way without having surgery.
- Therapy also can help someone with gender dysphoria cope with any issues the condition may cause. One way to gauge whether seeking treatment is needed is the presence of great distress and frequent unhappiness.

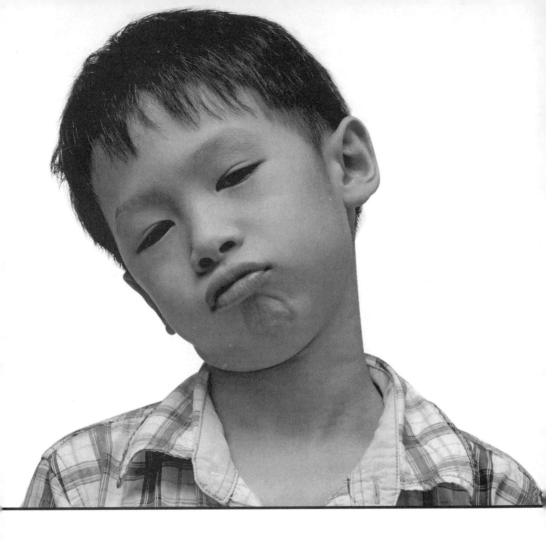

Oppositional Defiant Disorder
Intermittent Explosive Disorder
Conduct Disorder
Other Disruptive and Conduct Disorders
    Pyromania
    Kleptomania

*For a complete list of DSM-5 disorders, see Appendix A.*

CHAPTER 15

# Disruptive and Conduct Disorders

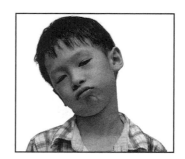

All children and teens misbehave at times. Stress may cause them to act out, such as when there is the birth of a sibling, a divorce, or a death in the family. *Disruptive and conduct disorders* are more severe problems that last a longer time than normal acting out. People with these disorders have a hard time controlling their angry feelings and may display hostile behaviors. These disorders can cause them to be aggressive toward other people or property, to break rules and laws, and to disobey or rebel against authority figures.

The disorders discussed in this chapter are *oppositional defiant disorder, intermittent explosive disorder, conduct disorder, pyromania,* and *kleptomania.* All of these disorders tend to begin in childhood or teenage years, and many are more common in boys than girls. Conduct disorder, for instance, is one of the most frequent mental disorders seen in teenage boys. Some of these disorders last into adult years or are first diagnosed then.

These conditions are often called *externalizing disorders* because the behaviors get attention and are "out there" for all to see. Distress is expressed by acting it out through angry behaviors that impact others. In contrast, people with *internalizing disorders*—such as *depressive* and *anxiety disorders*—keep distress inward and self-directed. These disorders are less likely to cause conflict with others.

Many factors can increase the risk for these disorders. These include harsh or inconsistent parenting, being neglected by parents, frequent changes in caregivers, physical or sexual abuse, lack of supervision, and parents with backgrounds in crime or addictions to drugs or alcohol. These disorders can occur with other mental disorders, such as a *depressive, bipolar,* or *substance use disorder,* or *attention-deficit/hyperactivity disorder* (ADHD).

# Treatment

Getting early treatment for these disorders will more quickly lessen distress and the impact of the problems in the child's or teen's life. The sooner treatment begins, the better the chances of improved symptoms and behavior. Treatment can be a challenge, however. Children and teens may resist therapy, not cooperate, and display fear and distrust of adults. Learning new attitudes and behavior patterns takes time and patience for all involved.

Behavior therapy and psychotherapy—either one-on-one or in a group or family setting—are needed to help children and teens express and control their anger. Therapy is aimed at helping young people be aware of their behavior and its effect on others. Parent training teaches skills to learn how best to support good behavior and relate with the child or teen. For children and teens who also have *ADHD* or a *depressive* or *bipolar disorder,* medications for these disorders may reduce the disruptive behaviors by bringing relief to some of the feelings that worsen them.

# Oppositional Defiant Disorder

Children or teens with *oppositional defiant disorder* display difficult behaviors such as tantrums, arguing, and angry or disruptive acts. On a frequent basis, they may argue with their parents, refuse to comply with adult requests or rules (such as cleaning their rooms or meeting curfews), and often are angry and resent others. These behaviors go beyond normal misbehavior when they last for at least 6 months and disrupt home and school life.

These behaviors are common among siblings and must be seen during contact with others. Symptoms often are displayed with adults or peers whom the child or teen knows well. The behaviors may not be shown during a visit with a doctor or a mental health care provider.

The symptoms of the disorder often reflect a pattern of problems in relating with others. People with this disorder tend not to see themselves as angry, oppositional (combative), or defiant. Instead, they often

- Children and teens who are combative or disruptive can be a special challenge for parents. It is normal for many younger children (ages 2–4 years) and teens to have stubborn or defiant behavior that they will out-grow. Remain calm and praise good behavior. Seek to connect with your child one-on-one.
- Misbehavior that is severe, persists, or disrupts family or school life should lead to seeking care from a mental health care provider who works with children and teens. Any behavior that harms or endangers others, such as other children or animals, requires urgent care.
- Older children and teens who misbehave need to learn that they are responsible for their own behavior and to accept the results of their actions and choices. Choose battles wisely and decide what rules are most helpful to enforce (such as rules for safety). Be steadfast to follow through on stated results.
- In some cases, parents can benefit from learning new skills to manage their child's misbehavior. Parents can promote and model healthy behavior and stand up to what is wrong.

justify their behavior as a response to unfair demands or events. The first symptoms tend to appear during the preschool years and rarely later than the early teens.

Parent management training has proved useful for oppositional defiant disorder and also may help improve *conduct disorder* symptoms. This method equips parents with behavior management techniques to improve how they respond when their child disobeys and obeys. It can help build the parent-child relationship and teaches ways to give clear instructions and results for behavior. Practice at home is key.

---

##  Oppositional Defiant Disorder

The disorder is diagnosed when the following occurs:

- There is a pattern of angry or irritable moods, arguing or defiant behavior, or spite or revenge lasting at least 6 months as shown by at least four symptoms from any of the following types. The behavior is shown during contact with at least one person who is not a sibling:

### Angry or Irritable Mood

- Often loses temper.
- Often touchy or easily annoyed.
- Often angry and resentful.

*Disruptive and Conduct Disorders*

### Arguing or Defiant Behavior

- Often argues with authority figures (or in children and teens, with adults).
- Often defies or refuses to follow the rules or requests from authority figures.
- Often annoys others on purpose.
- Often blames others for his or her own mistakes or misbehavior.

### Spite or Revenge

- Has been spiteful or sought revenge at least twice within the past 6 months.

The behavior causes distress for the person or others in his or her close daily life (such as family, peers, coworkers), or has a negative impact on social, school, work, or other key aspects of function. The behaviors are not due to any *psychotic, substance use, depressive,* or *bipolar disorder.*

# Intermittent Explosive Disorder

People with *intermittent explosive disorder* respond with quick, angry, forceful outbursts that are out of proportion to the situation—for instance, in response to a mild criticism from a loved one or friend. The outbursts often last for less than 30 minutes and can be in the form of temper tantrums, arguments, fights, or assault.

These symptoms can persist for many years. At risk are people with a history of physical and emotional trauma during the first 20 years of life. The disorder is common in people younger than age 35–40 years and in those who do not have a high school education.

Cognitive-behavior therapy is a helpful treatment for intermittent explosive disorder. It involves training in relaxation and coping skills, as well as changing thought patterns tied to anger and aggression.

Some medications also have been found to be helpful. These include the selective serotonin reuptake inhibitor (SSRI) antidepressants and mood stabilizers. (See Chapter 20, "Treatment Essentials," for more information on these medications.)

 **Intermittent Explosive Disorder**

The disorder is diagnosed when the following occurs:

- Frequent outbursts show a failure to control aggressive (angry, hostile, forceful) impulses as shown by either of the following:

- Verbal aggression (such as temper tantrums, rants, arguments) or physical aggression toward property, animals, or other people. Either occurs about twice a week for 3 months. The physical aggression does not damage property or injure others.
- Three outbursts that involve property damage, physical assault, or both. The physical assault causes physical harm to animals or other people. These acts have occurred within 1 year.
- The force of the outbursts is beyond the extent of what might have provoked the person or any stress the person has.
- The frequent aggressive outbursts are impulsive (not planned) and are not done to achieve a certain goal, such as money, power, or fear.
- The frequent aggressive outbursts cause much distress for the person, disrupt work function or relationships, or have legal or financial costs (such as arrests and fines).
- The person is at least 6 years old.

The frequent aggressive outbursts are not due to a medical condition or drug, alcohol, or medication use. Other mental disorders in which assault or aggressive behaviors are symptoms need to be ruled out. These include *bipolar disorder, psychotic disorders,* and *antisocial* or *borderline personality disorders.* A sudden behavior change along with such outbursts in someone who seems healthy may suggest a brain disorder or head trauma, which also needs to be ruled out.

---

### Sam's Story

Sam, a 32-year-old landscape architect, sought help from a mental health care provider to gain better control of his anger. His wife, who came with him to the appointment, said that Sam always had a temper. However, now he was angry so often that she worried that he would become violent with her or their two young children.

Their most recent quarrel began when Sam came home after a "hard day at work" to find that dinner was not on the table. When he entered the kitchen and saw his wife reading the paper, he exploded and launched into a rant about how "bad" a wife she was. When his wife tried to explain her own long day, Sam cursed at her and broke glasses and a kitchen chair. Frightened, Sam's wife ran out of the kitchen, gathered up their toddlers, and left for her mother's house a few miles away. The next day, she told Sam that he would need to get help right away or prepare for a divorce. She had reached the limit of what she could take.

Sam said his "blow-ups" began in childhood but did not become a problem for him until age 13. At about that time, he started having frequent fights with classmates that would at times result in visits to the principal's office. In between fights, he was a social and solid student.

Sam guessed that he had about four verbal outbursts a week in recent years, often in response to frustration, unexpected demands, or perceived insults. He also described violent acts about every 2 months. For instance, he threw a computer across the room when it started "acting up," he kicked a hole in a wall when one of his children would not stop crying, and he destroyed his mobile phone during an argument with his mother. He denied physical fights since his teens, although he came close to hitting a neighbor, a number of strangers, and the employees at his landscaping firm. His company had high turnover because of his quick temper. The idea that he might physically hurt someone scared Sam "to the core."

Sam described his angry episodes as short, reaching a peak within seconds, and rarely lasting more than a few minutes. Between episodes, he described feeling "fine." He was worried about his behavior and was sorry about his outbursts and actions toward his wife. Sam drank socially, but neither he nor his wife linked his outbursts to the alcohol.

Sam noted at least two other close family members with major "anger issues." His father was emotionally abusive and demanding, and his older sister had problems with her temper. Sam said her three divorces were caused by her emotionally abusive behavior.

Sam was diagnosed with *intermittent explosive disorder.* Treatment for Sam is a crucial issue not only for his marriage but also to stop the cycle of violence for his children.

# Conduct Disorder

*Conduct disorder* describes a pattern of frequent behavior in children or teens that involves grave and harmful breaking of rules or laws at home, school, and work. This can include using weapons, bullying, breaking into people's homes, and physical cruelty to people or animals. People with conduct disorders infringe on the rights of others. They may wrongly think others have a hostile intent against them and feel they are acting justly in response to perceived threats. They are likely to deny their behavior or downplay the degree of harm they caused.

Problems can start as early as the preschool years, but the first serious signs often appear during middle childhood through middle teenage years. For boys, the common signs are fighting, stealing, vandalism, and school discipline problems. Girls more often lie, skip school, or run away, and may become sexually active earlier than their peers. The disorder is rare after age 16.

*Antisocial personality disorder* has similar symptoms to those of conduct disorder and is diagnosed when a person is age 18 or older. The symptoms of antisocial personality disorder include deceit, hurting or mistreating others without any regret, and disregard for the rights of others (see Chapter 18, "Personality Disorders," for more detail). Conduct disorder is seen as the childhood warning sign for antisocial personality disorder—but it is vital to know that a young person with conduct disorder does not always go on to have antisocial personality disorder. Early diagnosis and treatment are key to helping learn healthy ways of thinking and acting and how to control angry feelings.

Helpful treatments for conduct disorders include parent management training (as described for *oppositional defiant disorder*) and functional family therapy (FFT). Either option lasts for about 12 weeks. FFT tackles unhealthy family beliefs about the problem, builds relationships and positive parenting skills, and helps plan use of community resources to prevent relapse.

---

 **Conduct Disorder**

Conduct disorder is diagnosed when the following occurs:

- A frequent and steady pattern of behavior that infringes on the basic rights of others or breaks social rules or laws, as shown by at least 3 of the 15 behaviors below in the past 12 months, with at least one behavior in the past 6 months:

### Aggression Toward People and Animals

- Often bullies, threatens, or intimidates others.
- Often starts physical fights.
- Has used a weapon that could cause serious physical harm to others, such as a bat, knife, brick, or gun.
- Has been physically cruel to people.
- Has been physically cruel to animals.
- Confronts and steals from a victim, such as mugging, purse snatching, armed robbery.
- Has forced someone into a sexual act.

### Destruction of Property

- Has set fires with the intent of causing great damage.
- Has destroyed other people's property on purpose.

### Deceit or Theft

- Has broken into someone's house, building, or car.
- Often lies to obtain goods or favors, or to avoid duties (cons others).
- Has stolen items without confronting a victim (such as shoplifting, but without breaking and entering).

### Serious Violations of Rules

- Often stays out at night despite parental rules against this.
- Has run away overnight at least twice from a parent's home, or once without coming back for a lengthy time.
- Often skips school, starting before age 13.

The behavior greatly impairs social, school, or work function. For the diagnosis to apply to someone age 18 years or older, the person must *not* meet the guidelines and standards for *antisocial personality disorder.* Some people with conduct disorder may show a lack of remorse or guilt for their actions, lack of concern for others' feelings, or lack of concern about their school or work duties and function. The disorder can be mild, moderate, or severe, based on the number of symptoms and degree of harm caused.

---

## Thomas's Story

Thomas was a 12-year-old boy who angrily agreed to see a mental health care provider after getting arrested for breaking into a grocery store. His mother said she was "worn out," adding that it was hard to raise a boy who "doesn't follow the rules."

As a young child, Thomas was often aggressive, bullying other children and taking their things. When confronted by his mother, stepfather, or a teacher, he would curse, punch, and show no concern for getting punished.

Thomas, his mother, and his teachers agreed that he was a loner and not well liked by his peers. There was no history of sexual or physical abuse.

The year before his arrest, Thomas had been caught stealing from school lockers (a cell phone, a jacket, a laptop computer). He also robbed a classmate of his wallet and was suspended after many physical fights with classmates. Thomas had no regret for his acts, blamed others for his stealing and fights, and did not care about others' feelings. When scolded about his behavior, he would say, "What are you going to do, shoot me?" Because of this pattern of behavior, Thomas was diagnosed with *conduct disorder.*

# Other Disruptive and Conduct Disorders

These disorders are marked by poor impulse control for certain behaviors that relieve inner tension. They include *pyromania* (fire setting) and *kleptomania* (stealing objects). These disorders are not due to *conduct disorder,* a manic episode (as in a *bipolar disorder*), a hallucination or delusion (as in a *psychotic disorder*), or *antisocial personality disorder.*

# Pyromania

*Pyromania* is the repeated setting of fires on purpose for pleasure or satisfaction. People with the disorder often have an unusual interest in or fascination with fire. They may set off false alarms, spend time at the local fire department, and often watch fires in their neighborhoods. Fire-setting behavior is more common in teenage boys, often in those with poor social skills and learning problems. Although the age that pyromania begins is unknown, more than 40% of the people arrested for arson in the United States are younger than age 18. Pyromania is diagnosed when the following occur:

- Fires are set on purpose more than once.
- Tension or excitement before the act.
- Fascination with, curiosity about, or attraction to fire.
- Pleasure, gratification, or relief when setting fires or watching their aftermath.

The fire setting is not done for financial gain, to express social or political views, to conceal a crime, to improve one's living condition, or as a result of impaired judgment.

Cognitive-behavior therapy that includes conflict- and problem-solving skills, parent education, and graphing is useful in stopping the behavior and its causes. *Graphing* involves mapping the event, feelings, and behavior on a graph with the person and family. It helps the person see the cause and effect of feelings and behaviors. It teaches the person to notice feelings and replace harmful behaviors done in response to those feelings. Fire-safety education and guided visits to burn units also have been shown to be helpful.

# Kleptomania

People with *kleptomania* do not resist their urge to steal objects that are not needed for personal use or for their monetary value. They know the act is wrong and senseless, but are not able to control the impulse. They often are afraid of getting caught stealing and may feel depressed or guilty about the thefts. Women are three times more likely to have kleptomania than men, and the disorder often begins in teenage years. Kleptomania is diagnosed when the following occur:

- Frequent failure to resist the impulse to steal objects that are not needed for personal use or that have little value.

- Increased tension right before stealing.
- Pleasure, gratification, or relief while stealing.

Treatment for kleptomania may include the medication naltrexone, which can reduce the impulse and pleasure of stealing. Psychotherapies include *exposure and response prevention therapy* (which includes practice thinking of stealing but not doing it), *covert sensitization* (which involves thinking of stealing and picturing a strong negative result, such as vomiting), and *cognitive-behavior therapy* (which involves changing thoughts that stealing will relieve distress).

## Key Points

- *Disruptive and conduct disorders* cross the line from normal misbehavior that occurs from time to time in children or teens or that is due to stressful life events. These are more severe problems in which people often do not control their angry feelings and display hostile behaviors. They may also act on impulse in ways that damage property or inflict financial cost on others.
- All of these disorders tend to begin in childhood or teenage years, and many are more common in boys. Some of these disorders last into adult years or are first diagnosed then. These disorders may reflect distress that is expressed by acting it out through angry behaviors that impact others.
- Many factors can increase the risk for these disorders. These include harsh or inconsistent parenting, neglect, frequent changes in caregivers, physical or sexual abuse, lack of supervision, parents with addictions to drugs or alcohol, and other mental disorders, such as a *depressive* or *bipolar disorder*, or *attention-deficit/hyperactivity disorder* (ADHD).
- Getting early treatment for these disorders will more quickly lessen distress and the impact of the problems in the child's or teen's life. The sooner treatment begins, the better the chances of improved symptoms.
- Behavior therapy and psychotherapy—either one-on-one or in a group—are needed to help children and teens express and control their anger. Therapy is aimed at helping young people realize and understand the effect their behavior has on others. Parent training teaches skills to learn how best to support good behavior and relate with the child or teen. For children and teens who also have depression or ADHD, medications for these disorders may reduce the disruptive behaviors by bringing relief to some of the feelings that worsen them.

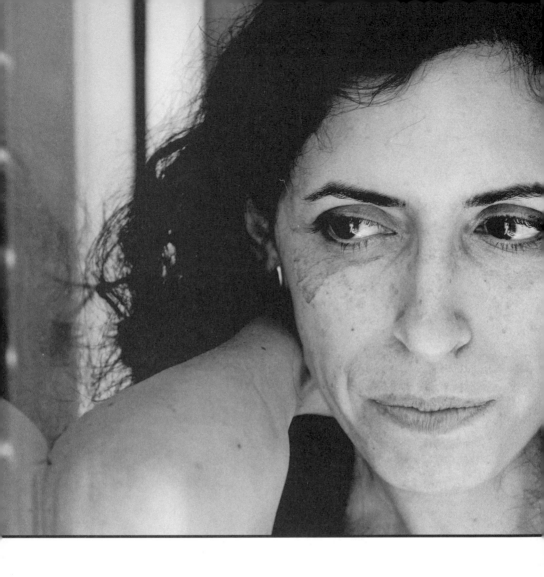

Substance Use Disorder

Substance Intoxication

Substance Withdrawal

Substance/Medication-Induced Mental Disorders

Gambling Disorder

*For a complete list of DSM-5 disorders, see Appendix A.*

# CHAPTER 16

# Addictive Disorders

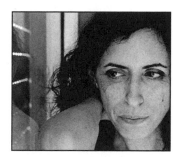

**D**rinking, other drug use, and gambling are often woven into the culture as social or fun pursuits. Alcohol, drugs, and gambling seem to quickly affect a portion of the brain called the *reward system*. This leads to intense pleasure (or a "high") and a craving to repeat that pleasure. A craving for the substance or behavior can send a message to both the brain and body that they must have the substance or these feelings of pleasure. What seemed harmless at first may become harmful. People with an *addiction* have an intense focus on using a certain substance (such as alcohol or drugs) or doing a certain activity (such as gambling) to the point that it takes over their life.

Those with *addictive disorders* spend a great deal of time and effort trying to obtain the substance to use or the money to gamble. This begins to outweigh the value of other people and duties in their lives. The addiction may cause them to have problems in their major roles (such as with their work or caring for children). Money and family problems often occur. Those with the most serious addictions sometimes break the law to satisfy their craving or urges. Some addictive drugs are illegal or obtained through illegal channels. People with the disorder may be aware of the problems caused by their addiction but cannot stop it on their own, even when they want to. The addiction causes concern and distress for those in their lives.

The addictive disorders included in this chapter are those caused by addictions to 10 different classes of substances (see Table 1). Addictive

| Table 1. Ten classes of substances | |
|---|---|
| **Substance** | **Examples** |
| Alcohol | Beer, wine |
| Caffeine | Coffee, cola |
| Cannabis (marijuana) | |
| Hallucinogens | Phencyclidine (PCP), LSD (acid), salvia |
| Inhalants (breathed in through the nose or mouth) | Paint thinners, glue, aerosol spray |
| Opioids | Heroin, painkillers such as codeine and oxycodone |
| Sedatives, hypnotics ("sleeping pills"), and anxio-lytics (medicines for anxiety, such as tranquilizers) | Barbiturates (such as Nembutal), benzodiazepines (such as Valium and Xanax), benzodiazepine hypnotics (such as Rohypnol or "roofies") |
| Stimulants | Cocaine, amphetamines ("uppers" such as methamphetamine or "meth") |
| Tobacco (nicotine) | Cigarettes |
| Other (or unknown) | Prescription medicines, over-the-counter medicines |

disorders include *substance use disorder, substance intoxication, substance withdrawal,* and *substance/medication-induced mental disorders.* For the first time, *gambling disorder* has been included in DSM as an addictive disorder (rather than as an impulse-control disorder).

The good news is that people can recover from an addiction. The first step on the road to recovery is to know there is a problem. Often this process is hindered by denial of the problem or a lack of knowledge about substance misuse and addiction. In these cases, the *intervention* of concerned friends and family can prompt treatment.

An intervention is a careful, planned meeting with the person with an addiction and his or her family, friends, and others concerned. These people gather to talk with the person about his or her addiction, express their concern, give examples of the behavior and problems that result from the addiction, outline a clear treatment plan, and state what each will do if the person will not get treatment. One person leads the planning and guides the meeting. Seeking advice and support from a mental health care provider before and after the meeting is crucial. (For more information, visit www.mayoclinic.org and search for "intervention," or see Appendix C, "Helpful Resources" for support groups that may be of help.)

People with an addiction are swept up in their behavior and cannot see as clearly as those who do not have the problem. They need people who care about them to get involved in healthy ways and be honest with them. Here are some ways to help:

- Preaching, blaming, and scolding won't help.
- Don't try to address the problem when the person is high, intoxicated, or engaged in gambling.
- Don't join in the activity or setting where the addiction occurs.
- Give feedback that is direct and focused on a certain behavior (such as, "You promised you would be there for our son's baseball game. When you didn't show up, I was worried—then upset when I learned you were at the bar drinking all night. Our son was sad you weren't there.").
- Learn as much as you can about the problem and its effects. Find resources for recovery and support in your area (see Appendix C, "Helpful Resources" for support groups). Seek help from a mental health care provider.
- Addictions cause painful problems with home, school, work, relationships, and finances—as well as brain and body effects. Pain causes those with addictions to seek help. If you remove the real result of their addiction, you remove a main reason for seeking change. Do not cover up the problem, give them money, make excuses for them, shield them from the results of their behavior, feel responsible for their addiction, or feel guilty for their behavior.
- Don't give up on showing care, concern, and emotional support. People with addictions need help to get better. Recovery is often a process without a quick fix.
- Realize that you cannot force people with addictions to stop. You can urge them to get help. Support them when they choose to get help and during the process of change.
- If the addiction impacts children, take steps to ensure that children are safe from harm and neglect.
- Seek help for yourself. Protect your finances, emotions, and health. Don't try to manage the problem of someone else's addiction on your own. Being alone can increase fear and loss of hope.

*Source.* Adapted from Missouri Department of Mental Health; National Council on Alcoholism and Drug Dependence.

# Treatment

Addiction is a life-long or chronic illness like heart disease, high cholesterol, or high blood pressure. Although people with an addiction are at risk of relapse, they can live full, healthy lives with treatment and support. *Relapse* occurs when someone has stopped use for a while and is getting back to daily life and doing well—but then resumes the addictive behavior, even just once. This return to drugs or gambling can pull the person back into the addiction. Relapse is not failure and can strengthen efforts for recovery. Learning to be aware of triggers for relapse can prevent it. Because addiction affects many aspects of a person's life, combined forms of treatment are often used. For most, a mix of medication and individual or group therapy works best.

Medications can help control drug cravings and relieve severe symptoms of *withdrawal* (how the body and brain respond when the substance or gambling is stopped or decreased). These medications include naltrexone and benzodiazepines, among for others (see Appendix B, "Medications"). Withdrawal symptoms differ for each drug and are described in the "Substance Intoxication and Withdrawal" section of this chapter.

Therapy can help those with addictions learn about their behavior and why they use the drug or gamble. It can help them learn to stop, rebuild their life without an addiction, build higher self-esteem, and cope with stress. Other treatments may be given in hospitals, outpatient programs, and community settings that provide a controlled, drug-free environment.

Self-help groups can provide support for those with an addiction. These programs often follow the 12 steps of treatment based on Alcoholics Anonymous. Sister organizations focus on those who abuse other substances (Cocaine Anonymous, Narcotics Anonymous), gambling (Gamblers Anonymous), and family members (Al-Anon, Gam-Anon, Nar-Anon Family Groups). These groups all provide a support system to those affected by addiction and help reinforce messages learned in treatment.

# Substance Use Disorder

People can develop a *substance use disorder* with any of the drugs listed in Table 1, except caffeine. (Substance use disorder with caffeine is not a current diagnosis. It is being studied further because of the many drinks and pills on the market with high caffeine content. A person can have *caffeine intoxication* or *caffeine withdrawal*, as shown in Table 2.) People with a substance use disorder have a mix of disturbed thinking, behavior, and body functions, and they keep using the substance when they know that problems will result.

These substances can cause harmful changes in how the brain functions. These changes can last well after the intoxication is over. *Intoxication* is recent use of the drug that can cause intense pleasure, calm,

## Tips to Help Recovery

The following tips have been adapted from the Web site **"Rethinking Drinking"** by the National Institute on Alcohol Abuse and Alcoholism (http://rethinkingdrinking.niaaa.nih.gov). These tips for problem drinking can apply to other addictions and can help prevent relapse once recovery has begun. The main goals are to stay in control, learn and use refusal skills, and build a new life without addiction.

- **Avoid triggers.** What triggers your urge toward your addiction? If certain people or places make you drink, use a drug, or gamble even when you don't want to, try to avoid them. If certain activities, times of day, or feelings trigger the urge, plan something else to do instead.
- **Plan to handle urges.** When you cannot avoid a trigger and an urge hits, try these options:
    - Remind yourself of your reasons for changing (it can help to carry them in writing or store them in an electronic message you can access quickly).
    - Talk things through with someone you trust.
    - Get involved with a healthy, distracting activity, such as physical exercise or a hobby that doesn't involve the addiction.
    - Instead of fighting the feeling, accept it and ride it out without giving in, knowing that it will soon crest like a wave and pass.
- **Be prepared to say "no."** You're likely to be offered a drink, a drug, or a chance to gamble at times when you don't want to or with old friends who joined you in your addiction. Have a polite, firm "no, thanks" ready. Review what might occur and script your response. The faster you can say "no" to these offers, the less likely you are to give in. If you hesitate, it allows you time to think of excuses to go along. In some cases, it may be best to avoid the setting or the people who cannot take "no" for an answer.
- **Rebuild your life without the addiction.** This may involve the following:
    - Let family and friends know about the problem and share information with them about the addiction. Enlist their support and let them know what helps you in the process of change and recovery.
    - Develop new interests and social groups.
    - Find rewarding ways to spend your time that don't involve the addiction.
    - Ask for help from others.
    - Decline taking on new demands, such as complex projects or new duties.
    - Consider joining a support group (see Appendix C, "Helpful Resources"). People in recovery who attend groups on a regular basis do better than those who do not. Groups can vary widely, so shop around for one that's comfortable. You'll get more out of it if you become involved by having a sponsor and reaching out to other members for help.

*Addictive Disorders*

## Drug Use and Teens

**Did you know…**

- About 24 million Americans over age 12 (or 9% of the population) have used an illegal drug (mostly marijuana) or abused a medication in the past month.
- Nearly 40% of 12th graders said they used alcohol and 21% had used marijuana in the past month.
- 60% of high school seniors do not view frequent marijuana use as harmful. The strength of marijuana has increased over the last few years, which means that daily use of today's marijuana may have a greater health impact than in the past.
- Prescription opioid pain relievers (such as Vicodin or Oxycontin) and over-the-counter cough and cold medicine with dextromethorphan are the most commonly abused substances (after marijuana and alcohol) by high school seniors.
- Most teens who abuse prescription drugs are given them for free by a friend or family member.

*Source.* National Institute on Drug Abuse; Substance Abuse and Mental Health Services Administration.

increased senses, or a high—as well as problems with function and behavior. (Intoxication symptoms differ for each drug and are described in the "Substance Intoxication and Withdrawal" section of this chapter.)

Changes to the brain and body are stronger in those with heavy or frequent drug use. The changes in the brain's wiring are what cause people to have intense cravings for the drug and make it hard to stop using the drug. The craving may be so strong that the person cannot think of anything else. Craving can be strongest in settings where the drug has been used before. Increased craving can be a warning sign for a relapse after recovery.

People with substance use disorders may spend a lot of time trying to get the substance, use the substance, or recover from its effects. In severe substance use disorders, the person's entire life revolves around the substance.

Over time, people with the disorder develop a *tolerance* for the substance. When this happens, they need a larger amount to feel high. Tolerance differs from person to person. It depends a great deal on the type of substance and a person's gender and weight.

Each drug shares the same checklist of symptoms for substance use disorder. The symptoms are grouped by the effects of substance use: impaired control, social problems, risky use, and drug effects. A person has a substance use disorder when he or she has the problem during a 12-month time frame. The degree of how severe the problem is depends on how many symptoms he or she has.

Understanding Mental Disorders

**Substance Use Disorder**

A problem of substance use leading to great impairment or distress, as shown by at least two of the following within 1 year:

## Impaired Control

- The substance is often taken in larger amounts or over a longer period than was planned.
- There is a constant desire or failed attempts to cut down or control substance use.
- A great deal of time is spent trying to get the substance, use the substance, or recover from its effects.
- There is a craving, or a strong urge to use the substance.

## Social Problems

- Regular substance use causes failure to complete major tasks at work, school, or home.
- Continued substance use despite having constant or regular social or personal problems caused or made worse by the effects of the substance.
- Important social, work, or leisure activities are given up or cut back because of the substance use.

## Risky Use

- The substance is often used in settings where it is unsafe.
- The substance keeps being used despite the known problems caused or made worse by the substance. These problems can be physical (linked to the body) or psychological (how someone thinks and feels), or both.

## Drug Effects

- Tolerance as defined by either of the following:
  - A need for larger amounts of the substance to get intoxicated or high.
  - The same amount of the substance gives fewer effects.
- Withdrawal, as evident by either of the following:
  - Symptoms of withdrawal (symptoms differ for each substance; see Table 2). These symptoms occur when the amounts of the substance in the body decline with stopping or less use.
  - The substance is taken to avoid or relieve withdrawal symptoms.

## Keith's Story

Keith, a 45-year-old plumber, was referred for a psychiatric evaluation after his family met with him to express their concern about his heavy drinking. Since making the appointment 3 days earlier, Keith denied having a drink.

For 20 years after high school, Keith drank 3–5 beers per evening, five times per week. Over the last 7 years, Keith drank almost daily, with an average of 6 beers on weeknights and 12 beers on weekends and holidays. His wife repeatedly voiced her concern that he was "drinking too much." Despite his efforts to limit his alcohol intake, Keith spent much of the weekend drinking, sometimes missing family get-togethers, and often passed out while watching TV in the evening. He remained productive at work and never called in sick. Keith was able to stop drinking twice for 1 month in the past 4 years. Both times, he said he had gone "cold turkey" in response to his wife's concerns. He denied having had symptoms of alcohol withdrawal either time.

Keith had been married for 18 years and had one 17-year-old daughter. He was a high school graduate with 2 years of community college. He owned a successful plumbing company and had never seen a psychiatrist.

Keith was diagnosed with *alcohol use disorder*. His lack of success in cutting down, overall time spent intoxicated or recovering from being intoxicated, missed family events, and frequent alcohol use despite problems all fit the criteria for the disorder.

## Stan's Story

Stan, a married 46-year-old pastor, was referred to the psychiatry outpatient department by his primary care doctor for depressive symptoms and misuse of opioids (painkillers) for his chronic right knee pain.

Stan injured his right knee playing basketball 17 months earlier. His mother gave him several tablets of hydrocodone-acetaminophen that she had for back pain, and he found this helpful. When he ran out of the pills and his pain continued, he went to the emergency room. He was told he had a mild sprain. He was given a 1-month supply of hydrocodone-acetaminophen. He took the pills as prescribed for 1 month, and his pain went away.

After stopping the pills, however, Stan began to have pain again in his knee. He saw an orthopedist (a doctor who treats bone and muscle problems), who ordered imaging scans and determined there was no major damage. He was given another 1-month supply of hydrocodone-acetaminophen. This time, however, he needed to take more than prescribed in order to ease the pain. He also felt sad and "achy" when he did not take the medication, and said he had a "craving" for more opioids. He returned to the orthopedist, who referred him to a pain specialist.

Stan was too embarrassed to go to the pain specialist. He believed that his faith and strength should help him defeat the pain. He found that he could not live without the pain medication, because of the pain and muscle

Understanding Mental Disorders

aches when he stopped the medication. He also began to enjoy the high and had intense craving. He began to frequent emergency rooms to get more opioids, often lying about the timing and nature of his right knee pain, and even stole pills from his mother on two occasions. He became fixed on trying to find more opioids, and his work and home life suffered. After a while, he told his primary care doctor about his opioid use and sadness, and that doctor referred him to the outpatient psychiatry clinic.

During the mental examination, Stan reported that his mood was "lousy." He denied symptoms of paranoia or hallucinations, or having any thoughts to harm himself or others.

Stan was diagnosed with *opioid use disorder.* The number of people who abuse prescription opioids ranks second among substance use disorders. Stan's use led to out-of-control opioid use that had a negative impact on his life.

# Substance Intoxication and Withdrawal

When people use the substances listed in Table 2, they can have substance intoxication or withdrawal. *Intoxication* occurs when the substance use was recent. *Withdrawal* occurs when the person stops or uses less of the substance.

When a person is intoxicated, he or she shows behavioral, physical, or psychological changes shortly after the substance is taken. Substance intoxication most often causes people to have problems with perception, staying awake, thinking, judgment, body movement, and personal behavior. The person may become aggressive or moody.

How people use a substance plays a part in how quickly it is absorbed into the bloodstream and how strongly they become intoxicated. For instance, smoking, snorting, or shooting a drug intravenously (into the vein) causes a more intense intoxication. These methods are also more likely to lead people to use the substance more often. Also, the substance can continue to have effects even after tests no longer detect the substance in the body.

---

 **Substance Intoxication**

Substance intoxication occurs when:

- Recent use of the substance has occurred.
- Major problems appear with behavior, body function, and thinking or feeling during or shortly after the substance is taken, due to the effect on the central nervous system.
- Certain symptoms appear after the substance is taken (see Table 2).
- Symptoms are not due to another medical condition or mental disorder.

---

When people stop using a substance—or use less of it—substance withdrawal can also occur. Withdrawal symptoms can cause problems with doing social, work, or other tasks. Most people who have substance withdrawal have the urge to start using the substance again to relieve the withdrawal symptoms.

---

 **Substance Withdrawal**

Substance withdrawal occurs when:

- The person stops or reduces use of the substance.
- Certain symptoms appear after the substance use is stopped or reduced (see Table 2).
- These symptoms cause great distress or problems with social, work, or other key, daily tasks.
- Symptoms are not due to another medical condition or mental disorder.

---

Compared to others in the general population, young people ages 18–24 have the highest rates of alcohol and another substance use disorder. Those between ages 12–17 who use alcohol and cigarettes are 15 times more likely to use drugs. Intoxication is often the first substance-related disorder to occur and often begins during the teen years. Withdrawal can happen at any age as long as the substance has been taken for a long time on a frequent basis.

People can have a wide range of symptoms when intoxicated or in withdrawal. Examples of intoxication and withdrawal symptoms for certain drugs are shown in Table 2.

# Substance/Medication-Induced Mental Disorders

Sometimes, the use of drugs and medications can bring on symptoms of certain mental disorders. These mental disorders often stop within days or weeks after the drug or medication was last used. For instance, *alcohol-induced depressive disorder* is a *depressive disorder* caused by alcohol.

Of the drugs in Table 1, tobacco causes the fewest mental disorders. Withdrawal from tobacco (quitting smoking) can cause sleep disorders (such as trouble sleeping).

The other drugs in Table 1 can cause more severe mental disorders. For example, intoxication from drugs that cause sedation (sleepiness)—such as sedatives, hypnotics, and alcohol—can lead to a *substance-induced psy-*

*chotic, bipolar, depressive,* or *sleep disorder* and *sexual dysfunctions.* Withdrawal from these same drugs can lead to *substance-induced panic* and *anxiety disorders.* Substances that cause stimulation (wakefulness)—such as cocaine and amphetamines—can cause *substance-induced psychotic, bipolar, depressive, sleep,* and *anxiety disorders* and *sexual dysfunctions.*

Using certain medications to treat some medical conditions can also carry a risk of developing a mental disorder. Neurocognitive problems (problems with how the brain processes thoughts and memory) can be caused by medications, such as anesthetics (used during surgery), antihistamines (for congestion and allergies), and antihypertensives (for high blood pressure). Neurocognitive problems can also be caused by alcohol, opioids, sedatives, and hypnotic drugs. Cardiovascular medications and steroids can cause psychotic symptoms.

Some people are more prone than others to develop a substance-induced mental disorder from using drugs. The risk of developing one of these disorders increases with frequent use and larger amounts taken. Some drugs can have a rapid, severe, and harmful impact on the brain and body even if used just once in a small amount.

 ## Substance/Medication-Induced Mental Disorder

The following are common features of this disorder:

- The disorder shows the same distinct symptoms of a certain mental disorder.
- There is proof from the person's health history, physical exam, or lab tests of both of the following:
  - The disorder began during or within 1 month of intoxication or withdrawal from the substance or from taking a medication.
  - The substance or medication can cause the mental disorder.
- The disorder is *not* due to a separate mental disorder (such as one that is not substance/medication-induced). Proof of a separate mental disorder could include the following:
  - The disorder symptoms started before the severe intoxication, withdrawal, or exposure to the substance or medication began.
  - The full mental disorder lasted for an ample amount of time (such as at least 1 month) after the severe withdrawal, intoxication, or exposure to the substance or medication ended.
- The disorder is not part of a *delirium* (confusion and reduced attention caused by a substance, medication, or medical condition).
- The disorder causes much distress and problems with social, work, or other daily functions.

| Table 2. Symptoms of intoxication and withdrawal | | |
|---|---|---|
| Substance | Intoxication symptoms | Withdrawal symptoms |
| **Alcohol** | Slurred speech, incoordination, unsteady walk, quick eye movements | Sweating or fast pulse, increased hand tremors, trouble sleeping, nausea or vomiting, hallucinations, anxiety |
| **Caffeine** | Restlessness, nervousness, excitement, trouble sleeping, flushed face, upset stomach, increased urination | Headache, fatigue or drowsiness, quickly annoyed or angry, sad mood, trouble staying focused |
| **Cannabis** | Red eyes, increased appetite, dry mouth, fast heart rate | Quickly annoyed or angry, nervousness, trouble sleeping, decreased appetite, restlessness |
| **Hallucinogens** | *With PCP:* quick eye movements up and down or side to side, fast heart rate, loss of muscle coordination *With other hallucinogens:* large pupils, fast heart rate, sweating, blurred vision, tremors | None |
| **Inhalants** | Feeling dizzy, quick eye movements, incoordination, slurred speech, unsteady walk, slow reflexes, blurred vision | None |
| **Opioids** | Small or large pupils, drowsiness or coma, slurred speech, impaired attention or memory | Sad mood, nausea or vomiting, muscle aches, large pupils |
| **Sedatives** | Slurred speech, incoordination, unsteady walk, quick eye movements, impaired attention or memory | Sweating or fast pulse, hand tremors, trouble sleeping, nausea or vomiting, hallucinations, anxiety, seizures |
| **Stimulants** | Fast or slow heart rate, large pupils, higher or lower blood pressure, sweating or chills, nausea or vomiting | Fatigue, trouble sleeping, vivid nightmares, increased appetite |

| Table 2. Symptoms of intoxication and withdrawal *(continued)* | | |
|---|---|---|
| Substance | Intoxication symptoms | Withdrawal symptoms |
| **Tobacco** | None | Quickly annoyed or angry, trouble keeping thoughts focused, increased appetite, restlessness, sad mood, trouble sleeping |

# Gambling Disorder

Gambling has occurred in almost every part of the world throughout time. People in many cultures gamble (or place bets) on games and sporting events, and most do it for fun and never have a problem with it. But for some people, gambling becomes an addiction that they find hard to resist. When that happens, it can lead to major problems that include family and marital discord (such as fighting over money or time away spent gambling), financial crises (such as not paying bills), and trouble at work (being late, missing work).

People with *gambling disorder* get the same effect from gambling as someone with an alcohol or other drug use disorder gets from having a drink or using a drug. The gambling changes their mood and they keep up the habit, trying to achieve that same effect. They may feel a sense of power, control, and confidence when gambling. Addicted gamblers then begin to crave gambling just as people begin to crave a substance. People who gamble also may abuse alcohol or other drugs.

People with a gambling disorder often get into a cycle of placing larger bets after they lose money on a bet. They then try to win back what they lost, which leads to an urgent need to keep gambling. This is called "chasing losses."

Those with a gambling disorder may see money as the source and answer to their problems. They may begin to lie to family members and others to conceal how much they gamble. They may slip into illegal behavior (such as forgery and theft) to obtain more money to keep gambling. They also may ask others to loan them money for gambling, to pay back debts, or to help in a financial crisis.

Younger persons with a gambling disorder tend to be male and to bet on active pursuits, such as card games or sports betting. Older people tend to bet using slot machines and playing bingo. Gambling in later life is more common among women, and the disorder can become more serious more quickly in this group.

Gambling can increase during times of stress. There may be times of heavy gambling that cause severe problems in life, followed by times of complete stops in gambling, and times of no problems with control when gambling. Some people with gambling disorder decide to fully stop on their own and do so with success. Others need help from a mental health care provider. Some others may think they are recovered and do not know their risk. After they gamble a few times without problems, they may assume they are immune and continue to gamble—only to return to a gambling disorder.

 ## Gambling Disorder

The disorder is diagnosed when:

- Frequent gambling leads to problems and distress, as shown when someone has at least four of the following symptoms in 1 year:
  - Needs to gamble with increasing amounts of money to get excited.
  - Is restless or quickly annoyed or angry when trying to cut down or stop gambling.
  - Has tried but cannot control, cut back, or stop gambling.
  - Has constant thoughts about gambling (for instance, thinks about past gambling times, plans the next venture, thinks about ways to get more money to gamble).
  - Often gambles when feeling stressed (helpless, guilty, depressed).
  - After losing money gambling, often returns another day to get even (chasing losses).
  - Lies to conceal the extent of the gambling habit.
  - Has placed at risk or lost a close relationship, job, or major school or career prospect because of gambling.
  - Relies on others to provide money to make up for money lost through gambling.
- The gambling behavior is not due to a *manic episode* (spells of high energy and mood that can occur in *bipolar disorder*).

How severe the gambling disorder is depends on how many symptoms a person has. A person can have a mild, moderate, or severe gambling disorder. Those with 4–5 symptoms on the list above have a mild gambling disorder. People with 6–7 symptoms have a moderate disorder, and those with the most severe form have 8 or all of the symptoms.

# Risk Factors

The following factors increase people's risk of gambling disorder:

- **Temperament.** People who begin gambling in childhood or early teenage years. Also those with *antisocial personality, depressive,* and *bipolar disorders.*
- **Genetics and physiology.** The disorder runs in families. This could be due to both genetics and environment (being exposed to gambling at home).

## Key Points

- Certain drugs—and gambling—seem to quickly affect a portion of the brain called the *reward system.* This leads to intense pleasure (or a "high") and a craving to repeat that pleasure. Those with *addictive disorders* spend a great deal of time and effort trying to obtain the substance to use or the money to gamble. This begins to outweigh the value of other people and duties in their lives.
- Addictions cause painful problems with home, school, work, relationships, finances, brain, and body. At the same time, the pain of addiction causes people to seek help. People with an addiction must choose to get better. They cannot be forced to change. People with the disorder often cannot stop it on their own, even when they want to. They must get proper help.
- Treatment can involve medications to help control drug cravings and relieve severe symptoms of withdrawal. Therapy can help those with an addiction learn about their behavior and why they engage in it, rebuild life without an addiction, build higher self-esteem, develop new and healthy coping skills, and cope with stress. Self-help or support groups play a major role in recovery for people with addictions. They also provide valued guidance and support for their loved ones.
- For those with an addiction and their loved ones, learning as much as they can about the problem and its effects is important. Loved ones and those with an addiction should seek help from others. It is best for loved ones not to cover up the addiction, make excuses for the addiction, or take responsibility for it.
- *Relapse* occurs when someone has stopped the addiction for a while and is getting back to daily life and doing well—but then resumes the addictive behavior. The following tips help to prevent relapse: learn what triggers the addiction, avoid those triggers, plan to handle urges for the addiction, be prepared to say "no" to offers to engage in the addiction, and replace the addiction with other rewarding activities and relationships.

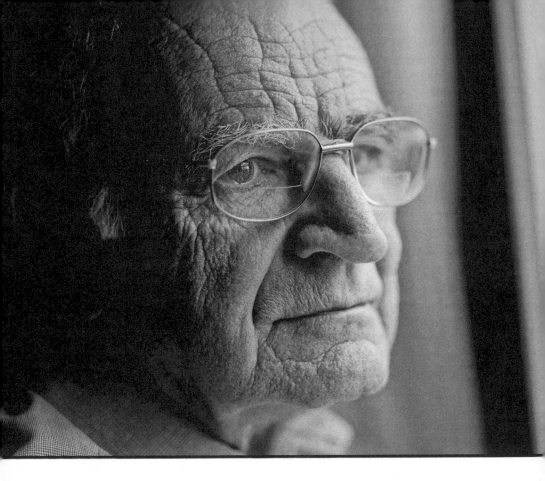

Delirium

Neurocognitive Disorder Due to Alzheimer's Disease

Neurocognitive Disorder Due to Traumatic Brain Injury

Neurocognitive Disorder Due to Parkinson's Disease

Frontotemporal Neurocognitive Disorder

Neurocognitive Disorder With Lewy Bodies

Vascular Neurocognitive Disorder

Other Dementia and Memory Problems

   Neurocognitive Disorder Due to HIV Infection

   Neurocognitive Disorder Due to Prion Disease

   Neurocognitive Disorder Due to Huntington's Disease

*For a complete list of DSM-5 disorders, see Appendix A.*

# CHAPTER 17

# Dementia and Other Memory Problems

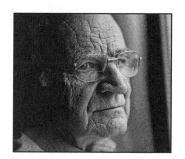

**D**ementia describes a decline of mental function that is severe enough to disrupt daily life. It can cause problems with people's memory and how well they think and plan. Dementia is not a disease itself, but a group of symptoms, such as memory loss and personality changes. These symptoms may be caused by different disorders, so there are different types of dementia based on the cause.

Emotional problems, such as stress, anxiety, or depression, can make a person more forgetful—which might be mistaken for dementia. For instance, someone who has recently retired or who is coping with the death of a loved one may feel sad, lonely, worried, or bored. Trying to deal with these life changes leaves some people confused or forgetful. These memory problems are often short-term and go away when the feelings fade. If these feelings and memory problems persist, seek help from a doctor or other mental health care provider.

Some memory problems are linked to health issues that may be treated. These include medication side effects, lack of vitamin $B_{12}$, and alcoholism. Some thyroid, kidney, or liver disorders also can lead to memory loss. A doctor should treat medical conditions like these as soon as possible. Some of these conditions may lead to dementia, and others do not. Early diagnosis and treatment can help limit and manage memory symptoms.

Alzheimer's disease is one of the most common causes of dementia. Dementia can also be caused by conditions such as stroke, Parkinson's disease, or a serious head injury. Dementia often gets worse over time. How quickly symptoms worsen differs from person to person.

In DSM-5, disorders that describe dementia and other memory problems are newly grouped as *neurocognitive disorders*. These disorders involve damage to parts of the brain that can affect memory, thinking, or reasoning (see Table 1 for brain functions that doctors assess). They include nine disorders named by their different medical causes: *Alzheimer's disease, frontotemporal degeneration, Lewy body disease, vascular disease, traumatic brain injury, HIV infection* (from AIDS), *prion disease, Parkinson's disease,* and *Huntington's disease.* A tenth disorder, called *delirium,* is a short-term state of confusion and reduced attention. Delirium can occur in someone who also has dementia. Unlike the other disorders, delirium is a temporary state that goes away, whereas the other neurocognitive disorders persist (although symptoms for some can be treated).

The nine neurocognitive disorders due to medical causes are diagnosed as either "major" or "mild" based on how severe symptoms are. The problems must occur when delirium is not present and are not the result of another mental disorder (such as *major depressive disorder* or *schizophrenia*). What marks the disorder as major or mild is defined as follows:

### Major Neurocognitive Disorder

- A major decline in at least one area of mental function—such as attention, ability to plan and make decisions, memory and learning, language, and motor skills. The decline is enough to cause concern from a loved one or a doctor, or is confirmed by testing.
- The major decline in mental skills impairs or disrupts the ability to do daily tasks such that help is required to perform them, such as paying bills or keeping track of medications to take.

### Mild Neurocognitive Disorder

- A slight decline in at least one area of a person's mental function—such as attention, ability to plan and make decisions, memory and learning, language, and motor skills—that causes concern from a loved one or a doctor, or is confirmed by testing.
- The slight decline in mental skills permits doing daily tasks without help, such as paying bills or keeping track of medications to take.

# Delirium

*Delirium* is a temporary state of confusion and reduced attention that is caused by a drug, alcohol, medication, toxin, or a medical condition, such as an illness or infection. Alcohol or drug intoxication or withdrawal can cause symptoms. People with delirium have problems staying focused or paying attention. Delirium occurs when normal brain signals are not working. It can start quickly, often within hours or a few days. One way to understand delirium is to think about what it is like to be "out of it," not being fully awake, having an illness with a high fever, or waking up from anesthesia.

People with delirium have disturbed mental function that causes a decreased awareness of their environment, memory problems, and confused thinking. They may be easily distracted and unable to answer questions. They can be sleepy during the day and awake at night. People with delirium may have other symptoms, such as anxiety, fear, depression, irritability, and anger. They may also call out, scream, curse, or moan, especially at night.

Any condition that requires a hospital stay, especially in intensive care, increases the risk of delirium. Between 14% and 24% of people admitted to the hospital develop delirium. In older people admitted to intensive care units, the rate is as high as 70% to 87%.

---

 **Delirium**

- Reduced attention and awareness. For instance, not able to stay focused on a topic or to change topics. Normal tasks take longer than before, and thinking is easier when other things don't compete for attention, such as the radio, TV, and other conversations.
- The problem develops over a short time (usually hours to a few days), tends to become more severe through the day, and worsens in the evening.
- A problem in mental function, such as memory loss, disorientation, language problems, and problems with judging shapes and sizes.

The first and third items above must not be due to another neurocognitive disorder. There must be evidence (for instance, from testing, physical exam, or report by self or others) of another medical condition, alcohol or drug intoxication or withdrawal, or exposure to a toxin or a medication that might have caused the symptoms. Delirium can last for hours, days, weeks, or months.

---

| Table 1. Brain functions (neurocognitive domains) | | |
|---|---|---|
| Domain (a type of thinking skill) | Examples of possible symptoms | |
| | Major | Mild |
| **Complex attention** | Quickly confused by other distractions in the surroundings (radio, TV, conversations). Has trouble holding new information in mind, such as a phone number just given. | Normal tasks take longer than before. Thinking is easier when other distractions are not present, such as radio, TV, and other conversations. |
| **Executive function** (includes planning, decision making, working memory) | Needs to focus on one task at a time. Needs others to help plan daily living tasks or make decisions. | Has more problems doing more than one task at once, or finishing a task after being interrupted by a visitor or phone call. May complain of being more tired from the extra effort needed to organize, plan, and make decisions. |
| **Learning and memory** (includes immediate, recent, and long-term memory) | Repeats self in conversation, often within same conversation. Cannot keep track of short list of items when shopping or of plans for the day. | Has problem recalling recent events and depends more on list making or calendar. May sometimes repeat self over a few weeks to the same person. |
| **Language** (includes naming objects, correct grammar, and understanding word definitions) | Uses vague phrases such as "that thing" and "you know what I mean," and uses general pronouns instead of people's names. Makes mistakes in grammar when talking, such as leaving out or using the wrong articles (such as *a, an, the*), prepositions (such as *in, to, of*), and verbs. | Has problem finding the correct words to use. May avoid using names of friends. |

| Table 1. Brain functions (neurocognitive domains) *(continued)* | | |
|---|---|---|
| Domain (a type of thinking skill) | Examples of possible symptoms | |
| | Major | Mild |
| **Perceptual-motor** (includes assembling items that require hand-eye coordination, and imitating gestures) | Has great problems with tasks that were once easy (such as using tools, driving a car), or getting around in familiar areas. | Needs to rely more on maps or others for directions. Takes more effort to do tasks such as assembly, sewing, or knitting. |
| **Social cognition** (recognizing other people's emotions or mental states) | Behaves outside social norms. Shows no awareness of what's proper to wear or say during religious, political, or sexual conversations. | Slight changes in behavior or personality appear. Less able to read facial expressions or feel empathy. |

## Risk Factors

The following factors increase the risk of delirium:

- **Environment.** Being immobile (not able to move), a history of falls, inactive lifestyle, and use of drugs and medications that change mood and behavior. These include alcohol, anticholinergics (medications for spasms or convulsions), antihistamines (for allergies), and asthma, sleep, and pain medications.
- **Genetics and biology.** Major and mild neurocognitive disorders can increase risk. Older people are at higher risk, as well as children who have an illness with fever.

## Treatment

While most people with delirium have a full recovery with or without treatment, early diagnosis and treatment can shorten the length of the illness. Delirium can progress to coma, seizures, or death if the cause for the symptoms remains untreated. The first goal of treatment is to address the underlying cause, such as stopping the use of a certain medication or substance. For that reason, the doctors will need to assess the possible causes of the delirium with a medical "workup." This involves a range of tests to check for possible causes. For instance, when an infection that causes a delirium is treated, it also will allow the delirium to end.

# Alzheimer's Disease

*Alzheimer's disease* is a condition that causes dementia by slowly killing nerve cells in the brain. It destroys memory and the ability to learn, reason, make judgments, communicate, and carry out daily tasks.

Alzheimer's disease is one of the most common forms of dementia, striking about 5.2 million Americans of all ages in 2014. This includes an estimated 5 million people over age 65 and about 200,000 people younger than age 65 who have a younger-onset (or early-onset) form of the disease. The Centers for Disease Control and Prevention (CDC) lists Alzheimer's disease as the sixth leading cause of death in the United States.

People with Alzheimer's disease first show slight symptoms of personality changes and memory loss that differ from normal changes that happen with age (see box). They may become upset or anxious more easily or withdraw from their usual hobbies and activities. They also do not cope well with change. For instance, they can follow their same daily routes, but travel to a new place confuses them and they quickly become lost. Another early sign of the disease is changes in judgment or decision making. For instance, they may pay less attention to grooming or keeping themselves clean.

In the early stages of the illness, people are often at risk of *depression*. Their condition also may be worsened by reactions to medications or changes in living arrangements. Because Alzheimer's disease happens late in life, the loss of a spouse or other close family members may increase the suffering of people with Alzheimer's disease.

As memory loss worsens, people with Alzheimer's disease may ask the same questions over and over and begin to forget the names of long-time friends. Social life becomes harder, and they may become more isolated. In the later stages of Alzheimer's disease, people with the illness begin to lose physical coordination and may need help dressing, bathing, and walking.

Most people with Alzheimer's disease are older adults. They may suffer from a number of medical conditions that can make diagnosing the disease more complicated. These other medical conditions also play a role in how quickly Alzheimer's disease may progress and the person's overall health worsens.

## Is It Alzheimer's Disease or Just Normal Aging?

While some changes in memory, thinking, and reasoning skills may be early warning signs of *Alzheimer's disease,* many changes are just a normal part of getting older. If you notice any of these signs of Alzheimer's disease, see a doctor right away for an evaluation.

| Signs of Alzheimer's disease | Normal age-related changes |
|---|---|
| Memory loss that disrupts daily life (forgetting recently learned information or important dates or events) | Sometimes forgetting names or appointments but can recall them later |
| Challenges in planning or solving problems (trouble following a familiar recipe or keeping track of monthly bills) | Sometimes making errors when balancing a checkbook |
| Problems completing familiar tasks at home, work, or leisure (managing a budget at work or knowing rules of a favorite game) | Sometimes needing help to use the settings on a microwave or to record a television show |
| Confused about time or place (losing track of the date or the season) | Forgetting the day of the week but can recall it later |
| Trouble making sense of visual images and spatial relationships (problems reading, judging distance, and knowing colors) | Vision changes from cataracts |
| New problems with words while writing or talking with others (repeating statements, calling items by the wrong name) | Sometimes having trouble finding the right word |
| Misplacing things and being unable to retrace steps to find them | Losing things from time to time |
| Decreased or poor judgment | Making a bad decision once in a while |
| No longer or seldom taking part in work or social functions | Sometimes feeling weary of work, family, and social duties |
| Changes in mood and personality (becoming confused, suspicious, depressed, or anxious) | Having certain ways of doing things and getting annoyed when a routine is changed |

*Source.* Alzheimer's Association.

## Neurocognitive Disorder Due to Alzheimer's Disease

- Symptoms of either major or mild neurocognitive disorder are present.
- The disease begins with few or no symptoms, and memory or thinking slowly become impaired.
- There may be signs of Alzheimer's disease from family history or genetic testing.
- All three of the following are present:
  - Proof of decline in memory, learning, and at least one other mental process (such as attention or language) based on health history or testing.
  - Progressive, gradual decline in mental processes.
  - No proof of another disease that may cause the mental decline.
- The disorder is not due to the effects of alcohol, drugs, or medication.

## Risk Factors

The following factors play a role in the development of Alzheimer's disease:

- **Environment.** Traumatic brain injury (serious head injury) increases the risk.
- **Aging.** Age is the greatest known risk factor for the disease. The odds of developing Alzheimer's disease doubles about every 5 years after age 65.
- **Genetics.** The disease also runs in families—having a first-degree blood relative (parent or sibling) with the disease increases a person's risk. A gene variation called *apolipoprotein E4* may increase the risk of developing Alzheimer's disease.

## Roger's Story

Roger, a 71-year-old man, was referred to a psychiatrist by his primary care doctor for symptoms of depression that had not responded to medication. Roger's wife reported that he had begun to change at age 68, about a year after his retirement. He had stopped playing golf and cards, which he had enjoyed for decades. He no longer looked forward to going out of the house, and he refused to socialize. Instead, he sat on the couch all day and watched TV or napped. His wife said he was sleeping 10–12 hours a day instead of his normal 7 hours.

His wife had become worried that retirement had left Roger depressed, and she had mentioned her concerns to their primary care doctor. Their doctor agreed and prescribed an antidepressant. Roger's symptoms did not improve on the medication, and the doctor then referred him for a psychiatric evaluation.

Roger's past psychiatric history was noted because one of his younger brothers had *major depression* that was treated with psychotherapy and antidepressant medication. His mother had developed *dementia* in her 70s.

Roger had graduated from college with a degree in business, had a successful career as a corporate manager, and retired at age 67. He and his wife had been married for 45 years, said there were no major marital problems, and had three children and four grandchildren, who were all in good health. Before this, he had been outgoing, energetic, and well organized.

Roger had high blood pressure and high cholesterol and was taking medication for these conditions. The exam showed he was alert and cooperative and had steady but slow speech. Roger had a limited range of emotional expression, denied feeling sad or guilty, but felt he had retired too early. He was aware that his wife was concerned and agreed that he had less energy and was less active than in the past. He blamed these changes on his retirement.

During the exam, Roger could name the year but not the month or day of the week for his appointment. He remembered one of three objects in 2 minutes, performed three of five subtractions correctly, named four common objects correctly, and repeated a complex sentence without error. He was able to draw the face of a clock and place the numbers correctly, but he was not able to correctly place the hands at 10 minutes after 2.

Roger was diagnosed with *Alzheimer's disease.* He had a 3-year history of gradual social withdrawal. He has a family history of depression in a brother and late-life dementia in his mother. The main symptoms were slowness, lack of concern about his decline, and increased sleep. The exam showed problems in memory, concentration, and math, as well as trouble with clock drawing.

# Treatment

While there is no cure for Alzheimer's disease, there are two types of medications that may help lessen the memory symptoms for a short time. Cholinesterase inhibitors often are prescribed in the early stages to treat symptoms such as memory loss, thinking, language, and judgment. About half the people who take the medication have a delay in their symptoms getting worse for about 6 to 12 months. Another medication, memantine, may help reduce the decline in memory, attention, reasoning, and ability to do simple tasks later in the disease. Antidepressants also may be used to treat mood symptoms or antipsychotic medications for hallucinations, agitation, and severe hostility.

Medications are not the only treatment for Alzheimer's disease. Patients and families also may need the help of support groups and counseling. Families can benefit from getting help with the care that is needed to maintain safety when a loved one has memory loss. Therapy can help family members learn ways to help their relative living with the disease to manage his or her illness. They also can learn coping skills to lessen the stress of caring for a loved one with Alzheimer's disease.

By taking advantage of group support and assistance in caregiving when needed, patients and their loved ones can prepare themselves for the disease and its progression. While the disease does not have a cure, quality of life can be greatly improved with support for patients and caregivers.

# Traumatic Brain Injury

A *traumatic brain injury* (TBI) is caused by an impact to the head or a rapid movement of the brain within the skull. Falls, vehicle accidents, and being struck in the head cause most TBIs.

TBIs can be mild, moderate, or severe, depending on how long the person lost consciousness, had amnesia, and remained confused after the injury. Collisions and blows to the head that happen during contact sports are considered a mild form of TBI. With mild TBIs, symptoms either go away or improve greatly within 3 months. Repeated mild TBIs may cause problems that last longer. Severe TBIs can cause seizures, emotional problems, weakness on one side of the body, and vision problems.

In the United States, 1.7 million TBIs occur each year, resulting in 1.4 million visits to hospital emergency rooms, 275,000 hospitalizations, and 52,000 deaths. Men suffer nearly 60% of the TBIs.

The following problems can occur as a result of TBIs:

- Emotional problems, such as quick frustration, irritability, moodiness, tension, and anxiety.
- Personality changes, such as aggression, lack of motivation, and suspiciousness.
- Physical symptoms, such as headache, fatigue, sensitivity to light, sleep problems, and dizziness.
- Mental challenges, such as slower thinking, problems staying focused, and reduced ability to perform usual activities.

## Neurocognitive Disorder Due to Traumatic Brain Injury

- Symptoms of either major or mild neurocognitive disorder are present.
- There is evidence of a traumatic brain injury, with one or more of the following:
  - Loss of consciousness.
  - Posttraumatic amnesia (loss of memory after a traumatic event).
  - Being disoriented and confused.
  - Signs of neurological problems (such as seizures, loss of smell, or weakness on one side of the body).
- The disorder starts right after the brain injury or right after the person regains consciousness and lasts past the acute post-injury period.

## Risk Factors

The following factors increase a person's risk:

- **For TBI:** Children younger than 4 years, older teens, and people older than 65 years. Falls are most common, with vehicle accidents being second. Sports concussions with older children, teens, and young adults also raise the risk of TBI.
- **For neurocognitive disorder after TBI:** Repeated concussions can lead to neurocognitive disorder.

# Olivia's Story

The parents of 19-year-old Olivia insisted she see a psychiatrist. "It's not me you want to see," Olivia proclaimed. "It's my insane parents who need your help." Olivia added, "Everything is going great in my life. I have plenty of friends, go out almost every night, and always have lots of fun."

Olivia agreed to have her parents join the session, and they told a different story. In tears, they disclosed that their daughter had become irritable, unproductive, and combative. In searching her room, they had found small amounts of marijuana, alprazolam (Xanax), cocaine, and prescription stimulants. The parents described major changes in Olivia's personality over the last few years. They also noted that Olivia's attitudes and behavior sharply differed from those of her family. Her sister went to a top university, and her younger brother excelled at a private high school. Her parents seemed to enjoy their careers as radiologists.

Her parents said that Olivia's sudden change began 4 years ago. At 15, she liked to study. She also had a lively sense of humor and a wide circle of "terrific friends." But "almost overnight," she began to shun her longtime friends in favor of "dropouts and malcontents" and began to get traffic tickets and school detentions. Her grades dropped from As to Ds. The parents were at a loss to explain the abrupt and dramatic change.

The change in school performance led the psychiatrist to ask Olivia to take a series of neuropsychological tests so the results could be compared with those of tests that she had taken when she had applied to a private high school several years ago. These involved two high school admissions tests that Olivia retook: the System for Assessment and Group Evaluation (SAGE), which tests a wide range of thinking skills, and the Differential Aptitude Tests (DAT), which focus on reasoning, spelling, and perception skills.

On the SAGE, her average scores dropped from the upper 10% for a 13-year-old to the bottom 20%. When Olivia took the DAT at age 13, she scored in the highest range for ninth graders across almost all measures. Upon repeating the test at age 19, she scored below the high school average in all measures.

A magnetic resonance imaging (MRI) brain scan displayed a clear "lesion" on the left side of the brain. This was a sign of prior injury to that area.

During more questions about the time in which she seemed to have changed, Olivia revealed that she had been in a traffic accident with her ex-boyfriend, Mark. Although Olivia did not recall much from this episode, she remembered that she hit her head and that she had bad headaches for many weeks thereafter. Because Olivia was not bleeding and there was no damage to the car, neither Mark nor Olivia reported the incident to anyone. With Olivia's permission, the psychiatrist contacted Mark, who remembered the incident well. "Olivia hit her head very, very hard on the dashboard of my car. She was not totally unconscious but very dazed. For about 3 hours, she spoke very slowly, complained that her head hurt badly, and was confused. For about 2 hours she didn't know where she was, what day it was, and when she had to get home. She also threw up twice. I was really scared, but Olivia didn't want me to worry her parents since they're so overprotective. And then she broke up with me, and we've hardly spoken since."

Olivia was diagnosed with *mild neurocognitive disorder due to traumatic brain injury* (TBI). The decision to retest Olivia's performance on high school aptitude and achievement examinations revealed the dramatic decline in her test scores. The questions about her history led to the discovery of the car accident that marked the start of Olivia's symptoms.

In the accident, Olivia suffered a TBI and had two of the four core symptoms for a TBI diagnosis: she was disoriented and confused for hours afterward, and she did not recall much about the accident (post-traumatic amnesia).

## Treatment

Treatment for most TBIs requires a short hospital stay or monitoring at home. More severe injuries need special hospital care that may take months. In Olivia's case, the symptoms from the TBI included both a change in personality and a change in thinking skills. Sometimes the personality changes can include anxiety or depression symptoms that require treatment. Other times they can include being impulsive, being easily angered, making poor decisions, or tending to abuse drugs or alcohol. The type of treatment varies by each person and is based on the type of symptoms from the injury.

# Parkinson's Disease

*Parkinson's disease* is a disorder of the nervous system that affects people's movement. It occurs when nerve cells in the brain stop making a chemical called dopamine, which helps control muscle movement. The disease progresses slowly and usually starts with a slight shaking or tremor in one hand. Over time, people with the disease may become stiff, move slowly, and have problems with balance and walking. They also may have confusion, slowed or quieter speech, and loss of thinking skills and facial expressions.

Each year in the United States, between 50,000 and 60,000 new cases of Parkinson's disease are diagnosed. About 1 million people currently have the condition, and the CDC ranked Parkinson's as the 14th leading cause of death in the United States. Symptoms of the disease often begin between ages 60–90.

When people have a neurocognitive disorder with Parkinson's disease, the loss of thinking skills often doesn't occur until years after the movement symptoms have been present. So when people are first diagnosed with Parkinson's disease, they don't have a neurocognitive disorder. When thinking problems do begin, the main problems involve slow thinking and taking a long time to process new information or learn new things. Problems with memory, planning, and keeping focused attention may also occur.

### Neurocognitive Disorder Due to Parkinson's Disease

- Symptoms of either major or mild neurocognitive disorder are present.
- The problem occurs with a diagnosis of Parkinson's disease.
- The disease begins with few or no symptoms and progresses with gradual impairment.
- The disorder is not due to another medical condition or mental disorder.

## Risk Factors

The following factors increase the risk of Parkinson's disease:

- **Environment.** Exposure to herbicides and pesticides.
- **Biology.** The risk of a neurocognitive disorder from Parkinson's disease increases with the person's age.

## Treatment

There is no cure for Parkinson's disease but treatment can help to reduce its symptoms. Treatment most often includes medication that helps replace the dopamine chemical in the brain that is lost with the disease.

These medications treat symptoms related to movement problems. One of the most effective is levodopa, which passes into the brain and converts to dopamine. A class of medications known as dopamine agonists may also be given that mimic the actions that dopamine has in the brain. Dopamine agonists include pramipexole and ropinirole. These medicines help with the movement problems but do not help with the neurocognitive (thinking) problems with Parkinson's disease. Sometimes the medicines that help increase dopamine can cause side effects when people lose thinking skills from Parkinson's disease, and too much dopamine agonist medicine can cause hallucinations or confusion.

Although less common, surgery also may be an option to help ease symptoms. A procedure known as *deep brain stimulation* involves placing electrical stimulators on areas of the brain that control movement. This treatment is only used when medications do not work. The surgery may help with movement problems, but not with changes in thinking skills that happen later with Parkinson's disease. There is no treatment to relieve the neurocognitive symptoms of Parkinson's disease. Occupational therapy may help with tasks used in daily life (such as getting dressed) and learning how to avoid falls.

# Frontotemporal Neurocognitive Disorder

*Frontotemporal neurocognitive disorder* is dementia caused by cell damage in the brain's frontal lobes (area behind the forehead) or temporal lobes (area of the brain that is just above the ears). These parts of the brain control a person's planning, judgment, emotions, and speaking, and some types of movement.

The disorder can cause severe changes in personality. For instance, someone who once had flawless manners may become profane or vulgar in public. People with the behavioral symptoms of the disorder may lose their sense of social skills, so that they may do awkward things, such as stand too close to people or make rude comments that are out of character for their personality. Others may lose their skill with language, such as showing problems with naming objects, using correct grammar, or finding words to say what they mean.

Frontotemporal dementia occurs in 2 to 10 of every 100,000 people This type of dementia can be seen often in people younger than age 65 years. Because its symptoms appear in people in their 60s or rarely even as early as age 30, the disorder can disrupt work and family life more often than the dementias that start later.

---

 **Frontotemporal Neurocognitive Disorder**

- Symptoms of either major or mild neurocognitive disorder are present.
- The disease begins with few or no symptoms and progresses gradually.
- A decline in thinking skills centers mainly on behavior control or language, with few or no problems with memory, learning, motor, or visual skills.
- The disorder is not due to another disorder or disease, such as strokes, or the effects of a medication, drug, or alcohol.
- Either a behavioral type or a language type is present:

### Behavioral Type

- At least three of the following behavioral symptoms:
  - Behavioral disinhibition (loss of social restraint).
  - Lack of emotion or interest.
  - Loss of sympathy or empathy.
  - Compulsive behavior.
  - Hyperorality (putting inappropriate objects in the mouth) and changes in diet, such as constant overeating or eating strange foods.
- Clear decline in social skills (such as decline in self-care, lack of interest in social interactions, less interest in personal responsibilities) and decline in ability to plan, organize, and make decisions.

### Language Type

- Clear decline in language, such as the ability to make words easily, name objects, or read and write.

---

## Risk Factors

About 40% of people with frontotemporal neurocognitive disorder have a family history of early-onset neurocognitive disorder. A number of gene mutations can increase the risk.

## Treatment

There is no treatment for frontotemporal neurocognitive disorder. Because the problem often causes changes in behavior or personality, the most important treatment involves counseling and support for families and caregivers to understand the illness. Often people with the disorder need supervision and care from their families. When there are severe behavior changes that involve irritability or hostility, antidepressant or antipsychotic medications may help those symptoms.

# Lewy Body Disease

*Neurocognitive disorder with Lewy bodies* (NCDLB) is a type of dementia caused by abnormal microscopic deposits in the brain that damage brain cells over time. The disorder is named after neurologist Frederick H. Lewy, M.D., who discovered the abnormal brain deposits in the early 1900s.

The damage caused to brain cells leads to a gradual decline in thinking and reasoning. The disease also causes confusion and degrees of alertness that change greatly through the day or from one day to the next. People with the disorder may fall often or have spells of lost consciousness. They may have problems feeding themselves and using the toilet. Symptoms tend to begin between ages 60–90.

Some symptoms of NCDLB can look like the symptoms of Parkinson's disease. People with NCDLB have the same motor problems that are seen in Parkinson's disease, such as a very slow walking gait, slow speech, and loss of facial expression.

People with the disorder may have two major symptoms not found in other dementia disorders: visual hallucinations (seeing things that are not there) and symptoms of *rapid eye movement (REM) sleep behavior disorder* (see Chapter 12, "Sleep-Wake Disorders," for details). Up to 50% of people with NCDLB also have severe reactions and side effects to antipsychotic medications, so a correct diagnosis of the condition is essential.

It is estimated that between 0.1% and 5% of elderly people have NCDLB. The disorder is thought to be the third most common cause of dementia after *Alzheimer's disease* and *vascular dementia,* making up as much as 30% of dementia cases.

---

 ## Neurocognitive Disorder With Lewy Bodies

- Symptoms for either major or mild neurocognitive disorder are present.
- The disease begins with few or no symptoms and progresses gradually.
- There is a range of severity for this disorder. See a doctor if at least one of the following symptoms is present:
  - Fluctuating cognition with noticeable changes in attention and alertness.
  - Frequent visual hallucinations that are clear and detailed.
  - Symptoms of Parkinson's disease (such as muscle tremors or stiffness) and decline in thinking abilities (such as understanding, judgment, and memory).
  - Symptoms of REM sleep behavior disorder.
  - Severe side effects to antipsychotic medications.
- The disorder is not due to another disorder or disease, such as strokes, or the effects of a medication, drug, or alcohol.

---

## Risk Factors

Several genes increase the risk of developing NCDLB. However, for most people with the disorder, there is not a family history for it. Men over age 60 may have a higher risk.

## Treatment

There are currently no treatments for NCDLB, although medications may be prescribed for some symptoms. As a rule, people with NCDLB are very sensitive to side effects from all types of medicines. For this reason, doctors must take great care with prescribed medication. Changes in alertness with NCDLB can worsen greatly with medications. For instance, sometimes dopamine-increasing medicines are used to help treat symptoms of stiffness and motor slowness, but these medicines can have the bad effect of making visual hallucinations worse. Sometimes the cholinesterase inhibitors used to treat the memory and thinking symptoms of Alzheimer's disease are prescribed for people with NCDLB, but it is not certain whether they are helpful. Careful prescribing to help with depression or sleep problems can be done with close watching for side effects.

Often the best help for NCDLB is to avoid things that may cause confusion. Keeping a home free of clutter and noise may help maintain focus and avoid distractions. Doing so may also lessen the risk for hallucinations. Setting routines can build structure into the day and keep tasks clear. Breaking down complex tasks into simple steps also helps.

# Vascular Neurocognitive Disorder

*Vascular neurocognitive disorder* is caused by reduced blood flow to the brain because of a problem with the blood vessels that supply it. Parts of the brain become damaged and die from a lack of oxygen and nutrients.

The most common cause of the disorder is *cerebrovascular disease* (brain problems due to diseased blood vessels that supply the brain). This includes stroke and transient ischemic attacks (ministrokes). Changes in thinking skills sometimes follow these episodes. While thinking problems may begin mildly, they can worsen over time as a result of multiple minor strokes or other conditions that affect smaller blood vessels. Personality changes, mood changes, depression, and slowed movements may also occur.

In the United States, estimates for vascular neurocognitive disorder range from 0.2% of people ages 65–70 years to 16% of those who are age 80 or older. Within 3 months of having a stroke, 20% to 30% of people are diagnosed with the disorder.

**Vascular Neurocognitive Disorder**

- Symptoms of either major or mild neurocognitive disorder are present.
- The symptoms reflect a vascular problem, as shown by either of the following:
  - Start of cognitive problems is related to at least once cerebrovascular event (such as stroke).
  - Decline in mental skills is shown in memory, problem solving, reasoning, and planning.
- Evidence of cerebrovascular disease is shown in the person's health history, from physical exam, or brain imaging.
- The disorder is not due to another brain disease or systemic disorder.

## Risk Factors

The following factors increase the risk of the disorder:

- **Environment.** How well people overcome the effects of vascular brain injury depends on how well their brain forms new connections after portions of the brain have died. Keeping up education, physical exercise, social interaction, and mental activity throughout life helps.
- **Genetics and biology.** Factors that lead to cerebrovascular disease increase the risk, such as high blood pressure, diabetes, smoking, high cholesterol, and obesity.

## Treatment

No medications have been approved to treat the symptoms of vascular dementia. The most important "treatment" is to prevent it. A healthy diet, exercise, weight control, and reducing stress can lower blood pressure, blood sugar, and cholesterol levels. These lifestyle changes can greatly reduce the risk of vascular dementia and also can reduce progress of the disease. Quitting smoking can also help. Sometimes the medicines used in *Alzheimer's disease* are prescribed for vascular dementia, but it is not certain if they offer any benefit.

# Other Dementia and Memory Problems

The following neurocognitive disorders are dementias caused by HIV infection, prion disease, and Huntington's disease. For a diagnosis, symptoms of either major or mild neurocognitive disorder must be present.

The disorders cannot result from another medical condition or mental disorder. There may be some medications that can treat the memory and thinking problems or mood symptoms for these disorders. The best care for all the dementias involves loved ones and care providers giving kindness, patience, respect, and dignity to those with these disorders.

## Neurocognitive Disorder Due to HIV Infection

*HIV disease* infects the body's immune cells and some people with the infection develop dementia symptoms, such as memory loss and problems with planning, decision making, and learning new information. Depending on the stage of the HIV disease, between 33% and 50% of people infected with HIV have at least mild neurocognitive problems. To prevent or reduce neurocognitive symptoms of HIV, seeking treatment with medications that cross the blood-brain barrier is key. (The *blood-brain barrier* protects the brain; it restricts passage of certain substances in the blood from reaching the brain, such as certain medications.) Symptoms of a neurocognitive disorder due to HIV infection are as follows:

- There is proven infection with HIV.
- The neurocognitive disorder is not better explained by non-HIV conditions, such as brain disease.

## Neurocognitive Disorder Due to Prion Disease

*Prion disease* describes a rare group of diseases that affect humans and animals. *Prions* cause infection in nerve tissue, with rapid brain damage and major neurocognitive disorder in as little as 6 months. The disease may begin with fatigue, anxiety, and problems with eating, sleeping, or keeping focus. After a few weeks, changes in vision, coordination, or walking occur, as well as jerking movements. The disease always causes death. Exposure to infected nerve tissue may cause the disease, but often it appears without a clear source of infection. One common type of prion disease is Creutzfeldt-Jakob disease, or "mad cow disease." Symptoms of a neurocognitive disorder due to prion disease are as follows:

- The disease begins with few or no symptoms and progresses rapidly.
- The presence of motor features of prion disease, such as muscle jerks or lack of muscle coordination.

# Neurocognitive Disorder Due to Huntington's Disease

*Huntington's disease* is a rare disease that is inherited within families, so people often know that they are at risk for it. It is diagnosed when people develop jerky movements that they cannot control. This movement problem is called *chorea*. Huntington's disease has been called "Huntington's chorea" in the past. People also have thinking problems and emotional changes with the disease. The range of symptoms may include rigid movements, fidgeting, problems with fine motor tasks (such as writing), trouble walking, irritability, anxiety, depression, increasing lack of motivation, impulsivity, and difficulty speaking, eating, and swallowing.

The average age when Huntington's disease is diagnosed is about 40 years—when most people begin to develop the first signs and symptoms. Symptoms of a neurocognitive disorder due to Huntington's disease are as follows:

- The disease begins with few or no symptoms and progresses gradually.
- There is clinically diagnosed Huntington's disease or a risk of the disease based on family history or genetic testing.

## Key Points

- Everyone forgets from time to time. Memory problems can be part of normal aging. They can also result from stress, grief, medication side effects, lack of vitamin $B_{12}$, drug or alcohol use, or medical problems. When the underlying cause is treated or the emotional event has passed, the memory problems often disappear.
- *Dementia* (or *neurocognitive disorder*) describes a decline in mental function that is severe enough to disrupt daily life. It can cause problems with people's memory and how well they think and plan. It is caused by different types of disorders or diseases. Alzheimer's disease is the most common cause of dementia.
- *Delirium* can occur in someone who also has dementia. Unlike the other neurocognitive disorders, delirium is a short-term state of confusion and lack of attention that goes away, while the other neurocognitive disorders persist. Treatment helps pinpoint the cause of delirium and quickens the end of symptoms.

- The neurocognitive disorders are diagnosed as either "major" or "mild" based on the level of decline in mental function. A *major neurocognitive disorder* occurs when someone can no longer do daily mental tasks without help, such as balancing a checkbook or keeping track of medicines. A *mild neurocognitive disorder* occurs when someone can still perform daily mental tasks, but may need extra time, structure, or reminders to complete them.
- Caring for a loved one with dementia can be stressful. It's helpful to know what resources are available; seek help from support groups, family, and friends; practice relaxation techniques; and take time for yourself. Giving kindness, patience, respect, and dignity to the person who has dementia is a key aspect of good care.

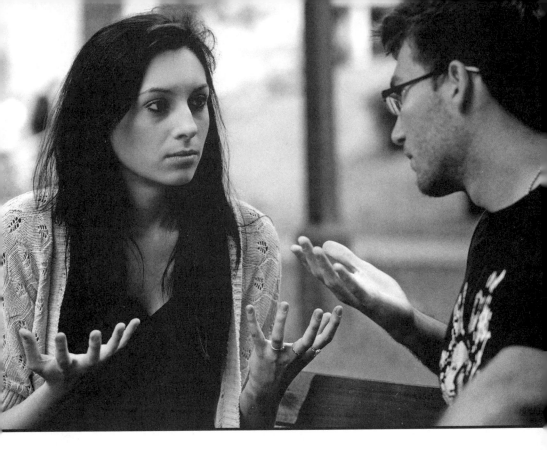

Borderline Personality Disorder

Antisocial Personality Disorder

Schizotypal Personality Disorder

Other Personality Disorders

    Paranoid Personality Disorder

    Schizoid Personality Disorder

    Histrionic Personality Disorder

    Narcissistic Personality Disorder

    Avoidant Personality Disorder

    Dependent Personality Disorder

    Obsessive-Compulsive Personality Disorder

*For a complete list of DSM-5 disorders, see Appendix A.*

# CHAPTER 18

# Personality Disorders

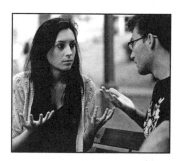

*ersonality* refers to how people behave, their thoughts and views, and how they relate to others. People with a *personality disorder* tend to be often rigid, extreme, and intense in their thoughts and in the way they act. They often are not able to respond in a healthy way to the changes and demands of life. They can be confused or unsure about how to define themselves, they have problems setting and meeting goals, and they find it hard to deal with other people in relationships, at work or school, and in social settings. Many people with these disorders do not realize they are not thinking or acting in a normal way, and they often blame other people for their problems.

All people have *personality traits* that make them unique and different from others. These traits are lasting patterns of how someone tends to think about and relate to his or her own world, others, and self. Some people are outgoing; others are shy. Some people are self-assured; others are more humble. These traits can serve each person well, but if strongly expressed, they can cause some trouble in relationships.

A *personality disorder* reflects deeper, more severe problems that can greatly impair how someone thinks, feels, lives, works, and perceives and loves others. People with personality disorders often have trouble trusting others, and they may ignore their own safety or risk the safety of others. They can behave in harmful ways, sometimes hurting themselves or breaking the law.

## Features of a Personality Disorder

All types of personality disorders have these **common features**:
- A pattern of disturbed behavior that is different in an extreme way from what is expected in a person's culture, as shown in at least two of the following areas:
  - Ways of thinking about self, others, and events.
  - Ways of having and showing feelings in diverse settings. This includes the range and strength of feelings.
  - Ways of relating to other people.
  - Ways of controlling feelings and conduct.
- The pattern is fairly constant across a range of personal and social settings.
- The pattern causes marked distress or problems in social life, work, and other parts of daily life.
- The pattern started in the teen or early adult years.

The behavior is not due to another mental disorder or the effects of a substance or another medical condition.

Personality disorders affect 10%–15% of people. They often begin to develop during childhood, and symptoms emerge during teenage or adult years.

In DSM-5 (as well as the prior DSM), personality disorders are grouped in clusters based on their features and symptoms (Table 1). The personality disorders covered in full detail in this chapter are *antisocial, borderline,* and *schizotypal personality disorders;* other personality disorders are reviewed briefly. Most people who have personality disorders will not have a single "pure" disorder, but will also have features of other personality disorders described in this chapter.

Many people with personality disorders get better over time with treatment. Some improve as they grow older. People with certain types of personality disorders seldom seek treatment on their own. When convinced to seek help, they can often benefit. Treating these disorders mostly involves forms of psychotherapy—often with both individual and group sessions. Many types of psychotherapy work well for people with *borderline personality disorder* (a condition that can be quite disabling and can involve high-risk behavior).

There are no medications approved as the main or sole treatment of any personality disorder. However, medications can be prescribed to treat some of the symptoms. These may include feeling depressed or prone to act on impulse, which are common in people with *borderline personality disorder.* Types of medications that may help symptoms of personality disorders include the following:

| Table 1.  Personality disorders by DSM-5 cluster | |
|---|---|
| **Cluster (or type) and key features** | **Personality disorders** |
| **Cluster A**—appear odd or eccentric (marked by odd or strange thoughts, feelings, or behavior) | Paranoid personality disorder<br>Schizoid personality disorder<br>Schizotypal personality disorder |
| **Cluster B**—appear dramatic, emotional, or erratic (marked by drama, extreme shifts in feelings, and frequent changes in behavior beyond what is normal) | Antisocial personality disorder<br>Borderline personality disorder<br>Histrionic personality disorder<br>Narcissistic personality disorder |
| **Cluster C**—appear anxious or fearful (marked by fear or worry) | Avoidant personality disorder<br>Dependent personality disorder<br>Obsessive-compulsive personality disorder |

- *Antidepressants* can help with low mood or feeling hopeless, guilty, or worthless.
- *Mood stabilizers* can help reduce extreme moods or mood swings from highs to lows.
- *Antipsychotics* may be used to help improve odd thinking, distrust of others, or false beliefs, such as in the case of *schizotypal personality disorder.*

There has been much debate about the concept of personality and how personality disorders are diagnosed. Finding the line between personality traits and personality disorders involves many questions. Personality disorders are complex and the subject of a growing field of research.

# Borderline Personality Disorder

People with *borderline personality disorder* suffer from extreme and frequent mood swings, poor self-image, and problems with relationships. They may have intense bouts of anger or anxiety that last a few hours, beyond the scope of the problem (such as a late friend or canceled meeting). They are not able to be just a *little* sad, a *little* angry, or a *little* worried. Each response is extreme. During these times, people with the disorder can be prone to act on impulse, bring harm to themselves, and ignore the safety of others. These behaviors are not easy for them to prevent or control.

Bonds with family and friends are also strained and stressful because of these extreme changes in mood and behavior. People with borderline personality disorder may profess intense love for someone that can quickly turn to intense anger and hate. This can occur when they believe (often falsely) that others find fault with or do not favor them.

Borderline personality disorder affects about 2% of people, and most of those (about 75%) diagnosed with the condition are women. The rate of those with the disorder may decrease in older age. Symptoms tend to lessen and become more stable in the 30s and 40s.

---

 **Borderline Personality Disorder**

Borderline personality disorder is diagnosed when a pattern of troubled relationships, extreme changes in self-image, and acting on impulse begins by early adulthood, as shown by at least five of the following:

- Frantic efforts to prevent someone from leaving him or her.
- Pattern of unstable and intense relationships (may switch between extremes of loving someone one moment and then hating that person the next).
- A self-image marked by extreme and frequent changes (may switch between great self-confidence and very poor self-esteem).
- Risky behavior prone to impulse and self-damage, such as spending sprees, risky sex, substance abuse, reckless driving, and binge eating.
- Pattern of suicidal behavior or self-injury.

- Intense bouts of sadness or being anxious that last a few hours and only rarely more than a few days.
- Often feeling empty (such as feeling bored, sense of having no meaning or purpose).
- Intense anger beyond the scope of the issue, or problems with anger control (such as frequent physical fights or displays of temper, constant anger).
- Fleeting, stress-induced paranoid thoughts or feelings (may suspect others have bad motives or plans against him or her), or feeling "unreal" or detached from self or the world.

## Risk Factors

Borderline personality disorder runs in families. The disorder is about five times more common among first-degree blood relatives (parent or sibling) of those with the disorder.

### Maria's Story

Maria, a single woman without a job, sought therapy at age 33 for treatment of depressed mood, chronic thoughts of killing herself, and having no social contact for many months. She had spent the last 6 months alone in her apartment, lying in bed, eating junk food, watching TV, and doing more online shopping than she could afford.

Maria was the middle of three children in a wealthy immigrant family. The father was said to value work success over all else. He often cursed at and hit all three children, Maria most of all. She felt alone through her school years and had bouts of feeling depressed. Within her family, she was known for angry outbursts. She had done well in high school but dropped out of college because of problems with a roommate and a professor. She had a series of jobs with the hope that she would return to college, but she kept quitting because "bosses are idiots." These "traumas" always left her feeling bad about herself ("I can't even succeed as a clerk!") and angry at her bosses ("I could run the place better than any of them").

She had dated men when she was younger but after a few weeks of "bliss at finding the perfect partner," she would feel hurt and angry when they did not pay enough attention to her or return her calls fast enough. She would end the relationship before they could "hurt me even more."

Maria sometimes cut herself (would make herself bleed using a knife on purpose) when she was feeling empty and depressed. She said that she was often "down and depressed," but that dozens of times for 1–2 days, she would act on impulse with great risk to her safety. This involved drug abuse and reckless driving. Doing these things would often make her feel better.

She had been in psychiatric treatment since age 17 and had stayed in a psychiatric hospital three times after overdoses. During the session, Maria described shame at her lack of job success. She believed she was very able and simply didn't know why she hadn't done better in life. Toward the end of the first session, she became angry with the doctor after he glanced at the clock (asking him, "Are you bored?"). In terms of social contact, she said she knew people who lived in her building, but most of them had become "frauds or losers." There were a few people from school who were "online friends" on social Web sites who were doing "big things all over the world."

Maria was diagnosed with *borderline personality disorder* and *major depressive disorder*. She could not stay at jobs or in school and has problems with anger control, reckless acts, self-harm (such as cutting), feeling empty, and paranoid thoughts. Maria refused prescribed medications, stating, "When I take those drugs, I have no feelings. I can't even cry at a sad movie." Instead, she was referred for a form of psychotherapy called *dialectical behavior therapy* or DBT. It helps people know and manage their thoughts and feelings and teaches calming methods. DBT helped Maria learn how to feel more in control of her extreme feelings, as well as when she felt empty or paranoid. She learned skills to stop judging herself and others. After many months, she was able to get and keep a job. She was slowly able to have more healthy friendships with both women and men, but still struggled at times to get along with others.

# Antisocial Personality Disorder

People with *antisocial personality disorder* ignore or infringe on the rights of others and may also break the law. Often from early childhood, they have had lives of abuse and neglect. They have learned to expect the world to be that way. They tend not to have remorse or regret for their actions—which can include fighting, lying, cheating, and stealing—because they see these acts as needed to survive.

In relationships, those with antisocial personality disorder often show contempt for others' feelings, hardships, and pain that they may have caused. They may abuse their partners, have many partners, and act without regard for safe sex. They may neglect their children, who may not receive enough food, clothing, bathing, or other care and comfort. They may be charming talkers but can also suffer from tension, boredom, and *depressive, anxiety, substance use*, and *gambling disorders*.

About 1% of adults in the United States have been diagnosed with antisocial personality disorder, and it is more common in men. More than 70% of those with *alcohol use disorder* or in prison may have this disorder. People with this disorder tend to show the most extreme behaviors when they are younger. They often have fewer symptoms as they get older—usually around age 40.

People with antisocial personality disorder often do not agree or believe that they have any problem. They often do not seek treatment. Their behaviors may be reduced in settings where there is great discipline, structure, and rules that prevent them from making bad choices.

 ## Antisocial Personality Disorder

Since age 15, a person with antisocial personality disorder ignores or breaches the rights of others as a common way of life, as shown by at least three of the following antisocial behaviors:

- Fails to follow social norms and laws, as shown by frequent acts that are grounds for arrest.
- Lies, uses fake names, or cons others for profit or pleasure.
- Lacks impulse control and fails to plan ahead.
- Is quickly annoyed, angry, and hostile, as shown by frequent fights or assaults.
- Lacks concern or care for the safety of self or others.
- Often shirks or ignores major duties, as shown by frequent failure to hold a job or pay debts.
- Lacks remorse (doesn't care about hurting, mistreating, or stealing from others).

In addition to the above, the person must meet each of these standards for the disorder:

- Is at least 18 years old.
- Shows signs of *conduct disorder* before age 15 (this involves breaking rules at home and school, or breaching the rights of others, such as skipping school, fighting, or stealing).
- Displays antisocial behavior outside an episode of *bipolar disorder* or *schizophrenia*.

# Risk Factors

Antisocial personality disorder runs in families. People with a first-degree blood relative (parent or sibling) with the disorder are at a higher risk. The risk appears to be greater for family members of women with the disorder compared to family members of men with the disorder.

# Liam's Story

Liam was a 32-year-old man referred for mental health treatment by the human resources (HR) department of a large construction firm where he had worked for 2 weeks. Before he began working there, Liam appeared very eager and gave proof of two carpentry school degrees that showed a high level of skill and training. Once Liam was employed, his boss noted he was often absent, argued with other workers, did poor work, and made mistakes that might have harmed others. When approached about these problems, Liam was not concerned, blaming the issues on "cheap wood" and "bad management" and said that if someone got hurt, "it's because they're stupid."

When the head of HR tried to fire Liam, he quickly pointed out that he had both attention-deficit/hyperactivity disorder (ADHD) and bipolar disorder. He said that if not granted a waiver under the law, he would sue. He demanded a psychiatric evaluation.

During the mental health exam, Liam focused on how the firm was unfair and on how he was "a better carpenter than anyone else there." Twice divorced, he claimed that his two marriages had ended because of his wives' envy and doubt. He said that they were "always thinking I was with other women," which is why "they both lied to judges and got restraining orders saying I'd hit them." As payback for the jail time because he broke the judges' orders, he refused to pay child support for his two children. He had no desire to see either of his two boys because they were "little liars" like their mothers.

Liam said he "must have been smart" because he made Cs in school despite showing up only half the time. He spent time in a jail for youth at age 14 for stealing "kid stuff, like tennis shoes and wallets that were almost empty." He left school at age 15 after being "framed for stealing a car" by his principal. Liam said he smoked marijuana as a teen and started drinking alcohol on a "regular basis" after he first got married at age 22. He denied that use of either substance was a problem.

Liam ended the exam by telling the doctor to write a note that he had "bipolar" and "ADHD." He said that he was "bipolar" because he had "ups and downs" and got "mad real fast." He learned about ADHD because "both of my boys got it." He ended the exam with a demand for medications, adding that the only ones that worked for him were the "stimulant" medicines that his sons also received for ADHD.

The head of HR did a background check during the psychiatric evaluation, which revealed that Liam had been expelled from two carpentry training programs and that both his degrees were fakes. He had been fired from one local construction firm after a fistfight with his boss and from a second firm after leaving a job site. A quick review of their records showed that he had given them the same false papers. There was also a report that he tried to sell prescribed medicines to his coworkers for cash.

Liam was diagnosed with *antisocial personality disorder.* He has been arrested twice for partner violence—once from each marriage—and has spent time in jail. Liam has faked his carpentry degrees and gives ample

Understanding Mental Disorders

proof of frequent fights and quickness to anger, both at work and within his relationships. He has no desire to see either of his young sons and neglects paying any child support. He shows no remorse for how his actions harm or deceive his family, coworkers, or employers. He often quits jobs and fails to plan ahead for his next one. He meets all seven symptoms for antisocial personality disorder.

# Schizotypal Personality Disorder

People with *schizotypal personality disorder* are often described as being odd, strange, or quirky. They tend to distrust others and have bizarre beliefs. For instance, they may believe they have special powers to control others, read other people's minds, or predict events before they happen. They may seem stiff or awkward to others because their feelings are hard for them to manage.

They have few, if any, close ties other than with their parents or siblings. They prefer to keep to themselves because they feel they do not "fit in." It is hard for them to pick up on social cues, such as eye contact. As they spend more time in a social setting, they tend not to become more relaxed around others. Instead, they grow more tense and have more distrust of those around them. As children or teens, they may be often alone, may attract teasing because they appear odd to others, may be prone to social anxiety, may do poorly in school, and may have strange thoughts, language, and daydreams. They may have unusual interests, such as learning about the paranormal (spirit world) or telepathy (using thoughts to communicate with other people).

About 1% of the population may have this disorder. The disorder can first appear in children or teens and may be slightly more common in males. Between 30% and 50% of people with schizotypal personality disorder also suffer from *major depressive disorder.*

Some cultures or faiths have customs that are normal and accepted within these groups but that might be seen as schizotypal traits by those from outside. These customs might include mind reading or speaking in tongues. In these settings, the disorder would not be diagnosed.

---

 **Schizotypal Personality Disorder**

Schizotypal personality disorder involves a lasting pattern of impaired social contact as shown by extreme unease with—and reduced capacity for—close bonds, and includes odd thoughts and behavior and an altered sense of what is real. The pattern starts by early adulthood and is present in a range of settings, as shown by at least five of the following:

- Thoughts that daily, chance events have special meaning or contain a certain message for oneself, when they do not.
- Odd beliefs that one has special powers (such as sensing events before they happen, reading other people's minds, controlling other people through one's own thoughts).
- Strange events perceived through the senses (such as sensing another person is in the room who is not, or hearing a voice saying one's name).
- Odd thinking and speech (such as speech that is vague or marked by tangents, strange phrasing or ways of linking words).
- Distrust of others or their motives (such as beliefs that others intend to harm oneself or damage one's status at work).
- Flat emotions or responses that do not fit the setting or event.
- Behavior or appearance that is outside social norms (such as not making eye contact, often wearing soiled or stained clothing when clean clothing exists).
- Lack of close friends outside close family.
- Extreme social anxiety that does not go away in known settings and is caused by distrust rather than downbeat judgments about oneself.

The pattern of behavior does not occur during the course of *schizophrenia* or a *bipolar, depressive, other psychotic,* or *autism spectrum disorder.*

## Risk Factors

Schizotypal personality disorder runs in families. People with a first-degree blood relative (parent or sibling) who has *schizophrenia* are at a higher risk.

# Other Personality Disorders

Other personality disorders can be diagnosed. These include *paranoid, schizoid, histrionic, narcissistic, avoidant, dependent,* and *obsessive-compulsive personality disorders.* These disorders are diagnosed when behaviors linked to the disorder begin by early adult years, are present in a range of home and social settings, and cause great distress or impair social, work, or other key aspects of function.

## Paranoid Personality Disorder

People with *paranoid personality disorder* distrust others and suspect their motives. They view the actions of other people as a threat, even those who are close to them or whom they see daily. Without any reason, they may question spouses, friends, and fellow workers to see if they can be trusted and are loyal. They can be hard to get along with and look for clues to support their fears. They may argue, complain, blame others for their own faults or mistakes, and try to control those around them. They can be guarded, hostile, and aloof, keeping their thoughts and feelings to themselves. The disorder is diagnosed when at least four of the following are present:

- Suspects, without reason, that others exploit, harm, or deceive him or her.
- Is fixed on needless doubts about whether friends or fellow workers are loyal.
- Is slow to confide in others due to needless fears of spiteful or unjust use of the information.
- Reads hidden insults or threats into harmless remarks or events.
- Holds lasting grudges (does not forgive insults or slights).
- Believes others attack his or her honor and standing when it is clear to others that this is not the case, and is quick to react with anger.
- Often suspects, without reason, that a spouse or sexual partner is cheating on him or her.

Symptoms do not occur during a time of *schizophrenia, bipolar* or *depressive disorder,* or another *psychotic disorder,* and are not due to another medical condition.

## Schizoid Personality Disorder

People with a *schizoid personality disorder* seem to lack a desire for close bonds with other people, are detached, and have a reduced range of feelings. They are the extreme loners. Praise or insults seem not to affect them. Anger may be hard for them to express, even if provoked. They may seem to drift through life without goals and seem passive to life events. They have few friends, often do not marry, and work well when they are left alone. They tend to seek out jobs where they have little contact with people, and they may do very well in these jobs. The disorder is diagnosed when at least four of the following are present:

- Neither desires nor enjoys close bonds with others, even if family.
- Almost always chooses to do things alone.
- Has little, if any, desire for sex with another person.
- Enjoys few, if any, activities.
- Lacks close friends other than first-degree blood relatives (parents, siblings).

- Appears not to care whether others praise, find fault, or insult him or her.
- Appears cold or detached, without any feelings.

Symptoms do not occur during a time of *schizophrenia, bipolar* or *depressive disorder*, another *psychotic disorder*, or *autism spectrum disorder*, and are not due to another medical condition.

## Histrionic Personality Disorder

People with *histrionic personality disorder* display frequent, extreme feelings and seek constant notice or attention. The word *histrionic* means "dramatic or theatrical." Those with this disorder seek constant approval and use their looks, flirting, and other means to draw notice to themselves. Although it can and does occur in men, histrionic personality disorder is diagnosed more often in women. People with this disorder are trapped in the present and consumed with getting just what they want, at the exact moment that they want it. They see their needs as more worthy than those of others. They may become depressed and upset when they are not the center of attention. The disorder is diagnosed when at least five of the following are present:

- Is not at ease or feels less valued when outside the center of attention.
- Relates to others by flirting or trying to seduce when it is not proper.
- Changes feelings quickly.
- Uses physical appearance to draw attention to himself or herself (such as spending much time and money on grooming, hair, makeup, fancy clothing).
- Has a style of speech that is very vague and lacks detail or facts.
- Acts with extreme feelings and public displays of emotion and drama even with people not known well (such as nonstop sobbing, temper tantrums).
- Is easily swayed by others, current fads, or changes in events.
- Thinks of ties with others as closer and of more value than they actually are (for instance, someone met just once is a "dear, dear friend").

## Narcissistic Personality Disorder

People with *narcissistic personality disorder* believe that they are more important and talented than other people and that other people should admire them. They tend to have little or no concern for the needs of other people. They expect to be praised and feel they are owed rewards that others may get. They tend to take more credit than they deserve for success, and they don't admit or give credit to those who deserve it. They may not be aware that their remarks can hurt others (such as boasting of health in front of someone who is sick). Despite high success, their work can suffer because they will not accept critiques to adjust or improve their work. The disorder is diagnosed when at least five of the following are present:

- Inflates talents and success and expects to be noticed as better than others.
- Is absorbed with notions of his or her own great and endless success, power, genius, beauty, or ideal love.
- Believes he or she is "special" and unique, and can only be known by or relate to other special or high-status people.
- Requires others to admire him or her on a constant basis.
- Believes he or she deserves or is owed special treatment (such as not needing to wait in lines) or that others should comply quickly with his or her demands.
- Exploits (takes advantage of) others to achieve his or her goals.
- Lacks concern or does not notice others' feelings or needs.
- Envies others' success or rewards, or believes that others envy him or her.
- Shows an arrogant (haughty, snobbish) behavior and/or attitude.

## Avoidant Personality Disorder

People with *avoidant personality disorder* have extreme shyness, often feel inadequate (not good enough), are quickly hurt by rejection (being unwanted or turned away), and shun closeness or contact with others because of these feelings and fears. When in social settings, a person with avoidant personality disorder may be afraid to speak up for fear of saying the wrong thing or being shamed, teased, or put down. They greatly desire to be liked and to enjoy social contacts, but their extreme fears and shyness keep them from reaching out to others. The disorder is diagnosed when at least four of the following are present:

- Avoids work that requires social contact because of fears that others will criticize (find fault) or reject him or her.
- Avoids getting involved with people unless certain of being liked.
- Is restrained in close relationships because of the fear of being shamed or mocked.
- Greatly concerned about being criticized or rejected in social settings.

- Shy in new settings because of feelings of inadequacy (not being good enough).
- Feels inept or inferior to others (low self-esteem).
- Doesn't take risks to engage in new social contacts or other pursuits (such as looking for a new job) for fear of being ashamed.

## Dependent Personality Disorder

People with *dependent personality disorder* have a constant and extreme need to be taken care of that leads to meek and clinging behaviors and fears of separation (being parted from another person). They have an extreme need for support and being nurtured. They are passive and have trouble making daily choices (such as what color shirt to wear to work) without getting advice from someone else. They believe they cannot function on their own and must depend on someone else. They rely on others to solve their problems and often do not learn skills to live on their own. From early adulthood, they have a profound fear that the person they depend on will leave them. The disorder is diagnosed when at least five of the following are present:

- Has problems making daily choices without getting advice and support from others.
- Needs others to take charge of most major areas of his or her life.
- Does not express thoughts that differ from others for fear of losing support or approval.
- Has problems starting projects or doing things on his or her own because of lack of self-confidence.
- Goes to extremes to get support and care from others (may offer to do unpleasant tasks or withstand abuse if doing so seems to secure desired care).
- Feels distressed or helpless when alone because of fears that he or she cannot care for himself or herself.
- Quickly seeks a new close relationship for care and support when the prior one ends.
- Maintains extreme focus on fears of being left to take care of himself or herself.

## Obsessive-Compulsive Personality Disorder

People with *obsessive-compulsive personality disorder* are obsessed with order, being perfect, and controlling their own thoughts and the behavior of others who relate to them. As a result, they cannot accept unplanned changes and are not open to help from others unless things are done their way. They can become angry when they are not in control. They are often unable to express warm or tender feelings. The disorder is diagnosed when at least four of the following are present:

- Is absorbed with details, rules, lists, order, and schedules to the extent that the major point of the task is lost.
- Hinders or stops a project because his or her extreme and strict standards are not met (for instance, staying so focused on making each detail perfect that the project is never finished).
- Consumed by work and productivity at the expense of leisure pursuits and friendships (for instance, does not take a day off to go on an outing, does not relax on the weekend).
- Holds extreme, high moral and ethical standards (and may force others to follow these rigid rules).
- Cannot throw away worn-out or worthless objects even when they have no sentimental value.
- Is slow to give tasks or work to others unless they follow his or her way of doing things.
- Adopts a stingy spending style (frugal with self and others) and lives far below what he or she can afford in case of future bad events.
- Is rigid and stubborn.

## Key Points

- *Personality* refers to how people behave, their thoughts and views, and how they relate to others. All people have *personality traits* that make each person unique. These traits are lasting patterns of how someone tends to think about and relate to his or her own world, others, and self. Personality traits can sometimes cause problems that need to be worked out to improve bonds with others.
- A *personality disorder* reflects deeper, more severe problems that can deeply impair how someone thinks, feels, lives, works, and perceives and loves others. Many people with these disorders do not realize they may be thinking or acting in harmful ways that are not normal. They often blame others for problems they have created.
- Many people with personality disorders get better over time with treatment. Some improve as they grow older. People with certain types of personality disorders seldom seek treatment on their own. When convinced to seek help, they can often benefit.
- Treating these disorders mostly involves forms of psychotherapy— often with both individual and group sessions. There are no medica-

tions approved as the main or sole treatment of any personality disorder. However, medications can be prescribed to treat some of the symptoms that a person with a personality disorder may have, such as feeling depressed or prone to act on impulse.

- A mental health care provider can also help people in close or frequent contact with someone who has a personality disorder. Therapy can help them to know themselves and the other person better, and find healthy ways to cope.

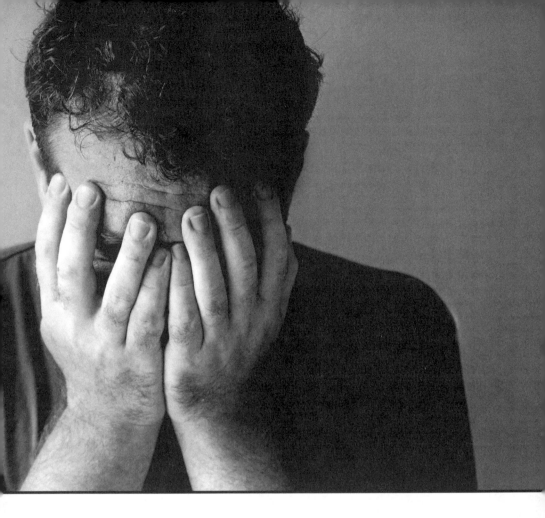

Voyeuristic Disorder

Exhibitionistic Disorder

Frotteuristic Disorder

Sexual Masochism Disorder

Sexual Sadism Disorder

Pedophilic Disorder

Fetishistic Disorder

Transvestic Disorder

---

*For a complete list of DSM-5 disorders, see Appendix A.*

# CHAPTER 19

# Paraphilic Disorders

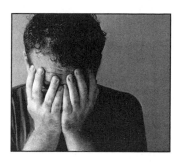

**P**eople who have a *paraphilia* have a sexual interest or preference outside the sexual norm (genital stimulation or fondling acts with a mature partner who gives consent). The paraphilia tends to exclude actual sexual intercourse and does not cause harm or distress to self or others. Many types of paraphilias exist, and a person can have more than one type. Having a paraphilia does not by itself lead to a paraphilic disorder.

People with *paraphilic disorders* have a paraphilia that causes distress; impairs work, social, or other key functions; or causes harm or risk of harm to self or others. These disorders often involve repeated, intense sexual fantasies and urges that the person then enacts in real life. Some of the paraphilic disorders are crimes because they risk harm to those who have not given consent for the action. Harm includes physical pain and mental anguish, torment, or distress. People with these disorders devote great time and energy to satisfying their sexual preference, and it may well cause problems in their job, marriage, and other aspects of life.

The eight paraphilic disorders in DSM-5 are discussed in this chapter:

- *Voyeuristic disorder* (watching others engage in private acts without their consent).
- *Exhibitionistic disorder* (exposing one's genitals to someone who has not given consent).
- *Frotteuristic disorder* (touching or rubbing against a person who has not given consent).
- *Sexual masochism disorder* (seeking pain or humiliation for sexual arousal).

- *Sexual sadism disorder* (causing hurt or humiliation for sexual arousal).
- *Pedophilic disorder* (forcing children to engage in sexual activities because of sexual arousal for children).
- *Fetishistic disorder* (using nonliving objects for sexual arousal or having a highly specific focus on nongenital body parts).
- *Transvestic disorder* (dressing in the clothes of the opposite gender for sexual arousal).

## Treatment

People with these disorders can receive treatment that helps improve their day-to-day function. Paraphilic disorders are mostly treated with psychotherapy to help the person be aware of his or her thoughts and behaviors and to regain control over them. This may involve cognitive-behavior therapy (CBT). CBT helps the person gain control over his or her interests and acts, and to achieve goals in healthy ways. Relaxation training is often a part of the therapy to help lower the anxiety and stress that the paraphilic disorder may cause. Relapse prevention techniques help the person avoid falling back into an unhealthy or harmful cycle of inappropriate sexual behavior. These techniques also may help target problems with eating, sleeping, and social function.

There are no medications approved to treat paraphilic disorders, but these disorders are often linked with depression or anxiety that may benefit from treatment. Treatment for these symptoms may include one of the selective serotonin reuptake inhibitor (SSRI) antidepressants. Because *depressive* or *anxiety disorders* may help fuel the paraphilic disorder, treating these disorders is an important first step in helping the person regain control over his or her desires and behavior. The SSRIs also may help to reduce the fantasies and urges that can fuel the paraphilic disorder. In some cases, medications that lower testosterone (hormone) levels are sometimes given to men whose sexual behavior is out of control and could cause harm to others.

## Voyeuristic Disorder

People with *voyeuristic disorder* are sexually aroused by spying on another person who is naked, undressing, or having sex. *Voyeurism* (or "peeping") is the most common law-breaking sexual behavior—about 12% of men and 4% of women have the disorder at some point in their lives. (Men are three times as likely as women to have the disorder.)

**Voyeuristic Disorder**

- For at least 6 months, there has been repeated and intense sexual arousal—as shown in fantasies, urges, or behaviors—from watching an unsuspecting person who is naked, undressing, or engaging in sexual activity.
- The person has acted on these sexual urges without consent of the person watched, or the sexual urges or fantasies cause much distress or impair social, work, or other key aspects of function.
- The person who is aroused or acting on the urges is at least 18 years old.

# Exhibitionistic Disorder

People with *exhibitionistic disorder* expose their genitals to strangers (children or adults) who have not given consent for this act. This is often referred to as "flashing." Those with exhibitionistic disorder make up about one-third of the sexual offenders who are referred for mental health treatment. About 2%–4% of men have the disorder, and it is rare in women. People with the disorder often are not dangerous and do not attempt sexual activity with the persons to whom they expose themselves.

 **Exhibitionistic Disorder**

- For at least 6 months, there has been repeated and intense sexual arousal—as shown in fantasies, urges, or behaviors—from exposing one's genitals to an unsuspecting (unaware) person.
- The person has acted on these sexual urges without consent of the other person, or the sexual urges or fantasies cause much distress or impair social, work, or other key aspects of function.

# Frotteuristic Disorder

People with *frotteuristic disorder* touch or rub against others without their consent. This often happens in crowded places, such as a busy sidewalk or subway car, and includes touching someone's genitals or breasts. Men ages 15–25 years who are often lonely and passive have higher rates of the disorder. The disorder is rare in women.

**Frotteuristic Disorder**

- For at least 6 months, there has been repeated and intense sexual arousal—as shown in fantasies, urges, or behaviors—from touching or rubbing against a person who has not given consent.
- The person has acted on these sexual urges without consent of the other person, or the sexual urges or fantasies cause much distress or impair social, work, or other key aspects of function.

# Sexual Masochism Disorder

*Sexual masochism disorder* involves getting sexually aroused when being beaten, bound, humiliated, or otherwise made to suffer. People with the disorder may also inflict pain on themselves by choking or pricking themselves with sharp objects. Sexual acts may occur with a partner and include being tied up, spanked, or whipped. One dangerous form of masochism involves cutting off oxygen by tying a noose around one's neck or putting a plastic bag over one's face. There is a risk of accidental death with these acts.

 **Sexual Masochism Disorder**

- For at least 6 months, there has been repeated and intense sexual arousal—as shown in fantasies, urges, or behaviors—from being humiliated, beaten, bound (tied up), or made to suffer in other ways.
- The fantasies, sexual urges, or behaviors cause much distress or impair social, work, or other key aspects of function.

# Sexual Sadism Disorder

People with *sexual sadism disorder* get sexually excited by causing pain, suffering, or humiliation in another person. The behavior may involve causing physical harm or mental anguish. People with sexual sadism disorder want complete control over a terrified victim or a partner who has not given consent.

**Sexual Sadism Disorder**

- For at least 6 months, there has been repeated and intense sexual arousal—as shown in fantasies, urges, or behaviors—from the physical or mental suffering of another person.
- The person has acted on these sexual urges without consent of the other person, or the sexual urges or fantasies cause much distress or impair social, work, or other key aspects of function.

# Pedophilic Disorder

People with *pedophilic disorder* have a strong sexual interest in or sexual preference for children and have acted on these urges. Most pedophiles are heterosexual. Use of pornography that features young children (generally age 13 years and younger) is a strong sign of the disorder, because it reflects sexual interest. When a person acts on this interest or urge and engages in sexual activity with a child, it is a criminal act.

 **Pedophilic Disorder**

- For at least 6 months, repeated, intense sexually arousing fantasies, sexual urges, or behaviors involving sexual activity with a child (generally age 13 years or younger) have been present.
- The person has acted on these sexual urges, or the sexual urges or fantasies cause much distress or relationship problems.
- The person is at least 16 years old and at least 5 years older than the child or children involved in the act.

# Fetishistic Disorder

People with *fetishistic disorder* become sexually excited by objects, such as women's underwear, rubber articles, and men's or women's shoes. A fetish (sexual fixation) also may involve a body part, such as feet, toes, and hair. Having contact with these objects (for instance, through holding, tasting, or rubbing) often leads to intense arousal and masturbation.

Some people with the disorder may have a large collection of desired objects. Sexual dysfunction may occur when the object is not present. The person may prefer sexual activity with the object more than sexual activity with a partner. It is rare for women to have this disorder.

##  Fetishistic Disorder

- For at least 6 months, there has been repeated and intense sexual arousal—as shown in fantasies, urges, or behaviors—from either using nonliving objects or a highly specific focus on nongenital body part(s).
- The fantasies, sexual urges, or behaviors cause much distress or impair social, work, or other key aspects of function.
- The fetish objects are not limited to articles of clothing used in cross-dressing or devices designed for genital stimulation (such as a vibrator).

 ## Leonard's Story

Leonard, a 65-year-old salesman for a large firm, had a psychiatric evaluation after his wife threatened to leave him. Although he said he was embarrassed to discuss his issues with a stranger, he described his sexual interest in women's undergarments in a matter-of-fact manner. This interest had begun several years earlier and had not been a problem until he was caught masturbating by his wife 6 weeks before the evaluation.

Upon seeing him dressed in panties and a bra, she "went nuts," thinking he was having an affair. After he clarified that he was not seeing anyone else, she "shut him out" and hardly spoke to him. When they argued, she called him a "pervert" and made it clear that she was considering divorce unless he "got help."

Leonard's habit began with his wife's severe arthritis and likely depression, both of which reduced her overall activity and interest in sex. His "fetish" was the bright spot during his frequent and otherwise dreary business trips. He also masturbated at home but waited until his wife was out of the house. He masturbated about twice weekly, using bras and panties that he had collected over several years. He said that intercourse with his wife had faded to "every month or two" but was mutually satisfying.

Leonard had been married for over 30 years, and the couple had two grown children. He had planned to retire comfortably later that year, but not if the two choices were either to "split the assets or to sit around the house and be called a pervert all day." He had made a show of throwing away a half dozen pieces of underwear, which had seemed to reassure his wife, but he had saved his "favorites" and "could always buy more." He did not want to end his marriage, but he saw nothing harmful in his fetish. "I'm not unfaithful or doing anything bad," he says. "It just excites me, and my wife certainly doesn't want to be having sex a few times a week."

Leonard denied any problems with his sexual function, adding that he could maintain erections and achieve orgasm without women's undergarments. He recalled being aroused when he touched women's underwear in his teenage years and had masturbated often to that experience. That fantasy had stopped when he became sexually active with his wife.

Leonard was diagnosed with *fetishistic disorder*. He has a several-year history of sexual arousal from women's underwear. His behavior caused him no problems until he was caught wearing women's underwear by his wife. At that point, Leonard began to feel distress. If his wife accepted or embraced his fetish and his own distress faded, he would likely no longer have a disorder.

Leonard was referred to an expert in sexual disorders. In therapy, Leonard learned that while the fetish harmed no one, it distressed his wife, who felt that he had lost interest in her. Leonard was encouraged to better communicate with his wife, and to focus on satisfying their mutual sexual needs. Leonard was still aroused by women's undergarments, but learned to make these fantasies a part of his sexual relationship with his wife.

# Transvestic Disorder

People with *transvestic disorder* become sexually aroused from dressing in the other gender's clothing (cross-dressing). It often involves a man wearing only one or two articles of women's clothing (such as underwear), or it can involve dressing completely in a woman's inner and outer garments, as well as wigs and makeup. Transvestic disorders tend to begin in childhood or early teenage years.

---

 **Transvestic Disorder**

- For at least 6 months, there has been repeated and intense sexual arousal—as shown in fantasies, urges, or behaviors—from cross-dressing.
- The fantasies, sexual urges, or behaviors cause much distress or impair social, work, or other key aspects of function.

---

# Key Points

- A *paraphilia* is an intense sexual interest or preference that differs from genital stimulation or fondling acts with a mature, consenting person. Many types of paraphilias exist and having a paraphilia does not by itself lead to a paraphilic disorder.

- People with *paraphilic disorders* have a paraphilia that causes distress; impairs work, social, or other key functions; or causes harm or risk of harm to self or others. These disorders often involve repeated, intense sexual fantasies and urges that the person then enacts in real life. Some of the paraphilic disorders are crimes because they risk harm to those who have not given consent for the action. Harm includes physical pain and mental anguish, torment, or distress.

- People with these disorders can receive treatment that helps improve their day-to-day function. Paraphilic disorders are mostly treated with psychotherapy to help the person be aware of his or her thoughts and behaviors and to regain control over them. This often involves cognitive-behavior therapy.

- For some paraphilic disorders, psychotherapy can help to focus on the other partner and satisfying the partner's sexual needs. A paraphilia may still exist, but in some cases it may be used as a healthy part of sexual relationships.

- There are no medications approved to treat paraphilic disorders, but these disorders are often linked with depression or anxiety that may benefit from treatment. Because *depressive* or *anxiety disorders* may help fuel the paraphilic disorder, treating these disorders is an important first step in helping the person regain control over his or her desires and behavior.

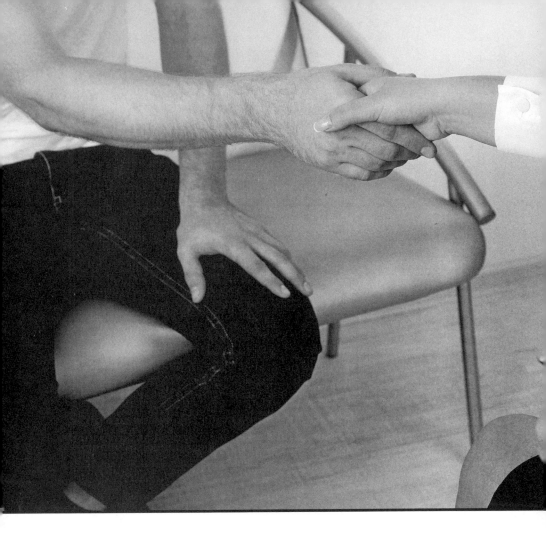

*For a complete list of DSM-5 disorders, see Appendix A.*

# CHAPTER 20

# Treatment Essentials

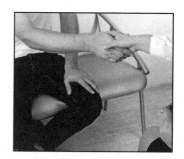

**M**ental illness, just like other medical disorders, can be treated with success. Treatment can bring relief from distress, improved symptoms, better coping with problems, and most of all, hope and support. All of the mental disorders in this book can be treated using one of the methods described in this chapter.

How does someone know when to seek help? A rule of thumb is to think about how much a problem has caused trouble or bothered someone, and how long it has lasted. When these problems cause great distress or disrupt work, social ties, or other key aspects of life, it is wise to seek help. What makes mental disorders differ from the normal problems of daily life is how extreme they are and how long they last. The quicker people know they have a problem that needs help (see box for warning signs) and seek treatment, the sooner their symptoms can improve and recovery can begin.

## Who Can Help

There are several types of mental health care and other health care providers who can help.

- *Psychiatrists* are licensed medical doctors who have finished medical school, as well as a 1-year internship that includes medicine and neurology (study of the human brain), and a 3-year psychiatric residency. The residency program gives in-depth training in psychopharmacology (how medicines work in the body and brain), psychotherapy ("talk therapy"), and patient care in hospitals and clinics. A psychiatrist can prescribe medication for patients and may suggest a psychologist, licensed clinical social worker, or marriage and family therapist for psychotherapy. People can have psychotherapy with the nonmedical mental health care provider but also consult the psychiatrist, who determines the need for medication, ensures that it is working, and monitors for side effects or medical complications.
- *Psychologists* have finished a graduate program, which includes clinical training, an internship, and postdoctoral clinical experience (client care) in various forms of psychotherapy and psychological testing. They cannot prescribe medications or admit people to hospitals in most states. States require that psychologists be licensed in order to treat clients. The degree is either a Ph.D. or Psy.D. Some specialize in treating children or families.

- *Licensed clinical social workers* have finished a 2-year graduate program in specialized training helping people with mental health problems in addition to conventional social work. Some social workers also have doctorate degrees. To practice, they must be licensed by a state.
- *Marriage and family therapists* are licensed in some, but not all, states and have a graduate or doctoral degree in psychology or a similar field. To practice, they must have at least 2 years of postdegree supervised clinical training with a focus on couples and family treatment. They must also pass a state or national exam.
- *Psychiatric nurses* have nursing degrees and have passed a state examination. They usually have special training and experience in mental health care although no special licensing or certification is required.
- *Nurse-practitioners* and *physician assistants* can treat patients and prescribe medications under the general supervision of a doctor.

To find a mental health care provider, ask for names from your doctor, other mental health care providers you may know, or friends who know of mental health care providers. Some of the support groups listed in Appendix C, "Helpful Resources," may be able to suggest names. If you have health insurance, you can ask for a list of mental health care providers who accept your insurance.

People may also seek help from their primary care doctor or a physician assistant when they have health problems. These health problems (such as problems with sleep) might be linked to a mental disorder. Primary care doctors and physician assistants may team up with mental health care providers to provide care and may also refer their patients to a mental health care provider.

# What Happens Next

The usual way of making first contact with a mental health care provider is to call his or her office to schedule an appointment. Some mental health care providers may want some background information before the visit.

## Interview

The first visit involves an "interview" with the mental health care provider. He or she will talk with you to learn about yourself and the problems you are having. Mental health care providers will ask questions to invite you to discuss your problem. Just as a doctor may ask patients about their health problems, a mental health care provider will have the same approach. This information helps the mental health care provider create a unique treatment plan for you. The first visit may last 45–90 minutes. Some common questions during a first visit include the following:

- What brings you here today?
- How have you been feeling?
- What do you think has caused your problem, if anything?
- What symptoms are bothering you?
- What problems have they caused?

Based on your problems and symptoms, mental health care providers also will ask about the following topics: family history, work history, education, leisure activities or hobbies, relationships, values, cultural background, medical history, past psychiatric history (if any, such as whether other mental health care providers were seen in the past), developmental history, and sexual history.

The mental health care provider may ask permission to obtain more information (such as medical records) and suggest psychological or lab tests. You may be asked to schedule a physical exam with your primary care doctor if prescribed medications for a mental disorder are needed—or if a medical disorder needs to be ruled out that may be causing the psychiatric symptoms. In some cases, a diagnosis or an initial assessment will require another one or two sessions, and sometimes the mental health care provider will request permission to interview a partner or family member.

## Diagnosis

The mental health care provider will diagnose the problem based on DSM-5 guidelines. The mental health care provider can then form a treatment plan. DSM-5 guidelines do not resolve whether a person needs or would benefit from treatment. The mental health care provider and the person seeking care make this decision.

More than one disorder may be diagnosed, such as *panic disorder* and *agoraphobia*. Many people with mental disorders often have a *substance use disorder*. People may turn to alcohol or drugs to ease the pain they feel. In some cases, the alcohol or drugs may cause a mental disorder, worsen its symptoms, hinder progress and efforts to get better, and disrupt effects of other medications taken for the disorder.

## Treatment

Treatment for mental health care and mental disorders is offered in a range of settings. The most common is an outpatient primary care or psychiatric clinic (that is, a mental health care provider's office or a clinic).

People who pose an urgent risk for harming themselves or others, or who are gravely disabled, may need care in a hospital. Sometimes this type of care is given involuntarily (against their will), often for a period of 3 days, for their or others' safety. This is allowed only if they are too ill to make safe decisions or accept needed care. After that time, a hearing in court with a judge and two doctors then decides if they should remain in the hospital or be discharged (this process may vary by state). If they remain gravely ill, or still are a threat to themselves or others, they may stay in the hospital involuntarily for a longer period of care and then are reevaluated in court. The hearing is in court to protect patients' civil liberties.

After hospital care, patients may be referred to a partial hospitalization service connected with an inpatient psychiatric unit. These programs provide daily treatment on a one-on-one basis with a psychiatrist and other mental health care providers, as well as group therapy. This type of care lasts until patients improve enough to be referred to a psychiatric outpatient clinic—often for about 2–4 weeks.

Left untreated, a mental disorder can increase the risk for suicide. For this reason, those who have these thoughts and feelings, their family members, and their loved ones should learn about suicide risk and warning signs. Thoughts and feelings about suicide should not be ignored. The following tips can help (see box).

# Forms of Treatment

There are many treatment options to help improve and relieve symptoms of mental disorders (Table 1). Treatment helps people cope with mental disorders and lead a full life. The main types of treatment include medication and psychotherapy ("talk therapy"). Medications and psychotherapy may be used alone or together. Psychotherapy can also help loved ones know how to better care for those with a disorder and to better cope with the impact of the disorder. Electroconvulsive therapy (ECT) and transcranial magnetic stimulation (TMS) are safe and helpful treatments when medications have not worked for severe symptoms of certain disorders.

For many disorders, medication can ease symptoms. As people start to improve with use of psychiatric medications, other problems may surface that may have been hidden or were not the main cause of concern in seeking treatment (such as how they relate to others). People may be able to give more focus to other behaviors they see that have added to their problems and need to change. Psychotherapy can help people learn how to better cope and think about their problems. In the process of treatment, even those who have endured trauma or years of suffering often discover within themselves strengths they may have never known. As they work toward recovery, they can learn more gratifying ways of living and acting and rebuild self-esteem.

## Psychotherapy

*Psychotherapy* ("talk therapy") refers to any type of counseling based on the exchange of words in the context of the unique relationship that develops between a mental health care provider and a person seeking help. The process of talking and listening can lead to new insights, relief from symptoms that cause distress, changes in unhealthy or maladaptive behaviors, and more effective ways of dealing with the world.

| Table 1. Treatments for mental disorders | |
|---|---|
| Psychotherapy<br>    Psychodynamic<br>        psychotherapy<br>    Interpersonal therapy<br>    Supportive psychotherapy<br>    Cognitive-behavior therapy<br>    Dialectical behavior therapy<br>    Behavior therapy<br>    Couples, marital, and<br>        family therapy<br>    Group therapy | Psychiatric medications<br>    Antidepressants<br>    Antipsychotics<br>    Sedatives, hypnotics, and<br>        anxiolytics<br>    Mood stabilizers and<br>        anticonvulsants<br>    Stimulants<br>Electroconvulsive therapy (ECT)<br>Transcranial magnetic stimulation<br>    (TMS) |

There are many different types of psychotherapy, and some are more effective for certain problems, or for certain people, than others. Most mental health care providers today are trained in a variety of techniques and tailor their approach to the problem, personality, and needs of the person seeking help. Because mental health care providers may combine different techniques in the course of therapy, the lines between the various approaches are often blurred. The relationship that grows between the person and the mental health care provider is called the *therapeutic alliance*. This working relationship allows them to work together in a trusting, cooperative manner. Anything shared in a session with a mental health care provider is kept private. Mental health care providers are bound by ethics not to divulge any information without the person's consent. The exception is if there is likely harm to the person or others.

## Psychodynamic Psychotherapy

*Psychodynamic psychotherapy* aims to help people gain insight into their problems and bring about change. This approach, also called *insight-oriented psychotherapy*, uses *free association*. This technique involves saying all thoughts that enter the mind as a way of finding and understanding unconscious conflicts that arose in childhood and have lasted into adult years. It involves face-to-face meetings with a mental health care provider, building a therapeutic alliance, and interpretation and clarification of what the person says. People most likely to benefit from this treatment are those who have enough knowledge and insight to have, express, and explore intense emotions. This includes people with certain *personality disorders* and certain chronic mental disorders (such as *depressive* or *anxiety disorders*). The therapy may be brief, with fewer than 25 sessions, or longer term, lasting for several years.

## Interpersonal Therapy

*Interpersonal therapy* is intended to enhance relationships and social interactions and improve interpersonal skills. It uses techniques such as reassurance and support, clarification of feelings, and improving interpersonal communication. People most likely to benefit are those with *major depression,* marital problems, or problems building relationships and interacting with others. The therapy often consists of 12–16 sessions, but may be longer for maintenance treatment (after problems are under control, therapy may go on to prevent relapse). This approach, first used for research into the treatment of depression, focuses on relationships to help deal with unrecognized feelings and needs and improve interpersonal and communication skills. Unlike other psychodynamic treatments, it does not deal with the psychological root of symptoms but focuses on current interpersonal problems.

## Supportive Psychotherapy

*Supportive psychotherapy* is the most common type of psychotherapy. It seeks to maintain or restore a person's highest possible level of function. It involves concern, advice, reassurance, suggestion, reinforcement (a technique that encourages desired response through a system of rewards and/or punishment), discussion of alternative behaviors, teaching of social/interpersonal skills, and help in problem solving. People most likely to benefit from this approach are those in highly stressful situations, those with severe medical illness, and those with mental disorders who do not benefit from other approaches. The timing may be brief (a single session or several sessions over a period of days or weeks) to very long term (over many years), based on the nature of the problem.

Any form of psychotherapy or counseling that offers reassurance, empathy, and education is supportive. The goal of supportive psychotherapy is to help people to adapt and to return to their normal or prior best level of function to the extent possible given personality, life events, ability, or illness.

## Cognitive-Behavior Therapy

The goal of *cognitive-behavior therapy* (CBT) is to identify and change distortions in thinking, as well as problem behaviors. It uses such techniques as identifying beliefs and attitudes; spotting negative thought patterns and unhelpful behaviors; education in other ways of thinking; cognitive rehearsal (reviewing in one's mind how to respond differently than in the past); and homework assignments. People most likely to benefit are those with *major depressive disorder* and *anxiety, eating, substance use,* and *trauma-related disorders.* The length of treatment often is brief, about 15–25 sessions.

## Dialectical Behavior Therapy

*Dialectical behavior therapy* (DBT) is a form of CBT. It helps people know and manage their thoughts and feelings and teaches calming methods. It can teach people to learn how to feel more in control of extreme feelings. At the same time, the mental health care provider coaches people to understand their own duty to change behavior that is risky and causes upset or problems.

DBT builds a strong and equal relationship between the person in treatment and the mental health care provider. The mental health care provider often reminds the person when behavior is not healthy or causes problems, such as when limits are broken. Needed skills are taught to better deal with future events. DBT involves both one-on-one and group therapy. One-on-one sessions are used to teach new skills, while group sessions provide the chance to practice these skills.

DBT has been helpful in the treatment of those who have *borderline personality disorder* and thoughts of suicide. It is also used for those with severe *depression, posttraumatic stress disorder, eating disorders, substance use disorders,* and traumatic brain injury.

## Behavior Therapy

*Behavior therapy* aims to replace unhealthy patterns of behavior with more healthy ways of behaving and coping with stress, fear, or worry. It uses a range of techniques to help people who want to change their behavior. People most likely to benefit are those who want to change habits and those with *anxiety disorders* (such as *phobias*), panic attacks, and *substance use* or *eating disorders.* The length of treatment often is brief and consists of less than 25 sessions.

The basic methods of behavior therapy include:

- *Behavior modification*, which focuses on a negative habit or behavior.
- *Systematic desensitization*, which teaches how to reduce or control fear triggered by certain things (such as animals or elevators) or settings (such as being out in public).
- *Relaxation training*, which helps individuals to control their physical and mental state.
- *Exposure therapy*, which involves gradual stages of direct exposure to a feared object or situation to control anxiety without the use of relaxation techniques. *Exposure and response prevention therapy* can be helpful for people with *obsessive-compulsive disorder*. This teaches them to stop doing a compulsion (a repeated act, such as hand washing) when exposed to the feared or unpleasant object.

- *Flooding,* which exposes people to what they fear most and keeps them exposed to the feared item or setting with the aid of the mental health care provider until their fear lessens.
- *Modeling,* in which a mental health care provider performs a desired behavior that the person seeking help can then copy.
- *Assertiveness training,* which teaches people to express their feelings and thoughts honestly and directly.

## Couples, Marital, and Family Therapy

*Couples, marital, and family therapy* seeks to change relationships, improve communications and interactions, and teach better ways to resolve conflicts. Those most likely to benefit are couples or families who want to change their basic ways of interacting, and children or teenagers with mental disorders or troubling behaviors. The treatment can last for weeks or months. In one-on-one psychotherapy, the focus is on the person within a couple or family. In couples, marital, and family therapy, all members and the way they relate or feel about the other is the focus. Depending on the nature of the problem, mental health care providers may suggest a mix of one-on-one and couples or family therapy.

Although some mental health care providers work with individuals as well as with couples and families, many specialize in marital and family therapy. It can be hard for couples or families to know when they should seek help for their problems. Their concerns may seem minor or petty, but even small things sometimes can be a sign of a greater underlying problem. As with individual symptoms, the key issue is to find out how severe or how long the problem has endured.

Couples with problems in their relationship may seek out a marital mental health care provider on their own. Sometimes mental health care providers treating one person may suggest couples or family therapy as a further form of treatment. Very often families do not seek family counseling themselves but are steered to therapy after a child is noted to have (or diagnosed with) a problem by the child's mental health care provider, school counselor, or doctor. Mental health care providers who work with a couple or a family look beyond one person's feelings or behavior to the impact of those feelings or behaviors on others.

Couples or marital therapy tends to be brief, lasting for weeks or months. Common issues include communication difficulties, sexual problems, and differing views of what partners expect from the relationship. The goal is to identify and resolve the issues as quickly as possible. Therapy begins with the partners identifying problems or areas in which they would like to see some change. A husband may report that his wife complains that he neglects his share of child care, while the wife may feel overwhelmed by the demands of their young children. The mental health care provider may help them pinpoint target behaviors that need to be changed and contract with each other to modify these behaviors in small, specific ways. The techniques are the same for opposite-sex and same-sex couples.

Family therapy involves treatment with one person who is the patient or client and at least one member of his or her family. Often the entire family is involved. The mental health care provider may meet with various family members separately, as well as with the entire family. The focus is on the *interaction* between people rather than on a single person's way of thinking or the content or nature of a certain problem. Common types of family therapy include the following: *Behavioral family therapy* views problem behaviors as the result of family attention and rewards, which support the behavior. *Structural family therapy* stresses the value of family structure for helping the family function as a whole, as well as its impact on the well-being of its members.

## Group Therapy

*Group therapy* seeks to change ways of relating with others and relieve distressing psychological symptoms. It provides a helpful way for mental health care providers to follow up with and monitor a group of patients or clients at the same time. It also provides patients or clients with a social environment (and peer group) that will help them learn new and healthier ways to interact with others in a controlled and supportive environment.

It uses basic approaches of supportive, cognitive-behavior, psychodynamic, interpersonal, or psychoanalytic therapy; self-disclosure and catharsis (the release of feelings through talking and expressing them); sharing of insight and information; and feedback from peers and the mental health care provider. Group therapy most often benefits those who have a similar mental or physical disorder (for instance, an *eating disorder* or *posttraumatic stress disorder*); teens; psychiatric patients in hospital care; and families of people with mental disorders. Group therapy has a brief or long-term time frame.

Groups take place in many settings such as psychiatric hospitals, community mental health centers, health maintenance organizations, teaching hospital clinics, and private offices. Mental health care providers in private practice may organize groups based on similar issues or needs. Psychotherapy groups that usually meet once a week can be a key part of treatment for a wide range of common mental health problems.

# Psychiatric Medications

Psychiatric medications can affect every aspect of a person's physical, mental, and emotional function, such as alertness, attention, coordination, energy, mood, judgment, sleep patterns, and interpersonal relationships. Some of these medications take effect at once; others do not have an effect right away. Some continue to exert their effects long after they are no longer being taken. Medications often used to treat mental health problems and shown to be helpful are listed in Appendix B, "Medications."

The doctor will take into account each person's needs and symptoms to prescribe the medications that have a good fit. Medications or doses can be changed to make sure they work. In prescribing these medications, psychiatrists and other doctors must consider many factors (see box below).

---

### What Doctors Review Before They Prescribe Medications

- **Allergies**—Allergies to certain chemicals in medications will rule out those medicines.
- **Lifestyle**—Some medications must be taken at certain times or have detailed rules for taking them.
- **Age**—This affects how medications are metabolized (or processed) in the body. Older adults may metabolize certain drugs more slowly or may be more prone to certain side effects.
- **Family history**—Presence of mental disorders in family members.
- **General medical health and history of medical problems**—Some illnesses can cause symptoms that mimic or bring on a mental health disorder. If not recent, a full physical exam is given, along with blood and laboratory tests, and if needed, brain-imaging scans.
- **Medication issues**—Benefits and risks of certain medications as they relate to the person seeking care:
  - Although most psychiatric medications are not habit forming, some can be addicting and must be prescribed with care.
  - Other medications may interact with those prescribed for mental disorders.
  - Many medications can cause side effects that range from mildly irritating (such as dry mouth) to more bothersome (dizziness or constipation) to life threatening (seizures or irregular heart rhythm). In general, side effects tend to be most common and troubling when the drugs are first taken and most tend to lessen or end after a few weeks.
  - Patients' concerns about side effects—often a different medication can be prescribed if certain side effects do not make the medication a good match for the patient.

---

## Tips to Help Medications Work Best

- Take the medication as the doctor directs.
- Ask if there are any foods to avoid with the medication.
- Ask if the medication should be taken with food or at certain times of day.
- Know what to expect with side effects. Ask questions and talk about any concerns with the doctor. Ask about how best to cope with side effects.
- Set a helpful routine to make sure the medications are taken every day.
- Do not stop a medication right away or decrease the dose without checking with the doctor first. If some medications are stopped right away or the dose is reduced, they may cause unhealthy and unpleasant symptoms—or can make the mental disorder worse.
- Pay close attention to how the medicines are working or not working, even as time passes. After a while, the body can adjust to medications, symptoms can improve or worsen, and the doctor may need to adjust the dose or switch medications.
- Even after you feel better and seem to have no symptoms—or if you dislike the side effects—know that medications will help you get and stay better.
- Seek your doctor's advice for any questions or concerns that you have about your medications.

People who take psychiatric medication should have follow-up visits with their doctor to see whether it is working, or perhaps causing side effects that are unhealthy or unpleasant (see box above on tips to help medications work best). The right medication and dose are needed to help resolve symptoms. This may take time as the dose is altered or another medication is tried. Trying different medications or doses may be needed to see what works best. The medications need to be taken long enough to work, and sometimes weeks or months must pass for the full effects to take hold.

For some mental disorders, people may need to take the medication every day for the rest of their lives, just as a person might take insulin or high blood pressure medicines every day. When this happens, a person is in *maintenance treatment*. This means a person's symptoms are under control or improved enough to function better in daily life when the dosage and medication that work best have been found. The person keeps taking the medication to preserve its effects, and the person checks in with the doctor at scheduled office visits from time to time. The doctor makes sure the medicine is still working, that no side effects are causing problems, that the person is doing well, and that the disorder symptoms are well controlled. This helps to prevent *relapse*—a return to harmful symptoms of the disorder and problems that can result.

## Antidepressants

Most of today's antidepressants work well with few side effects. The word "antidepressant" is somewhat misleading because these medications are used to treat many conditions other than depression. They can be effective in treating *panic disorder, posttraumatic stress disorder, generalized anxiety disorder, social phobia, obsessive-compulsive disorder, borderline personality disorder, bulimia nervosa,* irritable bowel syndrome, *attention deficit/hyperactivity disorder, autism spectrum disorder,* smoking cessation, chronic pain, and migraine headaches.

The types of antidepressants include selective serotonin reuptake inhibitors (SSRIs), serotonin-norepinephrine reuptake inhibitors (SNRIs), tricyclic antidepressants, tetracyclic antidepressants, and monoamine oxidase inhibitors (MAOIs). About 60%–70% of people who are prescribed a medication will improve. Combined treatment, which involves both drug therapy and psychotherapy, has proved most effective in treating depression and in lowering relapse rates.

Doctors weigh many factors in choosing an antidepressant, such as the person's medical status, history of manic or hypomanic episodes, prior bouts of depression, prior responses to an antidepressant, and the presence of symptoms such as increased sleep, weight gain, or anxiety, or psychotic symptoms, such as delusions or hallucinations.

Antidepressants do not work right away. A good response to these medications takes time. Although a few people may have some improvement, such as increased energy, by the end of the first week, most do not see major benefits for 3–4 weeks. Because doses are increased slowly for some medications, 5–6 weeks may pass from the time a person takes the first pill until the symptoms are relieved, and 8 weeks or longer until the medication has its full impact.

The various types of antidepressants produce different side effects. Many common side effects, such as dry mouth or nausea, subside after several weeks. Although bothersome, these effects do have a positive meaning: the drug is working and levels of the drug in the body are rising. Even when side effects are annoying, it is critical to keep taking the medication long enough for it to be of help and to keep increasing the dose as directed until symptoms improve.

## Antipsychotic Medications

*Antipsychotic medications* are used to treat psychotic symptoms, such as delusions and hallucinations. Antipsychotics are the preferred medications for the treatment of *schizophrenia* and other psychoses, and they have also been a key part in the treatment of manic and depressive symptoms in *bipolar disorder*. Antipsychotic medications are also used to treat psychotic symptoms linked with drug abuse, and behavior problems that may occur with *dementia* and *autism spectrum disorder*.

The choice of antipsychotic agents is based on their safety and how well side effects are tolerated. Some side effects are extreme but can be treated. One side effect is a symptom called *akathisia*, which is a feeling of restlessness in the lower limbs and inability to sit still. Other side effects are more serious. A rare but serious side effect is *neuroleptic malignant syndrome*. It causes someone to become rigid and develop fever, rapid heartbeat, abnormal blood pressure, rapid breathing, and changes in mental state ranging from confusion to coma. This condition is a medical emergency.

Antipsychotic medications may cause a drop in blood pressure, dizziness, increased blood lipids, increased blood glucose (sugar levels), high blood pressure, and weight gain. Like most other drugs, antipsychotic agents should be avoided if possible during pregnancy and when mothers are breast-feeding. This is a hard decision since the doctor must balance the low risk of birth defects in the child with the high risk of psychosis in the mother. Use of some antidepressants may increase or decrease the amount of antipsychotic medication to treat the underlying condition. Cigarette smoking can decrease the levels of some antipsychotic medications in the blood, thus making them less effective.

## Sedatives, Hypnotics, and Anxiolytics

*Sedatives* or *anxiolytic medications* are often used to treat anxiety and insomnia. *Hypnotic* agents are medications that are used to cause and maintain sleep.

In some cases, anxiolytics are used to treat *panic disorder* until the effects of the antidepressant medication take hold. *Benzodiazepines* are one class of anxiolytics. They have muscle relaxant and anticonvulsant features (that is, they help control seizures). They need to be used with care because they can be habit forming. Only a few of the benzodiazepines are approved for the treatment of insomnia, but almost all are used for this purpose. Alcohol should be used in moderation or avoided because its effects are increased with these medications.

All benzodiazepines have similar effects. The choice should be based on how long the medication stays in the blood, how fast it works, how it is processed in the body, and how potent it is. Major side effects of benzodiazepines are sedation, dizziness, and impairment in use of machinery, such as driving a car. Benzodiazepines are sometimes abused; in these cases, patients may be at risk for drug withdrawal if the medication is stopped too quickly. Withdrawal could include symptoms such as nausea, vomiting, tremors, and even seizures. Other common signs of withdrawal are increased blood pressure, rapid heartbeat, worsening of anxiety, panic attacks, and memory problems.

Another anxiolytic is buspirone. It does not interact with alcohol or benzodiazepines, affect the ability to complete tasks or operate machinery, or pose a risk of abuse. It is prescribed for the treatment of *generalized anxiety disorder,* but is not useful in the treatment of *panic disorder.* It is often used with antidepressants. Common side effects are nausea, nervousness, insomnia, and dizziness.

Hypnotic agents, or sleep medications, are prescribed for a brief time to help with sleep. They are short-acting drugs that produce a limited amount of daytime sleepiness. They should only be used in the short term, to decrease the risk of dependence. Another agent that causes sleep is ramelteon, which works on melatonin, a hormone that controls sleep and wake cycles.

## Mood Stabilizers

*Mood stabilizers* help reduce mood swings from highs and lows. These medications help in the treatment of *bipolar disorder.* Mood stabilizer medications include lithium, valproate, carbamazepine, lamotrigine, and antipsychotic medications. Some mood stabilizers include anticonvulsant medicines, which treat seizures but also help control moods. Mood stabilizers each vary in side effects, potential for drug interactions, and the way the body processes them.

- *Lithium* is effective for the acute and preventive treatment of both manic and depressive episodes in patients with *bipolar disorder.* It is also effective to prevent future depressive episodes in patients with recurrent *depression.* Lithium is the only mood stabilizer for which blood levels of the drug are measured to ensure it is within the needed range to help. As with most medications, lithium is started at a low dose and slowly increased over time. It may produce hypothyroidism, a change in the heartbeat, weight gain, tremors, decreased blood count, and stomach symptoms.
- *Valproate* is used to treat mania and other phases of *bipolar disorder.* Initial side effects of valproate are nausea, sedation, and hand tremor. Doctors may slowly increase the dose to reduce the side effects. Some people may start at a much higher dose. Valproate should not be used in someone with liver disease. Valproate also may produce changes in blood counts, heartburn, indigestion, weight gain, or drowsiness.
- *Carbamazepine and oxcarbazepine* are used to prevent and treat mania. The most serious side effects of carbamazepine are a major decrease

in white blood cell count and red blood cells (aplastic anemia) and the ability of the blood to clot. It also may affect the liver, cause a rash, and lower thyroid hormone levels in the blood. It also can produce drowsiness, dizziness, and difficulty walking. Oxcarbazepine does not require blood or liver tests and has fewer side effects than carbamazepine.

- *Lamotrigine* is used to prevent depression in people with *bipolar disorder*. A major side effect is a serious rash that may require treatment in a hospital. To lower the risk of a rash, doctors prescribe lamotrigine at a low dose and slowly increase it over a number of weeks.

## Stimulants

*Stimulants* are often prescribed for *attention-deficit/hyperactivity disorder* (ADHD), which is more common in boys than girls. These medications are mostly used to treat children but may be used in adults. They are often prescribed by pediatricians and primary care doctors.

There is a major concern in the United States that stimulants are being overused in children and adults with ADHD, and some who do not have the disorder. Most children with ADHD will respond to stimulant use, in terms of having improved focus to learn and do schoolwork. Nonstimulant medications can be prescribed to treat ADHD, such as atomoxetine or guanfacine.

Side effects of stimulants are specific to the age group. The principal side effects of stimulants are insomnia, irritable mood, and elevated blood pressure. Side effects such as excitability, increased activity, talkativeness, and irritability may be seen as the last dose of the day wears off or for several days if there is a sudden stop to the stimulant medication. The symptoms would be similar to the original ADHD symptoms. A small number of children being treated with stimulants may develop psychotic symptoms.

# Electroconvulsive Therapy

*Electroconvulsive therapy* (ECT)—the passage of a controlled electrical current through the brain to induce a brief seizure—is one of the best treatments for serious mental disorders, especially severe *depression*. As many as 80%–85% of depressed persons who undergo ECT improve.

The mild electrical stimulation affects many of the neurotransmitters and receptors in the brain involved in depression. Because anesthesia and muscle-relaxing drugs are used before the electrical current is given through electrodes attached to the scalp, patients do not feel any pain, and their muscles do not shake or jerk. Despite its well-known benefits as a safe, reliable, and effective treatment, ECT is still viewed with distrust by much of the general public. This attitude stems largely from outdated misperceptions of ECT as painful or even dangerous.

ECT is the treatment of choice for those with severe depression who are suicidal, for those who have psychotic symptoms, or for those whose disorder is life threatening, possibly because they refuse to eat and drink. Other people likely to benefit are men and women with depression who:

- Do not improve with other approaches, including psychotherapy and a trial of at least two antidepressant drugs.
- Have psychotic symptoms, such as delusions.
- Need a treatment that produces rapid results because of the danger of suicide or harm to themselves.
- Have had previous depressions that did not improve when treated with antidepressant drugs.
- Have improved with ECT in the past.

## Transcranial Magnetic Stimulation

Transcranial magnetic stimulation (TMS) of the brain is a new form of treatment for *depression* for those whose symptoms have not improved after trying two or three antidepressant medications. The treatment uses a device that creates an electronic pulse that is sent to certain areas of the brain. The pulse is sent through electrodes that are placed on the scalp. Patients report few side effects. In contrast to ECT, a seizure is not induced.

# Getting Better and Staying Healthy

Getting help from a mental health care provider is a great start toward getting better. Treatments take time to work and alone will not provide a total cure. Getting better depends on the nature of the problem, the therapy selected, the skill of the mental health care provider. More than anything else, the hard work of the person seeking help and the support of his or her loved ones are key. It takes courage to get better. Keep trying each day and don't give up. Here are some more things to do that can improve your health and treatment.

- Exercise has proven to be good not only for the body, but also for the mind. It is particularly beneficial for depression. It is also an effective means of reducing anxiety. Physical exercise can also relieve tension and enhance the sense of well-being and overall health.

- A healthy, well-balanced diet should be part of every treatment plan. This includes leafy greens, vegetables, fruit, beans, lean meats, fish, and whole grains. Poor eating habits such as skipping meals, eating too quickly, or eating too much junk food (lots of sugar, fast food) can make people physically uncomfortable and psychologically unwell. A healthful balanced diet can improve health and help someone feel better.
- High amounts of caffeine can cause anxiety or panic attacks and worsen these conditions. Alcohol can make problems worse.
- Avoid downbeat self-talk. Focus on things you like about yourself and those things that you do well.
- Create an optimistic point of view. When bad things happen to those with an optimistic view, they tend to see such setbacks or losses as specific and temporary incidents—not as judgments on themselves or their whole lives. The key to change is getting rid of the automatic negative thoughts that may flood your brain. Replace them with positive truths. Keep a list with you of your strengths and what you value in your life to remind yourself of what is important.
- Humor often allows us to express fears and negative feelings without causing distress to ourselves or others. It also may produce enhanced physical well-being. Since we laugh often with others, humor helps in forging supportive relationships.
- Build friendships to give and receive support. In relationships, people may find that some problems are easier to put into perspective. Reaching out to others is important.
- Doing good things enhances self-esteem and may relieve physical and mental stress. Find ways to help others that you enjoy or are linked to your hobbies.

- Peers or peer-support groups can offer empathy, build morale, and create a new social world for persons dealing with similar life issues. Talking with people who have similar problems is highly useful for those with mental disorders. Hospitals, community health centers, and local mental health organizations often sponsor support groups. By participating, people may develop a sense of connectedness with others who have similar problems.

## Key Points

- Seek help for mental health problems when they keep causing distress or problems with work, close ties, or other key aspects of life. Know the common warning signs for mental illness, such as eating or sleeping too much or too little, pulling away from people and usual activities, having low or no energy, and thinking of harming yourself or others.
- There are many types of qualified mental health care providers available. These include psychiatrists, psychologists, licensed clinical social workers, marriage and family therapists, and psychiatric nurses. These mental health care providers can also work with primary care doctors, nurse-practitioners, and physician assistants who prescribe medicines. Support groups can provide help and improve coping (see Appendix C, "Helpful Resources").
- Many treatments are available for nearly all the psychiatric disorders. Psychotherapy, medication, or a combination of the two can be used. Electroconvulsive therapy (ECT) is also a modern, proven, and safe treatment for certain mental disorders when other treatments have not worked.
- Treatment improves health and quality of life. Left untreated, mental disorders often get worse and lead to more problems and distress. Trying to relieve mental health symptoms with drugs or too much alcohol worsens mental disorders and raises the risk of other problems.
- You can improve and maintain your mental health by getting exercise, eating a healthy diet, avoiding too much caffeine or alcohol, keeping focused on positive truths, laughing often, building friendships, and helping others.

# Glossary

These terms can help build your knowledge about mental health disorders and mental health care. Many of these terms are defined in the book chapters where they appear. They are often used by mental health care providers.

**acting out**   Expressing feelings through actions rather than words.

**addiction**   A behavior pattern characterized by compulsion, loss of control, and continued repetition of a behavior or activity in spite of adverse consequences.

**affect**   External expression of emotion, feeling, or mood.

**aftercare**   Rehabilitation and other therapies after hospital care to help a person adjust to a new environment and to prevent relapse.

**agitation**   Excessive physical activity, usually associated with tension, such as an inability to sit still, fidgeting, pacing, or wringing of hands.

**agoraphobia**   Fear of open spaces, or being in places or situations in which escape may be difficult.

**akathisia**   Uncontrollable motor restlessness, commonly a side effect of certain medications.

**akinesia**   A state of reduced movement.

**amnesia**   Permanent or temporary loss of memory.

**analgesics**   Medications that relieve pain without inducing a loss of consciousness.

**anhedonia**   A loss of interest in once-pleasurable activities.

**antisocial behavior**   Actions performed without regard for another's rights, person, property, or societal norms.

**anxiety**   Apprehension or uneasiness about an anticipated or imagined danger.

**apathy**   Indifference, or lack of feeling, emotion, or interest.

**aphasia**   Impairment of the ability to use or to understand words, usually due to brain disease or trauma.

**assertiveness**   The ability to be open and direct in expressing needs, feelings, and rights.

**assertiveness training**   A form of behavior therapy that teaches people to express feelings and thoughts honestly and directly.

**avolition**   Lack of will, initiative, or motivation.

**behavior modification**   A method of changing behavior or eliminating a symptom by rewarding desired behavior and punishing unwanted behavior.

**behavior therapy**   A form of treatment that aims to change behavior by means of systematic desensitization, behavior modification, or aversion therapy.

**benzodiazepines**   A group of drugs used as anti-anxiety agents or sedatives.

**brief psychotherapy**   Any form of psychotherapy that is limited to a set number of sessions and to specific objectives or goals.

**burnout**   A state of physical, emotional, and mental exhaustion resulting from constant emotional pressure.

**catatonia**   A motionless state, characterized by muscle rigidity or inflexibility, seen in some types of psychosis.

**catharsis**   The release of emotions through talking and expressing feelings.

**chronic**   Persisting over a long period of time or recurring frequently.

**codependence**   An emotional and psychological behavior pattern of the spouse, partner, parents, or friends of people with addictive behaviors that "enables" these individuals to continue their destructive habits.

**cognitive**   Pertaining to the mental processes of thinking, understanding, perceiving, judging, remembering, and reasoning, in contrast to emotional processes.

**cognitive-behavior therapy**   A short-term form of psychotherapy whose goal is to enable the person to recognize and change specific conditions or symptoms, based on the interrelation of thoughts and behavior.

**commitment**   A legal process for the admission of a mentally ill person to a psychiatric treatment program.

**comorbidity**   The coexistence of two of more illnesses in a person.

**compulsion**   A repetitive behavior (e.g., hand washing) or repetitive mental process (e.g., counting) that serves no rational purpose.

**consciousness**   The aspects of mental functioning of which we are aware.

**contract**   An explicit agreement between a person and a therapist to follow a certain course of action.

**coping mechanism**   Ways of dealing with stress.

**counseling**   A general term for any interaction in which a person, who may or may not be a mental health professional, offers guidance or advice to another.

**crisis intervention**   Emergency action to address a threat of suicide, violence, or similar urgency.

**defense mechanism**   Any of several mental processes that work unconsciously to enable a person to cope with a difficult situation or problem, such as a major loss or trauma.

**delusion**   A false belief regarding the self or the world that a person holds despite clear evidence to the contrary.

**denial**   A defense mechanism that enables a person to deny the existence of a behavior, thought, need, feeling, or desire.

**depersonalization**   A strong sense of detachment from the self, as if observing one's body from the outside.

**depression**   A term that describes feelings of sadness, discouragement, and despair. It can be a normal and temporary reaction to events in a person's life, a symptom occurring in various physical and mental conditions, or a mental disorder in itself.

**derealization**   A feeling of detachment from one's environment, causing a person's view of objects, other people, or time to be distorted.

**detoxification**   A process that eliminates alcohol or addictive drugs from the body, usually combined with medication and supportive care.

**disorientation**   Loss of awareness of one's relation to space, time, or other persons.

**distractibility**   The inability to sustain attention or the tendency to shift focus from one activity or topic to another.

**drive**   A basic instinct or urge.

**drug interaction**    A change in the way the body reacts to a drug when two or more drugs are taken simultaneously.

**dual diagnosis**    The simultaneous occurrence of a psychiatric disorder and a substance use disorder in the same person at the time of diagnosis.

**dysfunctional family**    A family characterized by negative and destructive patterns of behavior between the parents or among parents and their children.

**dyskinesia**    Any disturbance of movement.

**etiology**    Cause, particularly of a disease.

**euphoria**    An exaggerated feeling of physical and emotional well-being.

**flashback**    Reexperiencing of a traumatic event.

**group psychotherapy**    The use of psychotherapeutic techniques by a therapist in a group setting.

**halfway house**    A specialized residence for people who do not require hospital care but are not yet ready to return to living on their own; it is often operated under the supervision of trained staff.

**hallucination**    A perception of sounds, sights, physical sensations, or smells that do not exist.

**homosexuality**    Sexual attraction to, and relationships with, people of the same sex.

**hyperactivity**    Excessive physical activity that may be purposeful or aimless.

**hypersomnia**    Prolonged sleep or excessive daytime drowsiness.

**hypnosis**    A state of intense concentration that makes someone suggestible and accepting of instructions. It is of therapeutic value in breaking undesirable habits (e.g., smoking, overeating) and in alleviating pain.

**hypnotic**    A drug used to induce relaxation or sleep.

**hypomania**    A state of abnormal mood that falls between euphoria and mania and that is characterized by unrealistic optimism, rapid speech and activity, and a decreased need for sleep.

**illusion**    Misperception of a real occurrence.

**impulse**    A sudden desire to act in a certain way to ease tension or feel pleasure.

**inhalants** Substances that produce vapors having psychoactive effects when inhaled.

**insomnia** A sleep-wake disorder that consists of difficulty in falling or staying asleep.

**institutionalization** Long-term placement of a person in a hospital, nursing home, residential center, or other care facility.

**interpersonal psychotherapy** A form of brief psychotherapy, originally developed for the treatment of depression, that focuses on relationship issues in order to help people improve their interpersonal and communication skills.

**interpretation** The process by which a therapist encourages a person to understand a particular problem.

**intimacy** A state of closeness between two people, characterized by the desire and ability to share their innermost feelings with each other in verbal and nonverbal ways.

**intoxication** The acute bodily effects of overdosage with a chemical substance.

**labile** Rapidly changing, as applied to emotions; unstable.

**magical thinking** A conviction that thinking about something can make it happen.

**maintenance therapy** The continuation of a treatment, whether psychotherapy, medication, or both, to prevent relapse or recurrence of a mental disorder.

**mania** A mood disturbance that occurs in bipolar disorder and that is characterized by excessive elation, inflated self-esteem, hyperactivity, agitation, and rapid and often confused thinking and speaking.

**marital therapy** A treatment intended to improve or work out problems that are impairing or threatening a primary relationship between two people.

**meditation** Any of a variety of approaches that use breathing and other techniques to achieve relaxation, improve concentration, and become attuned to one's inner self.

**mental disorder** A behavioral or psychological condition or syndrome that causes significant distress, disability, disturbed functioning, or increased risk of harm or pain to one's self or others.

**mental health**   A state of psychological and emotional well-being that enables someone to work, love, relate to others effectively, and resolve conflicts.

**mental status examination**   A process that evaluates psychological and behavioral functioning.

**modeling**   A technique used in behavior therapy in which a therapist performs a desired behavior that is then imitated by the patient.

**narcissism**   A tendency to overestimate one's abilities and importance.

**nystagmus**   Abnormal eye movements.

**obsession**   A recurrent, persistent, and senseless idea, thought, impulse, or image.

**orientation**   Awareness of self in relation to time, place, and person.

**outpatient**   A person who is receiving care or treatment at a hospital or other health facility without being admitted to the facility.

**panic attacks**   Sudden, unprovoked, emotionally intense experiences of impending doom, fear of dying, "going crazy," or losing control, marked by physical symptoms such as palpitations, dizziness, trembling, nausea, or shortness of breath.

**paranoia**   A tendency to view the actions of others as deliberately threatening or demeaning.

**paranoid ideation**   Suspiciousness about being harassed, persecuted, or unfairly treated.

**partial hospitalization**   A psychiatric treatment program for people who require hospital care only during the day, overnight, or on weekends.

**pastoral counseling**   The application of psychological principles by members of the clergy to assist persons in their congregations who have emotional problems.

**personality**   The characteristic way in which a person thinks, feels, and behaves.

**phase of life problem**   Difficulty in adapting to a particular developmental period in a person's life.

**phobia**   Fear of a particular object or setting. Phobias may be specific, such as fear of animals, insects, blood, airplane flights, heights, tunnels, or elevators.

**physical dependence**   The physiological attachment to, and need for, a drug, characterized by tolerance and withdrawal symptoms if the drug is stopped.

**play therapy**   A technique in the treatment of children in which the child's play is a medium for expression and communication between patient and therapist.

**polysomnography**   The all-night recording of brain waves, eye movements, muscle tone, respiration, heart rate, and penile tumescence (swelling) in order to diagnose sleep-related disorders.

**postconcussional disorder**   Physical symptoms and cognitive changes following head trauma and loss of consciousness.

**prognosis**   The prediction of the outcome of an illness.

**progressive relaxation**   A method of reducing muscle tension by contracting and then relaxing muscles in specific areas of the body in systematic order.

**projection**   A defense mechanism by which unacceptable feelings or impulses are attributed to someone else.

**psychedelic**   A term applied to any of several drugs capable of inducing hallucinations and altered mental states.

**psychiatry**   The medical science that deals with the etiology (origin), diagnosis, prevention, and treatment of mental disorders.

**psychoactive**   A term often used to describe both medications and illicit drugs that act on the brain to change feelings or emotions.

**psychodynamic psychotherapy**   Treatment based on an understanding of a person that takes into account the role of early experiences and unconscious influences in actively shaping his or her behavior.

**psychodynamics**   The knowledge and theory of human behavior and its motivations.

**psychomotor**   A term referring to combined physical and mental activity.

**psychomotor agitation**   Excessive motor activity associated with a feeling of inner tension.

**psychomotor retardation**   Slowing of physical and emotional reactions.

**psychopathology**   The study of the development and nature of mental disorders.

**psychosis**   A gross impairment of a person's perception of reality and ability to communicate and relate to others.

**psychosomatic**   A term often used to designate physical symptoms or conditions that have a mental or emotional component.

**psychotropic**   A term used to describe drugs that act in a particular way on the brain and affect the mind.

**recall**   The process of bringing a memory into consciousness.

**reinforcement**   A behavior therapy technique that involves the encouragement of a desired response through a system of rewards and/or punishments.

**response**   A behavior or an action compelled by a stimulus.

**ritual**   A repetitive activity, usually a distorted routine of daily life, that is used to relieve anxiety.

**sedative**   A general term applied to any quieting or sleep-producing agent.

**self-esteem**   A sense of self-worth; the valuing of oneself as a person.

**self-help group**   An assemblage of people with a common problem who together aid one another through personal and group support.

**sexual orientation**   The focus of a person's sexual attractions, whether to people of the opposite sex, the same sex, or both.

**side effect**   A drug response that accompanies the principal purpose of a medication.

**social phobia**   A persistent fear of finding oneself in situations that might lead to scrutiny by others and humiliation or embarrassment.

**somatic therapy**   In psychiatry, the biological treatment of mental disorders; examples are electroconvulsive therapy and psychopharmacological treatment.

**stress**   The nonspecific response of the body to any demands made upon it.

**stressor**   A specific or nonspecific agent, event, or situation that causes the body to experience a stress response.

**stupor**   A marked decrease in response to and awareness of the environment.

**supportive psychotherapy**   A type of therapy, which may be brief or long-term, that uses the therapist-patient relationship to help a person cope with specific crises or difficulties that he or she is currently facing.

**suppression**  The conscious inhibition of certain thoughts or impulses.

**syndrome**  A group of signs and symptoms that appear together, suggesting a particular cause.

**tardive dyskinesia**  A medication-induced movement disorder consisting of involuntary movements of the tongue, jaw, or extremities that develops with long-term use of antipsychotic medication.

**tic**  An involuntary, abrupt, rapid, and recurrent motor movement or vocalization.

**tolerance**  A characteristic of substance dependence marked by the need for increasing amounts of the substance to achieve the desired effect.

**trance**  A state of intensely focused attention in which a person becomes detached from the physical environment.

**tranquilizer**  A drug that decreases anxiety and agitation.

**transsexual**  A person whose psychological gender identify is the opposite of his or her biological sex.

**tremor**  A trembling or shaking of the body or any of its parts.

**visualization**  An approach to stress management that uses a technique of guided or directed imagery.

**withdrawal**  The symptoms and signs that develop within a short period of time after cessation or reduced use of an addictive substance. This may include sweating, rapid pulse, hand tremor, nausea or vomiting, agitation, anxiety, or hallucinations.

# Complete List of DSM-5 Disorders

These disorders are listed in the order and groupings found in DSM-5.

## Neurodevelopmental Disorders

### Intellectual Disabilities

Intellectual Disability (Intellectual Developmental Disorder)
Global Developmental Delay
Unspecified Intellectual Disability (Intellectual Developmental Disorder)

### Communication Disorders

Language Disorder
Speech Sound Disorder (previously Phonological Disorder)
Childhood-Onset Fluency Disorder (Stuttering)
Social (Pragmatic) Communication Disorder
Unspecified Communication Disorder

### Autism Spectrum Disorder

Autism Spectrum Disorder

### Attention-Deficit/ Hyperactivity Disorder

Attention-Deficit/Hyperactivity Disorder
Other Specified Attention-Deficit/Hyperactivity Disorder
Unspecified Attention-Deficit/ Hyperactivity Disorder

### Specific Learning Disorder

Specific Learning Disorder

### Motor Disorders

Developmental Coordination Disorder
Stereotypic Movement Disorder

### Tic Disorders

Tourette's Disorder
Persistent (Chronic) Motor or Vocal Tic Disorder
Provisional Tic Disorder
Other Specified Tic Disorder
Unspecified Tic Disorder

### Other Neurodevelopmental Disorders

Other Specified Neurodevelopmental Disorder
Unspecified Neurodevelopmental Disorder

## Schizophrenia Spectrum and Other Psychotic Disorders

Schizotypal (Personality) Disorder
Delusional Disorder
Brief Psychotic Disorder
Schizophreniform Disorder
Schizophrenia
Schizoaffective Disorder
Substance/Medication-Induced Psychotic Disorder
Psychotic Disorder Due to Another Medical Condition

## Catatonia

Catatonia Associated With
  Another Mental Disorder
Catatonic Disorder Due to
  Another Medical Condition
Unspecified Catatonia

Other Specified Schizophrenia
  Spectrum and Other Psychotic
  Disorder
Unspecified Schizophrenia
  Spectrum and Other Psychotic
  Disorder

## Bipolar and Related Disorders

Bipolar I Disorder
Bipolar II Disorder
Cyclothymic Disorder
Substance/Medication-Induced
  Bipolar and Related Disorder
Bipolar and Related Disorder Due
  to Another Medical Condition
Other Specified Bipolar and
  Related Disorder
Unspecified Bipolar and Related
  Disorder

## Depressive Disorders

Disruptive Mood Dysregulation
  Disorder
Major Depressive Disorder, Single
  and Recurrent Episodes
Persistent Depressive Disorder
  (Dysthymia)
Premenstrual Dysphoric Disorder
Substance/Medication-Induced
  Depressive Disorder
Depressive Disorder Due to
  Another Medical Condition
Other Specified Depressive
  Disorder
Unspecified Depressive Disorder

## Anxiety Disorders

Separation Anxiety Disorder
Selective Mutism
Specific Phobia

Social Anxiety Disorder (Social
  Phobia)
Panic Disorder
Panic Attack
Agoraphobia
Generalized Anxiety Disorder
Substance/Medication-Induced
  Anxiety Disorder
Anxiety Disorder Due to Another
  Medical Condition
Other Specified Anxiety Disorder
Unspecified Anxiety Disorder

## Obsessive-Compulsive and Related Disorders

Obsessive-Compulsive Disorder
Body Dysmorphic Disorder
Hoarding Disorder
Trichotillomania (Hair-Pulling
  Disorder)
Excoriation (Skin-Picking) Disorder
Substance/Medication-Induced
  Obsessive-Compulsive and
  Related Disorder
Obsessive-Compulsive and
  Related Disorder Due to Another
  Medical Condition
Other Specified Obsessive-
  Compulsive and Related
  Disorder
Unspecified Obsessive-
  Compulsive and Related
  Disorder

## Trauma- and Stressor-Related Disorders

Reactive Attachment Disorder
Disinhibited Social Engagement
  Disorder
Posttraumatic Stress Disorder
Acute Stress Disorder
Adjustment Disorders
Other Specified Trauma- and
  Stressor-Related Disorder
Unspecified Trauma- and Stressor-
  Related Disorder

## Dissociative Disorders

Dissociative Identity Disorder
Dissociative Amnesia
Depersonalization/Derealization
  Disorder
Other Specified Dissociative
  Disorder
Unspecified Dissociative Disorder

## Somatic Symptom and Related Disorders

Somatic Symptom Disorder
Illness Anxiety Disorder
Conversion Disorder (Functional
  Neurological Symptom Disorder)
Psychological Factors Affecting
  Other Medical Conditions
Factitious Disorder
Other Specified Somatic Symptom
  and Related Disorder
Unspecified Somatic Symptom
  and Related Disorder

## Feeding and Eating Disorders

Pica
Rumination Disorder
Avoidant/Restrictive Food Intake
  Disorder
Anorexia Nervosa
Bulimia Nervosa
Binge-Eating Disorder
Other Specified Feeding or Eating
  Disorder
Unspecified Feeding or Eating
  Disorder

## Elimination Disorders

Enuresis
Encopresis
Other Specified Elimination
  Disorder
Unspecified Elimination Disorder

## Sleep-Wake Disorders

Insomnia Disorder
Hypersomnolence Disorder
Narcolepsy

## Breathing-Related Sleep Disorders

Obstructive Sleep Apnea Hypopnea
Central Sleep Apnea
Sleep-Related Hypoventilation

Circadian Rhythm Sleep-Wake
  Disorders

## Parasomnias

Non–Rapid Eye Movement
  Sleep Arousal Disorders
Nightmare Disorder
Rapid Eye Movement Sleep
  Behavior Disorder

Restless Legs Syndrome
Substance/Medication-Induced
  Sleep Disorder
Other Specified Insomnia Disorder
Unspecified Insomnia Disorder
Other Specified Hypersomnolence
  Disorder
Unspecified Hypersomnolence
  Disorder
Other Specified Sleep-Wake
  Disorder
Unspecified Sleep-Wake Disorder

## Sexual Dysfunctions

Delayed Ejaculation
Erectile Disorder
Female Orgasmic Disorder
Female Sexual Interest/Arousal
  Disorder
Genito-Pelvic Pain/Penetration
  Disorder
Male Hypoactive Sexual Desire
  Disorder
Premature (Early) Ejaculation
Substance/Medication-Induced
  Sexual Dysfunction
Other Specified Sexual
  Dysfunction
Unspecified Sexual Dysfunction

## Gender Dysphoria

Gender Dysphoria
Other Specified Gender Dysphoria
Unspecified Gender Dysphoria

## Disruptive, Impulse-Control, and Conduct Disorders

Oppositional Defiant Disorder
Intermittent Explosive Disorder
Conduct Disorder
Antisocial Personality Disorder
Pyromania
Kleptomania
Other Specified Disruptive, Impulse-Control, and Conduct Disorder
Unspecified Disruptive, Impulse-Control, and Conduct Disorder

## Substance-Related and Addictive Disorders

### Substance-Related Disorders

*Alcohol-Related Disorders*

Alcohol Use Disorder
Alcohol Intoxication
Alcohol Withdrawal
Other Alcohol-Induced Disorders
Unspecified Alcohol-Related Disorder

*Caffeine-Related Disorders*

Caffeine Intoxication
Caffeine Withdrawal
Other Caffeine-Induced Disorders
Unspecified Caffeine-Related Disorder

*Cannabis-Related Disorders*

Cannabis Use Disorder
Cannabis Intoxication
Cannabis Withdrawal
Other Cannabis-Induced Disorders
Unspecified Cannabis-Related Disorder

*Hallucinogen-Related Disorders*

Phencyclidine Use Disorder
Other Hallucinogen Use Disorder
Phencyclidine Intoxication
Other Hallucinogen Intoxication
Hallucinogen Persisting Perception Disorder
Other Phencyclidine-Induced Disorders
Other Hallucinogen-Induced Disorders
Unspecified Phencyclidine-Related Disorder
Unspecified Hallucinogen-Related Disorder

*Inhalant-Related Disorders*

Inhalant Use Disorder
Inhalant Intoxication
Other Inhalant-Induced Disorders
Unspecified Inhalant-Related Disorder

*Opioid-Related Disorders*

Opioid Use Disorder
Opioid Intoxication
Opioid Withdrawal
Other Opioid-Induced Disorders
Unspecified Opioid-Related Disorder

*Sedative-, Hypnotic-, or Anxiolytic-Related Disorders*

Sedative, Hypnotic, or Anxiolytic Use Disorder
Sedative, Hypnotic, or Anxiolytic Intoxication
Sedative, Hypnotic, or Anxiolytic Withdrawal
Other Sedative-, Hypnotic-, or Anxiolytic-Induced Disorders
Unspecified Sedative-, Hypnotic-, or Anxiolytic-Related Disorder

*Stimulant-Related Disorders*

Stimulant Use Disorder
Stimulant Intoxication
Stimulant Withdrawal

Other Stimulant-Induced
Disorders
Unspecified Stimulant-Related
Disorder

***Tobacco-Related Disorders***

Tobacco Use Disorder
Tobacco Withdrawal
Other Tobacco-Induced Disorders
Unspecified Tobacco-Related
Disorder

***Other (or Unknown) Substance–
Related Disorders***

Other (or Unknown) Substance
Use Disorder
Other (or Unknown) Substance
Intoxication
Other (or Unknown) Substance
Withdrawal
Other (or Unknown) Substance–
Induced Disorders
Unspecified Other (or Unknown)
Substance–Related Disorder

## Non-Substance-Related Disorders

Gambling Disorder

## Neurocognitive Disorders

Delirium
Other Specified Delirium
Unspecified Delirium

## Major and Mild Neurocognitive Disorders

Major Neurocognitive Disorder
Mild Neurocognitive Disorder
Major or Mild Neurocognitive
Disorder Due to Alzheimer's
Disease
Major or Mild Frontotemporal
Neurocognitive Disorder
Major or Mild Neurocognitive
Disorder With Lewy Bodies
Major or Mild Vascular
Neurocognitive Disorder
Major or Mild Neurocognitive
Disorder Due to Traumatic
Brain Injury

Substance/Medication-Induced
Major or Mild Neurocognitive
Disorder
Major or Mild Neurocognitive
Disorder Due to HIV Infection
Major or Mild Neurocognitive
Disorder Due to Prion Disease
Major or Mild Neurocognitive
Disorder Due to Parkinson's
Disease
Major or Mild Neurocognitive
Disorder Due to Huntington's
Disease
Major or Mild Neurocognitive
Disorder Due to Another
Medical Condition
Major or Mild Neurocognitive
Disorder Due to Multiple
Etiologies
Unspecified Neurocognitive
Disorder

## Personality Disorders

### Cluster A Personality Disorders

Paranoid Personality Disorder
Schizoid Personality Disorder
Schizotypal Personality Disorder

### Cluster B Personality Disorders

Antisocial Personality Disorder
Borderline Personality Disorder
Histrionic Personality Disorder
Narcissistic Personality Disorder

### Cluster C Personality Disorders

Avoidant Personality Disorder
Dependent Personality Disorder
Obsessive-Compulsive
Personality Disorder

### Other Personality Disorders

Personality Change Due to
Another Medical Condition
Other Specified Personality
Disorder
Unspecified Personality Disorder

## Paraphilic Disorders

Voyeuristic Disorder
Exhibitionistic Disorder
Frotteuristic Disorder
Sexual Masochism Disorder
Sexual Sadism Disorder
Pedophilic Disorder
Fetishistic Disorder
Transvestic Disorder
Other Specified Paraphilic Disorder
Unspecified Paraphilic Disorder

## Other Mental Disorders

Other Specified Mental Disorder
  Due to Another Medical
  Condition
Unspecified Mental Disorder Due
  to Another Medical Condition
Other Specified Mental Disorder
Unspecified Mental Disorder

# Medications

The following medications are commonly used in the treatment of mental disorders.

| Generic | Common brand(s) | Medication class/use |
|---|---|---|
| acamprosate | Campral | mixed-action agent used to treat chronic alcohol use disorder |
| alprazolam | Xanax, Xanax XR | benzodiazepine used to treat anxiety |
| alprostadil injection | Caverject Impulse | prostaglandin inhibitor used to treat erectile disorder |
| amitriptyline | Elavil* (generic only) | tricyclic antidepressant |
| amoxapine | Asendin* (generic only) | tetracyclic antidepressant |
| amphetamine-dextroamphetamine | Adderall, Adderall XR | combination stimulant used to treat ADHD |
| aripiprazole | Abilify, Abilify Discmelt | second-generation antipsychotic |
| aripiprazole, intramuscular injection | Abilify Maintena | second-generation, long-acting antipsychotic |
| armodafinil | Nuvigil | stimulant used to treat narcolepsy and sleep apnea |
| asenapine | Saphris | second-generation antipsychotic |
| atomoxetine | Strattera | nonstimulant used to treat ADHD |

| Generic | Common brand(s) | Medication class/use |
|---------|-----------------|----------------------|
| avanafil | Stendra | phosphodiesterase inhibitor used to treat erectile disorder |
| benztropine | Cogentin | anticholinergic agent used to treat Parkinson's disease and abnormal movements induced by antipsychotic medications |
| buprenorphine | Subutex* | partial opioid agonist used to treat chronic opioid use disorder |
| bupropion<br><br>bupropion, long-acting | Wellbutin, Wellbutrin SR Wellbutrin XL, Zyban | mixed-action antidepressant also used to treat smoking cessation and ADHD |
| carbamazepine | Tegretol, Tegretol XR, Equetro | anticonvulsant also used to treat bipolar disorder and pain disorders |
| buspirone | BuSpar* (generic only) | anxiolytic used to treat anxiety |
| chlordiazepoxide | Librium* (generic only) | benzodiazepine used to treat anxiety and alcohol withdrawal |
| chlorpromazine | Thorazine* (generic only) | first-generation antipsychotic |
| citalopram | Celexa | SSRI antidepressant |
| clomipramine | Anafranil | tricyclic antidepressant that acts like an SSRI, used primarily for OCD |
| clonazepam | Klonopin | benzodiazepine used to treat anxiety and bipolar disorder |
| clonidine | Catapres | blood pressure medication also used to treat ADHD and PTSD |
| clorazepate | Tranxene | benzodiazepine used to treat anxiety and alcohol withdrawal |

| Generic | Common brand(s) | Medication class/use |
|---------|-----------------|----------------------|
| clozapine | Clozaril, FazaClo | second-generation antipsychotic |
| desipramine | Norpramin | tricyclic antidepressant |
| desvenlafaxine | Pristiq | mixed-action antidepressant |
| dexmethylphenidate | Focalin, Focalin XR | stimulant used to treat ADHD |
| dextroamphetamine | Dexedrine, Dextrostat* | stimulant used to treat ADHD |
| diazepam | Valium | benzodiazepine used to treat anxiety, seizures, and alcohol withdrawal |
| diphenhydramine | Benadryl | antihistamine used to treat movement disorder and insomnia |
| disulfiram | Antabuse | aldehyde dehydrogenase inhibitor used to treat chronic alcohol use disorder |
| donepezil | Aricept | cognitive enhancer used to treat dementia |
| doxepin | Sinequan,* Adapin,* Silenor | tricyclic antidepressant also used to treat insomnia |
| duloxetine | Cymbalta | mixed-action antidepressant also used to treat anxiety and pain disorders |
| escitalopram | Lexapro | SSRI antidepressant |
| eszopiclone | Lunesta | hypnotic used to treat insomnia |
| fluoxetine | Prozac | SSRI antidepressant |
| fluphenazine | Prolixin* (generic only) | first-generation antipsychotic |
| fluphenazine decanoate | Prolixin Decanoate* (generic only) | first-generation, long-acting depot antipsychotic |
| flurazepam | Dalmane* (generic only) | benzodiazepine used to treat insomnia |

| Generic | Common brand(s) | Medication class/use |
|---|---|---|
| fluvoxamine | Luvox, Luvox CR | SSRI antidepressant |
| gabapentin | Neurontin | anticonvulsant used to treat bipolar disorder and pain disorders |
| gabapentin enacarbil | Horizant | anticonvulsant used to treat restless legs syndrome |
| galantamine | Razadyne, Razadyne ER | cognitive enhancer used to treat dementia |
| guanfacine | Tenex, Intuniv | blood pressure medication also used to treat ADHD |
| haloperidol | Haldol | first-generation antipsychotic |
| iloperidone | Fanapt | second-generation antipsychotic |
| imipramine | Tofranil, Tofranil-PM | tricyclic antidepressant |
| isocarboxazid | Marplan | MAOI antidepressant |
| lamotrigine | Lamictal, Lamictal XR | anticonvulsant also used to treat bipolar disorder and depression |
| levomilnacipran | Fetzima | mixed-action antidepressant also used to treat fibromyalgia and neuropathy |
| lisdexamfetamine | Vyvanse | stimulant used to treat ADHD |
| lithium carbonate | generic only | mood stabilizer used to treat bipolar disorder |
| lithium carbonate, extended release | Lithobid, Eskalith* | mood stabilizer used to treat bipolar disorder |
| lithium citrate | lithium liquid (generic only) | mood stabilizer used to treat bipolar disorder |
| lorazepam | Ativan | benzodiazepine used to treat anxiety |

| Generic | Common brand(s) | Medication class/use |
| --- | --- | --- |
| loxapine | Loxitane | first-generation antipsychotic |
| lurasidone | Latuda | second-generation antipsychotic |
| maprotiline | Ludiomil* (generic only) | tetracyclic antidepressant |
| melatonin | generic available | synthetic hormone used to treat insomnia |
| memantine | Namenda, Namenda XR | cognitive enhancer used to treat dementia |
| methylphenidate | Methylin, Ritalin | stimulant used to treat ADHD |
| methylphenidate, extended release | Concerta, Ritalin SR, Ritalin LA, Metadate CD, Methyline ER | long-acting stimulants used to treat ADHD |
| methylphenidate, topical patch | Daytrana | topical stimulant used to treat ADHD |
| milnacipran | Savella | mixed-action antidepressant also used to treat fibromyalgia and neuropathy |
| mirtazapine | Remeron | mixed-action antidepressant also used to treat insomnia |
| modafinil | Provigil | stimulant used to treat narcolepsy, sleep apnea, and ADHD |
| naloxone | Narcan* (generic only) | narcotic antagonist used to reverse opioid effects from overdose |
| naltrexone | ReVia, Vivitrol | narcotic antagonist used to treat chronic opioid and alcohol use disorders |
| nefazodone | Serzone* (generic only) | mixed-action antidepressant |
| nortriptyline | Pamelor | tricyclic antidepressant |

| Generic | Common brand(s) | Medication class/use |
|---|---|---|
| olanzapine | Zyprexa, Zyprexa Zydis | second-generation antipsychotic |
| olanzapine, intramuscular injection | Zyprexa Relprevv | second-generation, long-acting depot antipsychotic |
| olanzapine-fluoxetine | Symbyax | combination antipsychotic-antidepressant |
| oxazepam | Serax* (generic only) | benzodiazepine used to treat anxiety and alcohol withdrawal |
| oxcarbazepine | Trileptal | anticonvulsant also used to treat bipolar disorder |
| oxybate | Xyrem | used to treat cataplexy due to narcolepsy |
| paliperidone | Invega | second-generation antipsychotic |
| paroxetine | Paxil, Paxil CR, Pexeva | SSRI antidepressant |
| perphenazine | Trilafon* (generic only) | first-generation antipsychotic |
| phenelzine | Nardil | monoamine oxidase inhibitor antidepressant |
| pimozide | Orap | first-generation antipsychotic used to treat Tourette syndrome |
| pramipexole | Mirapex, Mirapex ER | dopamine agonist used to treat Parkinson's disease and restless legs syndrome |
| pregabalin | Lyrica | anticonvulsant also used to treat fibromyalgia and neuropathy |
| protriptyline | Vivactil | tricyclic antidepressant |
| quetiapine | Seroquel, Seroquel XR | second-generation antipsychotic |
| ramelteon | Rozerem | melatonin agonist used to treat insomnia |

| Generic | Common brand(s) | Medication class/use |
|---------|-----------------|----------------------|
| risperidone | Risperdal, Risperdal M-Tab | second-generation antipsychotic |
| risperidone, long-acting | Risperdal Consta | second-generation, long-acting antipsychotic |
| rivastigmine | Exelon, Exelon Patch | cognitive enhancer used to treat dementia |
| ropinirole | Requip, Requip XL | dopamine agonist used to treat Parkinson's disease and restless legs syndrome |
| rotigotine, topical patch | Neupro | dopamine agonist used to treat Parkinson's disease and restless legs syndrome |
| selegiline | Eldepryl | MAOI antidepressant |
| selegiline, topical patch | Emsam | MAOI antidepressant |
| sertraline | Zoloft | SSRI antidepressant |
| sildenafil | Viagra | phosphodiesterase inhibitor used to treat erectile disorder |
| tadalafil | Cialis | phosphodiesterase inhibitor used to treat erectile disorder |
| temazepam | Restoril | benzodiazepine used to treat insomnia |
| thioridazine | Mellaril* (generic only) | first-generation antipsychotic |
| topiramate | Topamax | anticonvulsant also used to treat bipolar disorder |
| tranylcypromine | Parnate | MAOI antidepressant |
| trazodone | Desyrel*, Oleptro | mixed-action antidepressant also used for insomnia |
| triazolam | Halcion | benzodiazepine used to treat insomnia |

| Generic | Common brand(s) | Medication class/use |
|---|---|---|
| trifluoperazine | Stelazine* (generic only) | first-generation antipsychotic |
| trihexyphenidyl | Artane* (generic only) | anticholinergic agent used to treat Parkinson's disease and abnormal movements caused by antipsychotic medications |
| trimipramine | Surmontil | tricyclic antidepressant |
| valproate | Depakene, Depakote, Depakote ER | anticonvulsant also used to treat bipolar disorder |
| vardenafil | Levitra | phosphodiesterase inhibitor used to treat erectile dysfunction |
| varenicline | Chantix | nicotinic agonist used to treat smoking cessation |
| venlafaxine | Effexor, Effexor XR | mixed-action antidepressant also used to treat anxiety, panic disorder, and pain disorders |
| vortioxetine | Brintellix | mixed-action antidepressant |
| zaleplon | Sonata | hypnotic used to treat insomnia |
| ziprasidone | Geodon | second-generation antipsychotic |
| zolpidem | Ambien, Ambien CR | hypnotic used to treat insomnia |

*This original or leading brand was discontinued.
ADHD=attention-deficit/hyperactivity disorder; CD=extended-release capsules; CR=controlled-release; ER=extended-release; LA=long-acting; MAOI=monoamine oxidase inhibitor; M-Tab=orally disintegrating tablets; OCD=obsessive-compulsive disorder; PM=imipramine pamoate; PTSD=posttraumatic stress disorder; SR=sustained-release; SSRI=selective serotonin reuptake inhibitor; XL=extended-release tablet; XR=extended-release.

# Helpful Resources

## General Mental Health

### American Academy of Child and Adolescent Psychiatry
**www.aacap.org**

This Web site for child and adolescent psychiatrists provides Facts for Families and other resources for seeking help and understanding mental illnesses.

### American Psychiatric Association
**www.psychiatry.org**

The Web site for the world's largest psychiatric organization provides an online resource about mental health topics, wellness, coping with disasters, and other issues for the general public. It includes videos, ways to find help, a blog and treatment locator, warning signs of mental illness, and information for caregivers.

### American Psychiatric Foundation
**www.americanpsychiatricfoundation.org**

The American Psychiatric Foundation seeks to educate the public that mental illnesses are real and that effective treatment options exist. It offers programs and information about mental health in schools, military, workplace, and the criminal justice system. Its Web site provides resources to get help.

### American Psychological Association
www.apa.org

This Web site features Psychology Topics and a Psychology Help Center—an online consumer resource featuring articles and information related to psychological issues affecting daily physical and emotional well-being, free brochures, and Find a Psychologist.

### Brain & Behavior Research Foundation
http://bbrfoundation.org

The Brain & Behavior Research Foundation awards grants that will lead to advances and breakthroughs in scientific research. Its Web site provides information on mental illnesses, cutting-edge research, and stories of recovery.

### Centers for Disease Control and Prevention
www.cdc.gov

The Centers for Disease Control and Prevention (CDC) works to fight disease. Its Web site provides general health information on wellness, safety, and disorders.

### Eunice Kennedy Shriver National Institute of Child Health and Human Development
www.nichd.nih.gov

This institute supports research in human development across the lifespan, focusing on developmental disabilities, reproductive health of men and women, and medical rehabilitation interventions. Its Web site contains A–Z topics and a Resources link for parents, patients, and caregivers.

### MedlinePlus
www.nlm.nih.gov/medlineplus

MedlinePlus is the National Institutes of Health Web site for patients and their families and friends. It contains information about diseases, conditions, treatments, drugs and supplements, wellness issues, and meanings of words in everyday language.

### Mental Health America
www.mentalhealthamerica.net

This Web site provides mental health screens, tips for working with a mental health care provider, mental health wellness and illness information, a crisis line, and more.

### National Alliance on Mental Illness (NAMI)
www.nami.org

NAMI is the largest grassroots mental health organization in the United States dedicated to building better lives for the millions of Americans affected by mental illness. NAMI's Web site offers information on mental illness and treatment, as well as free education, support, and awareness programs.

### National Federation of Families for Children's Mental Health
www.ffcmh.org

This family-run organization focuses on advocacy and offers families a voice in the formation of national policy, services, and supports for children with mental health needs and their families.

### National Institute of Mental Health (National Institutes of Health)
www.nimh.nih.gov

The National Institute of Mental Health aims to transform the understanding and treatment of mental illnesses through research, paving the way for prevention, recovery, and cure. Health Topics on its Web site contain information about mental illnesses, their causes, and treatment.

### National Kidney and Urologic Diseases Information Clearinghouse (National Institute of Diabetes and Digestive and Kidney Diseases)
www.kidney.niddk.nih.gov

The National Kidney and Urologic Diseases Information Clearinghouse provides information about elimination disorders and sexual dysfunctions.

## Addictive Disorders

### Above the Influence
http://abovetheinfluence.com

Teenagers who need help facing the pressure to use drugs, pills, and alcohol can learn the facts about these substances and how other teens handled the same problems at the Web site.

### Alcoholics Anonymous (AA)
www.aa.org

An international support group for people who have a drinking problem, AA helps its members quit drinking through its Twelve Steps recovery program.

### Gamblers Anonymous
www.gamblersanonymous.org

This Web site is built on the same 12-step recovery program as Alcoholics Anonymous.

### National Institute on Drug Abuse:
### Seeking Drug Abuse Treatment: Know What to Ask
www.drugabuse.gov/publications/seeking-drug-abuse-treatment

This free online treatment guide offers guidance in seeking drug abuse treatment and lists five questions to ask when searching for a treatment program.

### Rational Recovery
**https://rational.org**

This Web site provides information on independent recovery from addiction through planned, permanent abstinence; FAQs; and information for friends and family.

### Rethinking Drinking
**http://rethinkingdrinking.niaaa.nih.gov**

This Web site provides user-friendly tools and information to assess and address drinking habits, such as How Much Is Too Much, Is Your Drinking Pattern Risky, What's the Harm, Strategies for Cutting Down, Support for Quitting, Resources, and more.

### Substance Abuse and Mental Health Services Administration
**www.samhsa.gov**

This Web site provides links to find alcohol and drug abuse treatment or mental health treatment facilities and programs around the United States.

## Anxiety, Bipolar, and Depressive Disorders

### Anxiety and Depression Association of America
**www.adaa.org**

Anxiety and Depression Association of America brings together researchers, clinicians, and patients to improve lives through research, training, and education. It helps adults and children with anxiety disorders, depression, obsessive-compulsive disorder, and PTSD find treatment and resources.

### The Balanced Mind Parent Network
**www.thebalancedmind.org**

This Web site offers answers, support, and connection to families raising children with mood disorders, such as depression and bipolar disorder. It offers information on treatment, school accommodations, cutting-edge scientific research, and more through its Online Support Communities and Family Helpline.

### Depression and Bipolar Support Alliance
**www.dbsalliance.org**

The Depression and Bipolar Support Alliance provides in-person and 24/7 online peer support; current, readily understandable information about depression and bipolar disorder; and empowering tools focused on an integrated approach to wellness.

### Families for Depression Awareness
**http://familyaware.org**

Families for Depression Awareness helps families recognize and cope with depressive disorders to get people well and prevent suicides.

### International Bipolar Foundation
http://ibpf.org

The International Bipolar Foundation strives to improve understanding and treatment of bipolar disorder through research, to promote care and support resources for individuals and caregivers, and to erase stigma through education.

### Juvenile Bipolar Research Foundation
www.bpchildresearch.org

The Juvenile Bipolar Research Foundation Web site contains information about bipolar disorder in children and questions to help assess a child's symptoms for bipolar disorder.

### Postpartum Support International
www.postpartum.net

This Web site features a help line, Get the Facts, Get Help, information for friends and family, and links to resources.

### Right Direction
http://rightdirectionforme.com

This Web site defines depression, lists warning signs, provides a quick test to assess whether you have depression, provides resources for help, and lists answers to frequent questions about depression.

## Attention-Deficit/Hyperactivity Disorder (ADHD)

### Attention Deficit Disorder Association
www.add.org

The Attention Deficit Disorder Association provides information, resources, and networking opportunities to help adults with ADHD lead better lives.

### Children and Adults With Attention-Deficit/Hyperactivity Disorder
www.chadd.org

CHADD provides education, advocacy, and support, including training for parents and teachers, educational Webinars, evidence-based ADHD information, local support groups, and information specialists to support the ADHD community.

## Autism Spectrum

### Academic Autistic Spectrum Partnership in Research and Education (AASPIRE)
http://aaspire.org

AASPIRE brings together the academic community and the autistic community to develop and perform research projects relevant to the needs of adults on the autism spectrum.

### Autism National Committee
www.autcom.org

The Autism National Committee aims to protect and advance the human rights and civil rights of all persons with autism and related differences of communication and behavior.

### Autism Science Foundation
http://autismsciencefoundation.org

The Autism Science Foundation supports autism research, provides information about autism to the general public, and serves to increase awareness of autism spectrum disorders and the needs of individuals and families affected by autism.

### Autism Society
www.autism-society.org

The Autism Society strives to improve the lives of all affected by autism. It advocates for appropriate services across the life span and provides the latest information on treatment, education, research, and advocacy.

### Autism Speaks
www.autismspeaks.org

Autism Speaks funds research for autism, raises public awareness about autism and its effects, and works to bring hope to all who deal with the hardships of this disorder.

### Autistic Self Advocacy Network
http://autisticadvocacy.org

The Autistic Self Advocacy Network seeks to organize the community of autistic adults and youth to advocate for a world in which autistic people enjoy the same access, rights, and opportunities as all other citizens.

### Centers for Disease Control and Prevention
www.cdc.gov/vaccinesafety/Concerns/Autism/Index.html

The article "Concerns About Autism" discusses the issue of childhood vaccinations and provides information for parents.

## Dementia and Other Memory Problems

### Alzheimer's Association
www.alz.org

The Alzheimer's Association offers information about many dementia-related conditions and other helpful resources, such as a community resource finder, 24-hour help line, virtual library, and caregiver center.

### National Institute on Aging (NIA):
### Alzheimer's Disease Education and Referral Center
www.nia.nih.gov/alzheimers

The NIA is the main federal agency for Alzheimer's disease research. Its Web site provides information on Alzheimer's disease and other dementias, as well as practical information for caregivers and health care providers.

### National Parkinson Foundation
www.parkinson.org

The National Parkinson Foundation aims to improve the quality of care through research, education, and outreach. Its Web site provides information about the disease, warning signs, questions to ask doctors, treatment information, and resources for patients and caregivers.

## Eating Disorders

### National Association of Anorexia Nervosa
### and Associated Disorders
www.anad.org

The National Association of Anorexia Nervosa and Associated Disorders promotes eating disorder awareness, prevention, and recovery through supporting, educating, and connecting individuals, families, and professionals.

### National Eating Disorders Association
www.nationaleatingdisorders.org

The National Eating Disorders Association supports individuals and families affected by eating disorders, and serves as a catalyst for prevention, cures, and access to quality care.

## Elimination Disorders

### American Academy of Child and Adolescent Psychiatry:
### Facts for Families
www.aacap.org/cs/root/facts_for_families/bedwetting

This fact sheet contains information for parents about bed-wetting in children.

### FamilyDoctor.org: Stool Soiling and Constipation in Children
http://familydoctor.org/familydoctor/en/kids/toileting/stool-soiling-and-constipation-in-children.html

This Web site contains information on the causes of stool soiling and toilet training tips.

# Gay and Lesbian Mental Health and Advocacy

### Human Rights Campaign
www.hrc.org

The Human Rights Campaign works to achieve equality for lesbian, gay, bisexual, and transgender (LGBT) Americans, invests strategically to elect fair-minded individuals to office, and educates the public about LGBT issues.

### Parents, Families, and Friends of Lesbians and Gays
www.pflag.org

Parents, Families, and Friends of Lesbians and Gays works to advance equality and societal acceptance of LGBT people. It provides support, education, and advocacy.

### The Trevor Project
www.thetrevorproject.org

The Trevor Project provides crisis intervention and suicide prevention services to LGBT and questioning young people ages 13–24.

# Gender Dysphoria

### Accord Alliance
www.accordalliance.org

Accord Alliance promotes comprehensive and integrated approaches to care that enhance the health and well-being of people and families affected by disorders of sex development.

### National Center for Transgender Equality
http://transequality.org

The National Center for Transgender Equality is devoted to ending discrimination and violence against transgender people through education and advocacy on national issues of importance to transgender people.

# Intellectual Disability

### American Association on Intellectual and Developmental Disabilities
http://aaidd.org

The American Association on Intellectual and Developmental Disabilities promotes progressive policies, sound research, effective practices, and universal human rights for people with intellectual and developmental disabilities. Its Web site provides information about intellectual disability.

**National Association for the Dually Diagnosed**
http://thenadd.org

The National Association for the Dually Diagnosed promotes the development of appropriate community-based policies, programs, and opportunities in addressing the mental health needs of persons with intellectual and developmental disabilities.

# Learning Disabilities

**Learning Disabilities Association of America**
ldaamerica.org

The Learning Disabilities Association of America aims to create opportunities for success for all people affected by learning disabilities and to reduce the incidence of learning disabilities in future generations.

**National Center for Learning Disabilities**
www.ncld.org

The National Center for Learning Disabilities improves the lives of all people with learning difficulties and disabilities by empowering parents, enabling young adults, transforming schools, and creating policy and advocacy impact.

# Military Mental Health and Support

**Disabled American Veterans**
www.dav.org

Disabled American Veterans ensures that veterans and their families can access the full range of benefits available to them and provides structure through which disabled veterans can express their compassion for their fellow veterans through a variety of volunteer programs.

**DoD Safe Helpline**
www.safehelpline.org
877-995-5247

This Web site provides sexual assault support for the Department of Defense community and features 24/7 help that is secure, worldwide, and confidential in a variety of formats.

**Give an Hour**
www.giveanhour.org

This organization provides free mental health services to the military and their family members affected by current conflicts in Afghanistan and Iraq. The site provides a link to resources and includes Search for a Provider.

## Iraq and Afghanistan Veterans of America
http://iava.org

Iraq and Afghanistan Veterans of America provides programs in four key impact areas: health, education, employment, and building a lasting community for vets and their families. It offers assistance to veterans and their families.

## National Center for PTSD
## (and the U.S. Department of Veterans Affairs)
www.ptsd.va.gov

The National Center for PTSD strives to advance the clinical care and social welfare of America's veterans and others who have experienced trauma, or who suffer from posttraumatic stress disorder. It conducts research, education, and training in the science, diagnosis, and treatment of PTSD and stress-related disorders.

## National Military Family Association
www.militaryfamily.org

The National Military Family Association pursues the goal that all military families deserve comprehensive child care, accessible health care, spouse employment options, great schools, caring communities, a secure retirement, and support for widows and widowers.

## Vietnam Veterans of America
http://vva.org

Vietnam Veterans of America works to promote and support the full range of issues important to Vietnam veterans.

## Wounded Warrior Project
www.woundedwarriorproject.org

The Wounded Warrior Project helps injured service members aid and assist each other and provides unique, direct programs and services to meet the needs of injured service members.

# Obsessive-Compulsive and Related Disorders

## International OCD Foundation
www.ocfoundation.org

The International OCD Foundation provides resources and support for those affected by OCD and related disorders, including those with OCD, their family members, friends, and loved ones.

### Trichotillomania Learning Center
www.trich.org

The Trichotillomania Learning Center aims to end the suffering caused by hair pulling disorder, skin picking disorder, and related body-focused repetitive behaviors. Guided by a scientific advisory board of leading researchers and clinicians, it provides treatment referrals, support groups, educational events, and more.

## Personality Disorders

### National Education Alliance for Borderline Personality Disorder
www.borderlinepersonalitydisorder.com

The National Education Alliance for Borderline Personality Disorder works with families and persons in recovery, raises public awareness, promotes research, and advocates to enhance the quality of life for those affected by this serious but treatable mental illness.

### Treatment and Research Advancements:
### National Association for Personality Disorder
www.tara4bpd.org

This organization fosters education and research in the field of personality disorder, specifically but not only borderline personality disorder; advocates to reduce stigma and increase awareness of personality disorder; and provides information on causes and treatment.

## Schizophrenia and Other Psychotic Disorders

### Schizophrenia and Related Disorders Alliance of America
www.sardaa.org

Schizophrenia and Related Disorders Alliance of America promotes improvement in the lives of people with schizophrenia-related illnesses and their families by providing support, hope, and awareness so that early diagnosis, treatment, and community services increase recovery.

## Sexual and Other Violence

### Centers for Disease Control and Prevention
www.cdc.gov/violenceprevention

This Web site contains facts-at-a-glance, prevention tips, and resources on child maltreatment, elder abuse, global violence, intimate partner violence, sexual violence, and youth violence. The sexual violence page contains a hotline for rape, abuse, and incest survivors.

**RAINN (Rape, Abuse & Incest National Network)**
https://rainn.org
National Sexual Assault Hotline: 1-800-656-HOPE (4673)

RAINN is the nation's largest anti-sexual violence organization; it carries out programs to prevent sexual violence, help victims, and ensure that rapists are brought to justice.

**Womenshealth.gov**
www.womenshealth.gov/violence-against-women

The Web page "Violence Against Women" contains helpful information, such as Am I Being Abused, Types of Violence Against Women, Mental Health Effects of Violence, and hotlines for different types of violence against women (such as domestic violence, teen dating, and sexual assault).

## Sleep-Wake Disorders

**American Sleep Association**
www.sleepassociation.org

The American Sleep Association promotes public awareness about sleep disorders, sleep health, and sleep medicine research.

**National Heart, Lung, and Blood Institute**
www.nhlbi.nih.gov

This Web site provides information on sleep disorders, including causes, risk factors, signs and symptoms, treatments, coping tips, research trials, and links to more information.

**National Sleep Foundation**
http://sleepfoundation.org

The National Sleep Foundation Web site provides information on sleep health, sleep problems and disorders, sleep tools and tips, and a sleep professional locator.

## Suicide Awareness and Prevention

**Active Minds**
www.activeminds.org

Active Minds was founded by a college student as the result of the suicide of her older brother. It aims to remove the stigma on college campuses that surrounds mental health issues, and it supports help seeking for mental health.

**American Foundation for Suicide Prevention**
www.afsp.org

The American Foundation for Suicide Prevention works with those who have been personally touched by suicide to understand, prevent, and help heal the pain it causes. It provides research support, education, community, and advocacy.

### The Jed Foundation
http://jedfoundation.org

The Jed Foundation works to promote emotional health and prevent suicide among college and university students. It helps build knowledge of warning signs, foster help-seeking, build coping skills, protect at-risk students, and raise the importance of mental health services and policies.

### National Organization for Persons of Color Against Suicide
http://nopcas.org

The National Organization for Persons of Color Against Suicide helps to decrease life-threatening behaviors in minority communities. It aims to develop prevention, intervention, and postvention support services to the families and communities impacted by violence, depression, and suicide.

### National Suicide Prevention Lifeline
www.suicidepreventionlifeline.org
**1-800-273-TALK (1-800-273-8255)**

The National Suicide Prevention Lifeline is a 24-hour, toll-free, confidential suicide prevention hotline for anyone in suicidal crisis or emotional distress. Its Web site contains information on mental health and suicide prevention and links for more help for veterans and young adults.

### Suicide Awareness Voices of Education
www.save.org

Suicide Awareness Voices of Education strives to prevent suicide through public awareness and education, reduce stigma, serve as a resource to those touched by suicide, and support the need for professional assessment and treatment.

## Tourette's Disorder

### National Tourette Syndrome Association
www.tsa-usa.org

The National Tourette Syndrome Association offers resources and referrals to help people and their families cope with the problems that occur with Tourette syndrome.

## International Mental Health Organizations

These organizations are based outside the United States and promote mental health wellness, support services, and advocacy.

## ABRATA
## (Associação Brasileira de Familiares, Amigos e Portadores de Transtornos Afetivos; Brazilian Association of Family, Friends, and Patients With Affective Disorders)
www.abrata.org.br

ABRATA works in Brazil to raise awareness about mood disorders and increase psychosocial support for patients with depression and bipolar disorder, as well as their families and friends.

## Global Alliance of Mental Illness Advocacy Networks (GAMIAN)—Europe
www.gamian.eu

Global Alliance of Mental Illness Advocacy Networks, a patient-driven pan-European organization, represents the interests of persons affected by mental illness and advocates for their rights.

## *Australia and New Zealand*

## The Australian Association for Infant Mental Health
www.aaimhi.org

This organization represents professionals from many fields who work with infants and their families. Its Web site provides position statements to support infant mental health for professionals and parents.

## Australian and New Zealand Mental Health Association
http://anzmh.asn.au

Available to professionals, patients, and carers, this organization provides knowledge about mental health to the public; teaches mental health skills to interested citizens such as patients, consumers, and carers; and advocates for improved mental health and mental health services.

## Australian Psychological Society
www.psychology.org.au

This Web site for the largest professional association for psychologists in Australia provides information for the public such as Psychology Topics, Find a Psychologist, and Areas of Psychology.

## *beyondblue*
www.beyondblue.org.au and www.beyondblue.org.au/getsupport

Learn more about anxiety, depression and suicide prevention, or talk through your concerns with our Support Service. Our trained mental health professionals will listen and provide information and advice.

## Black Dog Institute
www.blackdoginstitute.org.au

The Black Dog Institute is a world leader in the diagnosis, treatment, and prevention of mood disorders, such as depression and bipolar disorder. Its Web site contains helpful information on these disorders and ways to get help in Australia.

### Headspace—National Youth Mental Health Foundation
http://www.headspace.org.au

Headspace helps young people who are going through a tough time. The Web site provides information for young people, parents, carers, and professionals and features a Kids Help Line and a link to find Headspace Centres for young people ages 12–25.

### Mental Health Council of Australia
http://mhca.org.au

Devoted to changing perceptions about mental illness, this organization has a Web site with links to a range of groups that can help those with mental illness.

### Mental Health Foundation of New Zealand
www.mentalhealth.org.nz

This Web site provides mental health topics from A to Z, wellness information, and links to information and resources in New Zealand.

### mindhealthconnect
www.mindhealthconnect.org.au

Find trusted mental health and well-being information, online programs, help lines, and news on this site.

### New Zealand Psychological Society
www.psychology.org.nz

This Web site for psychologists in New Zealand features Find a Psychologist and useful links for the public.

### The Royal Australian and New Zealand College of Psychiatrists
www.ranzcp.org

This Web site features Find a Psychiatrist, About Psychiatry, Guides for the Public, crisis information, links to online resources, and more for the public.

## United Kingdom

### Carers UK
www.carersuk.org

This Web site offers expert advice, information, and support for carers; a help and advice phone line; links to topics of concern; and ways to connect with other carers.

### Centre for Mental Health
www.centreformentalhealth.org.uk

The Centre for Mental Health focuses on criminal justice, employment, mental health at work, recovery, and children, with supporting work on broader mental health and public policy.

## Mental Health Foundation
www.mentalhealth.org.uk

This organization helps people to survive, recover from, and prevent mental health problems. Its Web site contains mental health topics from A to Z, free publications, an e-mail newsletter, a blog, well-being apps and podcasts, and more.

## MIND (for Better Mental Health)—United Kingdom
www.mind.org.uk

MIND provides advice and support to empower anyone with a mental health problem. Goals include helping people to stay well, make informed choices, get the right services, participate in society, and gain equality of treatment.

## SANE
http://sane.org.uk

SANE works to improve the quality of life for anyone affected by mental illness, offers emotional support and information to anyone affected by mental health problems through a help line, and offers an online support forum where people share their feelings and experiences.

## Time to Change
www.time-to-change.org.uk

This Web site contains facts and myths to challenge mental health stigma and discrimination; information for work managers, parents, and young people; tips on how to help a friend with mental illness; and answers to the question "What is mental health?"

## Together
www.together-uk.org

Together offers a wide range of support to help people deal with the personal and practical impacts of mental health issues. The Web site provides a service finder and a link to peer support.

## Young Minds
www.youngminds.org.uk

This Web site provides practical information for children, young people, parents, and professionals, including a help line for parents of those ages 0–25.

# Index

*Page numbers printed in **boldface** type refer to tables or figures.*

Bell-and-pad method, 161
Benzodiazepines
  anxiety disorders and, 77, 90
  overview of, 303–304
  parasomnias and, 178
  PTSD and, 114
  restless legs syndrome and, 183
  side effects of, 303
Bilevel positive airway pressure
    (BiPAP), 177
Binge-eating disorder, 153–154
Binge-eating/purging type, of
    anorexia nervosa, 149
Bingeing, and bulimia nervosa, 151–
    152
Biochemistry, and risk factors for
    major depressive disorder, 61
Biofeedback
  acute stress disorder and, 120
  factitious disorder and, 141
Bipolar disorders, 45–57
  description of, 45
  key points on, 57
  other conditions and,
      gambling disorder, 235
      major depressive disorder, 61
      narcolepsy, 172
      persistent insomnia, 169
  substance-induced, 231
  treatment of, 302, 304–305
Bipolar I disorder
  description of, 46
  diagnosis of, 46–48
  other conditions and, 46
  risk factors for, 48
  story about, 48–49
  treatment of, 49–51
Bipolar II disorder
  description of, 51–52
  diagnosis of, 52–53
  other conditions and, 52
  risk factors for, 53
  story about, 53–54
  treatment of, 54
Bizarre delusions, 30, 39

Bladder retraining exercise, 161
Blood-brain barrier, and HIV
    infection, 256
Body dysmorphic disorder, 98–99
Body image, and eating disorders,
    147, 150
Body mass index (BMI), **147, 148,**
    149, 150
Borderline personality disorder
  description of, 263–264
  diagnosis of, 264–265
  dialectical behavior therapy for,
      297
  risk factors for, 265
  story about, 265–266
  treatment of, 297, 302
Brain. *See also* Brain injury;
    Traumatic brain injury
  addictive disorders and, 226
  frontal lobes of, 251
  functions assessed of,
      **240–241**
Brain injury, and intellectual
    disability, 17. *See also* Traumatic
    brain injury
Breathing-related sleep disorders,
    174–178
  central sleep apnea, 176–177
  obstructive sleep apnea
      hypopnea, 174–176
  sleep-related hypoventilation,
      177–178
Brief psychotherapy
  for adjustment disorder, 121
  for erectile disorder, 192
Brief psychotic disorder, 41
Bulimia nervosa, 151–153

Caffeine, 77, 224, **232,** 307
Cannabis, **232**
Caregivers, of those with
  dementia, 246, **247,** 252, 258
  schizophrenia, 37
  trauma and stress disorders, 122,
      123

Collecting, and hoarding disorder, 100

Combined treatment, with drug therapy and psychotherapy, 302

Combined type, of ADHD, 12

Communication. *See also* Communication disorders; Language
autism spectrum disorder and, 5, 6, **7**
intellectual disability and, 15
sexual health and, **198**

Communications disorders, 20–22, 33
language disorder, 5, 20
social communication disorder, 21–22
speech sound disorder, 20–21
stuttering, 21

Community support programs, for schizophrenia, 36

Complex attention, and brain functions, **240**

Compulsions, and obsessive-compulsive disorders, 93, 94–95, 105

Conceptual functions, and intellectual disability, 16, **18–19**

Concussions, and traumatic brain injury, 247

Conduct disorder
antisocial personality disorder and, 214–215, 216, 267
description of, 214–215
diagnosis of, 215–216
encopresis and, 162
parent management training and, 211
story about, 216

Confusion
Alzheimer's disease and, **243**
Lewy body disease and, 254

Consciousness, loss of and traumatic brain injury, 247

Constipation, and encopresis, 161–162

Continuous amnesia, 129

Continuous positive airway pressure (CPAP) device, 176, 177

Conversion disorder, 136, 138–139

Coping, and coping skills. *See also* Caregivers
in adults with autism spectrum disorder, 5
for children exposed to trauma, **115**
for families of those with autism spectrum disorder, 10
PTSD, **115**
for parents of those with ADHD, 14
disruptive mood dysregulation disorder, 71

Counseling
Alzheimer's disease and, 246
frontotemporal neurocognitive disorder and, 252

Couples therapy. *See also* Family therapy
goals and applications of, 298–299
marriage and family therapists, 291
sexual dysfunctions and, 197

Covert sensitization, and kleptomania, 218

Cravings, and addictive disorders, 226

Creutzfeldt-Jakob disease, 256

Cross-dressing. *See* Transvestic disorder

Culture
diagnosis of schizophrenia or psychotic disorders and, 31
dissociative identity disorder and, 129
eating disorders and, 145, 150
schizotypal personality disorder and, 269
sexual dysfunctions and, 187

Cyclothymic disorder, 54–56

Gambling disorder, 222, **223,** 233–235, 266
Gender dysphoria, 201–207
  diagnosis of, 203–204
  key points on, 206–207
  overview of, 201–202
  risk factors for, 204
  story about, 204–205
  treatment of, 205–206
Generalized amnesia, 129
Generalized anxiety disorder
  anxiolytic medications for, 304
  description of, 82
  diagnosis of, 83
  other conditions and, 82, 87
  risk factors for, 83
Generalized sexual dysfunction, 188, 191
Genetics, and risk factors
  for acute stress disorder, 118
  for ADHD, 12
  for agoraphobia, 82
  for Alzheimer's disease, 244
  for anorexia nervosa, 150
  for autism spectrum disorder, 8
  for bulimia nervosa, 153
  for delirium, 241
  for female orgasmic disorder, 194
  for gender dysphoria, 204
  for generalized anxiety disorder, 83
  for hoarding disorder, 101
  for insomnia disorder, 170
  for intellectual disability, 17
  for major depressive disorder, 61
  for non-REM sleep arousal disorders, 180
  for OCD, 96
  for panic disorder, 79
  for persistent depressive disorder, 66
  for premenstrual dysphoric disorder, 69
  for PTSD, 112
  for schizophrenia, 33

for separation anxiety disorder, 88
for social anxiety disorder, 87
for specific phobia, 85
Genito-pelvic pain/penetration disorder, 196
Glossary, 309–317
Grandiose delusions, 30
Graphing, and pyromania, 217
Grief
  as distinct from major depressive disorder, **62**
  hoarding disorder and, 100
Grossly disorganized behavior, in context of schizophrenia, 31
Group homes
  intellectual disability and, 17
  schizophrenia and, 37
Group therapy
  for adjustment disorder, 121
  for eating disorders, 146, 156
  goals, approaches, and methods of, 299
  for major depressive disorder, 63
  for somatic symptom disorders, 136–137

Habit reversal, and hair-pulling disorder, 104
Hair-pulling disorder, 103–104
Hallucinations
  as key feature of psychotic disorders, 30
  Lewy body disease and, 253, 254
  narcolepsy and, 172
Health and health care. *See* Hormone treatments; Hospital; Lifestyle; Medical conditions; Medical examination; Primary care physicians
Health insurance, and lists of mental health care providers, 291
Histrionic personality disorder, 272
HIV infection, neurocognitive disorder due to, 256
Hoarding disorder, 100–103

Understanding Mental Disorders

Hormone treatments. *See also* Testosterone replacement therapy
 premenstrual dysphoric disorder and, 69
 sex reassignment surgery and, 206
Hospital
 and suicide prevention, in emergency room, **294**
 as treatment setting, 293
Humor, and healthy lifestyle, 307
Huntington's disease, neurocognitive disorder due to, 257
Hyperactive/impulsive type, of ADHD, 12
Hyperactivity, and ADHD, 10, 12
Hypersomnolence disorder, 182
Hypervigilance
 acute stress disorder and, 118
 PTSD and, 110, 112
Hypnosis, and PTSD, 114. *See also* Self-hypnosis
Hypnotic agents, 303, 304
Hypocretin, 172
Hypomanic episodes, and bipolar disorders, 46, 47–48, 51–52
Hypopnea, definition of, 174

IDEA. *See* Individuals with Disabilities Education Act
Illness anxiety disorder, 136, 140
Impaired control, and substance use disorder, 227
Impulsivity, and ADHD, 10, 12
Inattention, and ADHD, 10, 11–12
Inattentive type, of ADHD, 12
Individual factors, in sexual dysfunctions, 187
Individuals with Disabilities Education Act (IDEA), 10, 15, 17, 26
Infection
 and delirium, 241
 HIV disease and, 256

Inflammatory bowel disease, and agoraphobia, 81
Insight, and OCD, 94
Insight-oriented psychotherapy, 295
Insomnia disorder, 169–171
Intellectual disability
 changes in DSM-5 and, 4
 description of, 15
 diagnosis of, 16–17
 intelligence quotient and, 16
 other conditions and, 5, 24
 range of levels in, 16, **18–19**
 risk factors for, 17
 rumination disorder and, 155
 treatment of, 17
Intermittent explosive disorder, 212–214
Internalizing disorders, 209
Interpersonal psychotherapy, 63, 296
Interpersonal and social rhythm therapy, and bipolar I disorder, 50
Interventions, and addictive disorders, 222
Interview, as first step in treatment, 291–292
Intoxication, and drug use, 224, 226, 229, 230, **232**
IQ, and definition of intellectual disability, 16

Kegel exercises, 161
Kleptomania, 217–218

Language. *See also* Communication; Language disorder; Speech; Speech and language therapy
 Alzheimer's disease and, **243**
 brain functions and, **240**
 frontotemporal neurocognitive disorder and, 251, 252
Language disorder, 5, 20
Learning, and brain functions, **240.** *See also* Specific learning disorder

Lewy body disease, 252–253
Life goals program, and bipolar I
    disorder, 50
Lifelong sexual dysfunction, 188, 191
Lifestyle, healthy
    anxiety disorders and, 77, 90
    bipolar I disorder and, 51
    eating disorders and, 147
    erectile disorder and, 192
    improving health and treatment
        through, 306–308
    major depressive disorder and,
        64–65
    narcolepsy and, 173
    obsessive-compulsive disorders
        and, 94, 105
    obstructive sleep apnea and, 176
    premenstrual dysphoric disorder
        and, 69–70
    PTSD and, 116
    review of for prescription of
        medication, **300**
    sleep-wake disorders and, 185
    vascular neurocognitive disorder
        and, 255
Light therapy, and circadian rhythm
    sleep-wake disorders, 183
Localized amnesia, 129

"Mad cow disease," 256
Maintenance treatment
    for major depressive disorder, 64
    medications and, 301
Major depressive disorder
    description of, 60
    diagnosis of, 60–61
    grief compared to, **62**
    healthy lifestyle and, 64–65
    other conditions and, 60, 82, 86,
        269
    risk factors for, 61
    schizotypal personality disorder
        and, 269
    story about, 62
    treatment of, 62–64, 296, 302

Major neurocognitive disorder, 238,
    **240–241,** 258
Male hypoactive sexual desire
    disorder, 197
Mania and manic episodes, and
    bipolar disorders, 46, 47, 61, 304
Manic-depressive disorder. *See*
    Bipolar I disorder
MAOIs (monoamine oxidase
    inhibitors), 63, 189, 302
Marijuana, **232**
Marriage and family therapists, 291.
    *See also* Couples therapy; Family
    therapy
Measles-mumps-rubella (MMR)
    vaccine, 8
Medical conditions. *See also*
    Infection; Medical emergency;
    Medical examinations; Physical
    symptoms; Seizures; Surgery
    agoraphobia and, 81
    caused by eating disorders, 146,
        156
    delirium and, 239
    elimination disorders and, 159,
        163
    female orgasmic disorder and, 194
    illness anxiety disorder and, 140
    memory problems and, 237
    mental disorders and, 5, 16
    prescription of medications and,
        **300**
    risk factors for intellectual
        disability and, 17
    sleep-wake disorders and, 184
    somatic symptom disorders and,
        135, 137
Medical emergency
    catatonia as, 40, 42
    suicide crisis as, **294**
Medical examinations. *See also*
    Medical conditions
    delirium and, 241
    eating disorders and, 146
    schizophrenia and, 35

Medications, 300–305, 325–332. *See also* Antidepressants; Antipsychotic medications; Mood stabilizers; Over-the-counter medications; Side effects; Stimulants; Treatment; *specific disorders*

abuse of prescription drugs and, **226**

anxiolytic medications, 303–304

hypnotic agents, 303, 304

sedatives, 77, **232,** 303–304

overview of, 300–301

tips for most effective use of, **301**

tranquilizers, 77

Memory. *See also* Dementia

acute stress disorder and, 117

Alzheimer's disease and, 242, **243**

brain functions and, **240**

dissociative amnesia and, 129, 130

health issues and, 237

Lewy body disease and, 253

normal aging and problems with, 257

PTSD and, 108, 109, 111

Mental retardation. *See* Intellectual disability

Mild intellectual disability, 16, **18**

Mild neurocognitive disorder, 238, **240–241,** 258

Mild traumatic brain injury, and PTSD, 109. *See also* Traumatic brain injury

Military, and PTSD, 109, **115**

Modeling, and behavior therapy, 298

Moderate intellectual disability, 16, **18**

Monoamine oxidase inhibitors (MAOIs), 63, 189, 302

Mood. *See also* Emotional problems

acute stress disorder and negative, 117

Alzheimer's disease and, **243**

bipolar disorders and episodes, 45

oppositional defiant disorder and, 211

Mood stabilizers

bipolar I disorder and, 49

bipolar II disorder and, 54

cyclothymic disorder and, 56

overview of, 304–305

personality disorders and, 263

Motor behavior, disorganized or abnormal, and psychotic disorders, 30–31

Motor disorders, 23–25

developmental coordination disorder, 5, 23–24

stereotypic movement disorder, 24–25

tic disorders, 25

Multiple personality disorder. *See* Dissociative identity disorder

Narcissistic personality disorder, 272–273

Narcolepsy, 172–173

National Alliance on Mental Illness, 65, 71

National Association of Anorexia Nervosa and Associated Disorders, 147

National Eating Disorders Association, 147

National Institute on Alcohol Abuse and Alcoholism, **225**

National Suicide Prevention Lifeline, **294**

Negative symptoms, of schizophrenia, 31

Neurocognitive disorders. *See* Dementia

Neurocognitive problems, caused by medications, 231.

Neurodevelopmental disorders. *See* Disorders that start in childhood

Neuroleptic malignant syndrome, 303

Neurological problems, and traumatic brain injury, 247

Nightmare disorder, 180–181

Premature (early) ejaculation, 191, 192–193
Premenstrual dysphoric disorder (PMDD), 68–70
Premenstrual syndrome (PMS), 68
Pretraumatic factors, and PTSD, 112
Primary care physicians
  autism spectrum disorder and, 6–7
  mental health care providers and, 291
Primary enuresis, 160
Primary sex features, **202**
Prion disease, neurocognitive disorder due to, 256
Problem solving, and Alzheimer's disease, **243**
Profound intellectual disability, 16, **19**
Provisional tic disorder, 25
Psychiatric nurses, 291
Psychiatrists, 290. *See also* Therapeutic alliance
Psychodynamic psychotherapy, 295
Psychologists, 290
Psychosis. *See also* Psychotic disorders
  definition of, 29
  substance-induced, 230–231
Psychotherapy, 294–299. *See also* Behavior therapy; Cognitive-behavior therapy
  combined treatment and, 302
  definition of, 294–295
  and treatment of,
    bipolar I disorder, 50
    bipolar II disorder, 54
    cyclothymic disorder, 56
    delusional disorder, 40
    disruptive and conduct disorders, 210
    disruptive mood dysregulation disorder, 71
    eating disorders, 156
    elimination disorders, 160
    gender dysphoria, 206
    language disorder, 20
    major depressive disorder, 63

male hypoactive sexual desire disorder, 197
paraphilic disorders, 280
persistent depressive disorder, 67
personality disorders, 275
premenstrual dysphoric disorder, 69
psychotic disorders, 43
schizophrenia, 34
stereotypic movement disorder, 24
types of,
  brief psychotherapy, 121, 192
  couples therapy, 197, 298–299
  dialectical behavior therapy, 297
  family therapy, 50, 56, 63, 122, 146, 156, 215, 291, 298, 299
  group therapy, 63, 121, 136–137, 146, 156, 299
  insight-oriented psychotherapy, 295
  interpersonal psychotherapy, 63, 296
  psychodynamic psychotherapy, 295
  supportive psychotherapy, 63, 120, 141, 296
Psychotic disorders, 29–43
  features of, 29–31
  key points on, 43
PTSD. *See* Posttraumatic stress disorder
Purging, and bulimia nervosa, 151–152
Pyromania, 217

Rapid cycling, and bipolar I disorder, 46
Rapid eye movement (REM) sleep, 168
Rapid eye movement (REM) sleep behavior disorder, 181–182
Reactive attachment disorder, 122

Reading, and specific learning
disorder, 23
Receptive language, 20
Recurrent insomnia, 169
Referential delusions, 30
Rehabilitation programs, and
schizophrenia, 36
Relapse
addictive disorders and, 224, **225,**
235
medications and, 301
paraphilic disorders and
prevention techniques for,
280
Relationship factors, in sexual
dysfunctions, 187
Relaxation techniques, 297
acute stress disorder and, 120
Alzheimer's disease and, **247**
anxiety disorders and, 77
depersonalization/derealization
disorder and, 132
insomnia disorder and, 171
obsessive-compulsive disorders
and, 94
Religion
dissociative identity disorder
and, 129
sexual dysfunctions and, 187
REM (rapid eye movement) sleep,
168
REM (rapid eye movement) sleep
behavior disorder, 181–182
Repetitive behaviors, and autism
spectrum disorder, 6, **7**
Resources, **307,** 333–348
Restless legs syndrome, 183
Restricted behaviors, and autism
spectrum disorder, **7**
Restricting type, of anorexia nervosa,
149
Revenge, and oppositional defiant
disorder, 212
Reward system, and addictive
disorders, 221, 235

Risk factors, for mental disorders.
*See* Childbirth complications;
Environment; Genetics;
Temperament; *specific disorders*
Rumination disorder, 155

Safety
hoarding disorder and, 100
narcolepsy and, 172
plans for suicide prevention and,
**294**
Schedules, and autism spectrum
disorder, 10
Schizoaffective disorder, 38–39
Schizoid personality disorder, 271–
272
Schizophrenia
age of onset in, 31
course of, 31–32
description of, 31
diagnosis of, 32–33
key support options for, 36–37
as most common of psychotic
disorders, 29
risk factors for, 33
schizotypal personality disorder
and, 270
story about, 33–34
treatment of, 34–36, **37,** 302
Schizophreniform disorder, 41–42
Schizotypal personality disorder,
269–270
Script
and OCD, 97
and relapse prevention, **225**
Secondary enuresis, 160
Secondary sex features, **202**
Sedatives, 77, **232,** 303–304
Seizures, and conversion disorder,
138
Selective amnesia, 129
Selective serotonin reuptake
inhibitors (SSRIs)
depersonalization/derealization
disorder and, 132

Sleep-wake disorders, 167–185. *See also* Sleep
    cyclothymic disorder and, 55
    key points on, 184–185
    overview of, 167–169
    substance-induced, 231
Sleepwalking, 178, 179
Snoring, and sleep apnea, 174
SNRIs (serotonin-norepinephrine reuptake inhibitors), 63, 302
Social anxiety disorder, 85–87
Social (pragmatic) communication disorder, 21–22
Social cognition, and brain functions, **241**
Social contact, and social skills. *See also* Social skills training
    autism spectrum disorder and, 5, 6, **7**
    avoidant personality disorder and, 273–274
    frontotemporal neurocognitive disorder and, 251, 252
    healthy lifestyle and, 307
    major depressive disorder and, 65
    narcolepsy and, 172
    schizotypal personality disorder and, 269, 270
    substance use disorder and, 227
    trauma and stress disorders and, 122
Social functions, and intellectual disability, 16, **18–19**
Social phobia. *See* Social anxiety disorder
Social skills training, and autism spectrum disorder, 9
Social workers, 291
Somatic delusions, 30
Somatic symptom disorder, 136, 137–138
Somatic symptom disorders, 135–142
    key points on, 141–142
    overview of, 135–136
    treatment of, 136–137

Somatization. *See* Somatic symptom disorder
Specific learning disorder, 11, 22–23
Specific phobia. *See also* Agoraphobia; Social anxiety disorder
    description of, 83–84
    diagnosis of, 84–85
    risk factors for, 85
    separation anxiety disorder and, 87
Speech, disorganized as feature of psychotic disorders, 30. *See also* Communication; Language; Speech and language therapy; Speech sound disorder
Speech and language therapy
    autism spectrum disorder and, 9
    language disorder and, 20
    speech sound disorder and, 21
    stuttering and, 21
Speech sound disorder, 20–21
Spite, and oppositional defiant disorder, 212
SSRIs. *See* Selective serotonin reuptake inhibitors
Standardized tests
    intellectual disability and, 16
    specific learning disorder and, 22
Stereotypic movement disorder, 24–25
Stimulants
    ADHD and, 14
    narcolepsy and, 173
    overview of, 305
    sleep hygiene and avoidance of, **184**
    symptoms of intoxication and withdrawal, **232**
Stories about
    acute stress disorder, 118–119
    ADHD, 13
    Alzheimer's disease, 244–245
    anorexia nervosa, 150–151

Understanding Mental Disorders

Support groups. *See also* Resources
  addictive disorders and, 224, 235
  ADHD and, 15
  Alzheimer's disease and, 246
  anxiety disorders and, 77
  autism spectrum disorder and, 10
  bipolar I disorder and, 51
  disruptive mood dysregulation
    disorder and, 71
  eating disorders and, 147
  healthy lifestyle and, 308
  major depressive disorder and, 65
  mental health care providers and,
    291
  PTSD and, 116
  schizophrenia and, 36, 37
  substance use disorder and, **225**
Supportive housing
  intellectual disability and, 17
  schizophrenia and, 37
Supportive psychotherapy
  acute stress disorder and, 120
  definition and applications of, 296
  factitious disorder and, 141
  major depressive disorder and, 63
Surgery. *See also* Medical conditions
  gender dysphoria and sex
    reassignment, 206, 207
  genito-pelvic pain/penetration
    disorder and, 196
  obstructive sleep apnea and, 176
  Parkinson's disease and, 250
Symptoms, xi–xii, xvi–xviii. *See also*
  Diagnosis; Dissociative
  symptoms; Negative symptoms;
  Physical symptoms; *specific*
  *disorders*
Systematic desensitization, 297
Systemized amnesia, 129
TBI. *See* Traumatic brain injury
Temperament, as risk factor. *See also*
  Personality
  for agoraphobia, 82
  for anorexia nervosa, 150
  for bulimia nervosa, 152

  for female orgasmic disorder, 194
  for gender dysphoria, 204
  for generalized anxiety disorder,
    83
  for hoarding disorder, 101
  for insomnia disorder, 170
  for major depressive disorder, 61
  for OCD, 96
  for panic disorder, 79
  for persistent depressive
    disorder, 66
  for PTSD, 112, 113
  for social anxiety disorder, 86
  for specific phobia, 85
Temper tantrums, and intermittent
  explosive disorder, 212
Testosterone replacement therapy,
  197. *See also* Hormone
  treatments
Theft
  conduct disorder and, 215
  kleptomania and, 217–218
Therapeutic alliance, 136, 295
Thinking and thoughts
  psychotic disorders and, 30
  PTSD and, 108
  schizotypal personality disorder
    and, 270
  somatic symptom disorder and,
    138
  traumatic brain injury and, 246
Tic disorders, 25
Tobacco, withdrawal from, 230, **233.**
  *See also* Cigarette smoking
Tolerance, and substance use
  disorder, 226, 227
Tourette's disorder, 25
Tranquilizers, 77
Transcranial magnetic stimulation
  (TMS), 293, 306
Transient ischemic attacks, and
  vascular neurocognitive
  disorder, 254
Transexualism, 206
Transvestic disorder, 280, 285